New Advances in Neurosurgery: Clinical Diagnosis, Treatment and Prognosis

New Advances in Neurosurgery: Clinical Diagnosis, Treatment and Prognosis

Guest Editor

Janez Ravnik

MDPI

Basel • Beijing • Wuhan • Barcelona • Belgrade • Novi Sad • Cluj • Manchester

Guest Editor
Janez Ravnik
Department of Neurosurgery
University Medical Centre
Maribor
Maribor
Slovenia

Editorial Office
MDPI AG
Grosspeteranlage 5
4052 Basel, Switzerland

This is a reprint of the Special Issue, published open access by the journal *Diagnostics* (ISSN 2075-4418), freely accessible at: https://www.mdpi.com/journal/diagnostics/special_issues/TLHTJ6F037.

For citation purposes, cite each article independently as indicated on the article page online and as indicated below:

Lastname, A.A.; Lastname, B.B. Article Title. *Journal Name* **Year**, *Volume Number*, Page Range.

ISBN 978-3-7258-5043-3 (Hbk)
ISBN 978-3-7258-5044-0 (PDF)
https://doi.org/10.3390/books978-3-7258-5044-0

Contents

About the Editor vii

Janez Ravnik
Editorial for "New Advances in Neurosurgery: Clinical Diagnosis, Treatment and Prognosis"
Reprinted from: *Diagnostics* **2025**, *15*, 2000, https://doi.org/10.3390/diagnostics15162000 1

Peter Spazzapan and Tomaz Velnar
Isolated Sagittal Craniosynostosis: A Comprehensive Review
Reprinted from: *Diagnostics* **2024**, *14*, 435, https://doi.org/10.3390/diagnostics14040435 4

Peter Spazzapan, Tomaz Velnar, Nina Perosa, Andrej Porcnik and Borut Prestor
Results of Surgical Treatment of Occult Spinal Dysraphisms—A Single Centre Experience
Reprinted from: *Diagnostics* **2024**, *14*, 703, https://doi.org/10.3390/diagnostics14070703 22

Janez Ravnik, Hojka Rowbottom, Carl H. Snyderman, Paul A. Gardner, Tomaž Šmigoc, Matic Glavan, et al.
The Impact of Surgical Telementoring on Reducing the Complication Rate in Endoscopic Endonasal Surgery of the Skull Base
Reprinted from: *Diagnostics* **2024**, *14*, 1874, https://doi.org/10.3390/diagnostics14171874 35

Tomislav Felbabić, Tomaž Velnar and Tomaž Kocjan
Hypopituitarism, Diabetes Insipidus, and Syndrome of Inappropriate Antidiuretic Hormone Secretion after Pituitary Macroadenoma Surgery with Indocyanine Green Dye
Reprinted from: *Diagnostics* **2024**, *14*, 1863, https://doi.org/10.3390/diagnostics14171863 51

Andreas Filis, Kay Engellandt, Sergio M. F. Romualdo, Ibrahim El-Battrawy, Dino Podlesek, Tareq A. Juratli, et al.
The Impact of Magnetic Resonance Imaging Findings in Predicting Neurological Status Pre- and Post-Treatment of Spinal Dural Arteriovenous Fistulas: A 22-Year Experience in a Neurovascular and Spine Center
Reprinted from: *Diagnostics* **2024**, *14*, 581, https://doi.org/10.3390/diagnostics14060581 63

Huanwen Chen, Matthew K. McIntyre, Mihir Khunte, Ajay Malhotra, Mohamed Labib, Marco Colasurdo and Dheeraj Gandhi
Minimally Invasive Surgery Versus Conventional Neurosurgical Treatments for Patients with Subcortical Supratentorial Intracerebral Hemorrhage: A Nationwide Study of Real-World Data from 2016 to 2022
Reprinted from: *Diagnostics* **2025**, *15*, 1308, https://doi.org/10.3390/diagnostics15111308 73

José Pablo Martínez Barbero, Francisco Javier Pérez García, Paula María Jiménez Gutiérrez, Marta García Cerezo, David López Cornejo, Gonzalo Olivares Granados, et al.
The Value of Cerebral Blood Volume Derived from Dynamic Susceptibility Contrast Perfusion MRI in Predicting IDH Mutation Status of Brain Gliomas—A Systematic Review and Meta-Analysis
Reprinted from: *Diagnostics* **2025**, *15*, 896, https://doi.org/10.3390/diagnostics15070896 83

Yusuf Sukru Caglar, Murat Buyuktepe, Emre Yagiz Sayaci, Ihsan Dogan, Melih Bozkurt, Elif Peker, et al.
Hybrid Positron Emission Tomography and Magnetic Resonance Imaging Guided Microsurgical Management of Glial Tumors: Case Series and Review of the Literature
Reprinted from: *Diagnostics* **2024**, *14*, 1551, https://doi.org/10.3390/diagnostics14141551 106

Kruthajn Rajesh, Helen Shen and Sonu M. M. Bhaskar
Seizures Following Carotid Endarterectomy: A Comprehensive Meta-Analysis of 69,479 Patients and Evidence-Based Recommendations for Perioperative Care
Reprinted from: *Diagnostics* **2025**, *15*, 6, https://doi.org/10.3390/diagnostics15010006 . . . . . . **115**

Jure Pešak, Andrej Porčnik and Borut Prestor
Captive Bolt Gun-Related Vascular Injury: A Single Center Experience
Reprinted from: *Diagnostics* **2024**, *14*, 977, https://doi.org/10.3390/diagnostics14100977 . . . . . **134**

Tomaž Šmigoc, Hojka Rowbottom and Janez Ravnik
The Impact of Class III Obesity on Outcomes for Vestibular Schwannoma Surgery: A Case Report
Reprinted from: *Diagnostics* **2025**, *15*, 888, https://doi.org/10.3390/diagnostics15070888 . . . . . **142**

Serghei Covantsev, Anna Bumbu, Anna Sukhotko, Evghenii Zakurdaev, Ivan Kuts and Andrey Evsikov
Neck Schwannoma Masking as Thyroid Tumour: Into the Deep of Diagnostics and Anatomy
Reprinted from: *Diagnostics* **2024**, *14*, 2332, https://doi.org/10.3390/diagnostics14202332 . . . . **152**

About the Editor

Janez Ravnik

Janez Ravnik, MD, PhD, is a consultant neurosurgeon and Head of the Department of Neurosurgery at the University Medical Centre Maribor, Slovenia. He graduated from the Faculty of Medicine in Ljubljana and also earned a degree in Psychology from the Faculty of Arts in Ljubljana. He completed his specialization in neurosurgery at the University Medical Centre in Ljubljana and obtained his PhD from the Faculty of Medicine in Ljubljana. Dr. Ravnik is an Assistant Professor in the Faculty of Medicine in Maribor, where he serves as the Course Director for Neurosurgery. His clinical and research interests are primarily focused on brain tumor surgery, skull base surgery, and endoscopic neurosurgery.

diagnostics

MDPI

Editorial

Editorial for "New Advances in Neurosurgery: Clinical Diagnosis, Treatment and Prognosis"

Janez Ravnik

Department of Neurosurgery, University Medical Centre Maribor, 2000 Maribor, Slovenia; janez.ravnik@ukc-mb.si

Neurosurgery represents one of the most rapidly evolving disciplines in modern medicine. Technological innovations, novel imaging modalities, and emerging treatment strategies have significantly enhanced both the understanding and management of disorders affecting the brain, spine, and peripheral nervous system.

The routine application of high-resolution preoperative imaging, intraoperative neuronavigation, fluorescence-guided resection, intraoperative imaging, and neurophysiological monitoring have markedly improved the safety and efficacy of brain tumor surgery [1]. These advancements have facilitated more extensive resections of malignant primary brain tumors [2]. In particular, the integration of 5-aminolevulinic acid (5-ALA) and intraoperative imaging have become the standard of care in many neurosurgical centers. Furthermore, endoscopic endonasal approaches have seen considerable refinement in recent years [3], offering enhanced safety profiles and becoming the preferred approach for an increasing number of tumors located at or near the skull base [3].

Endovascular techniques have undergone transformative progress, now allowing for the minimally invasive management of a wide range of cerebrovascular and spinal vascular pathologies [4]. Despite these advances, traditional open microsurgical approaches continue to play a critical role, particularly in complex cases, supported by minimally invasive strategies, novel instrumentation, and detailed patient-specific anatomical planning [5].

The combination of sophisticated imaging technologies, precise neuronavigation, intraoperative visualization, and refined surgical tools has enabled neurosurgical interventions to become increasingly less invasive [6]. Contemporary procedures often require only a small cranial opening and utilize narrow operative corridors to access deep-seated intracranial and spinal lesions, reducing patient morbidity and enhancing recovery.

Pediatric neurosurgery continues to pose unique challenges due to the complexity and heterogeneity of childhood neurological disorders. Significant strides have been made in understanding the biological underpinnings of various pediatric diseases. Nonetheless, treatment outcomes for certain conditions, particularly malignant pediatric brain tumors, remain suboptimal, underscoring the need for continued research and innovation [7].

Advanced multimodal monitoring has become increasingly widespread in the management of TBI. Given that brain trauma remains a leading cause of morbidity and mortality worldwide, optimal outcomes are best achieved through care delivered in specialized, high-volume centers equipped with the necessary expertise and infrastructure [8].

In this Special Issue, we present a range of innovative solutions across various neurosurgical domains. The benefits of minimally invasive surgery in the treatment of spontaneous intracerebral hematomas are highlighted, alongside advancements in endoscopic endonasal approaches detailed in two contributions. We introduce telementoring as a promising strategy to enhance surgical outcomes in low-volume centers. Within pediatric

https://doi.org/10.3390/diagnostics15162000

neurosurgery, we explore surgical outcomes for sagittal craniosynostosis and occult spinal dysraphisms, demonstrating that specialized care in dedicated centers yields superior results. A comprehensive retrospective study spanning more than two decades offers insights into the management of spinal dural arteriovenous fistulas, emphasizing the predictive value of MRI findings on neurological outcomes. Two studies showcase the critical role of advanced imaging in optimizing treatment strategies for glial tumors. Additionally, two case reports illustrate the challenges encountered in the management of vestibular and cervical schwannomas. Another large-scale study investigates seizure management strategies during carotid endarterectomy. Finally, a detailed anatomical study provides novel insights into vascular injuries sustained in firearm-related brain trauma.

Although outcomes for benign cranial tumors have improved significantly, the management of malignant brain neoplasms, particularly primary gliomas, remains a formidable challenge. The limitations of conventional microsurgical resection underscore the need for a dual approach: continued refinement of surgical technologies and a deeper understanding of the molecular and biological mechanisms driving disease progression. A similar paradigm applies to vascular neurosurgery. While endovascular interventions have become safer and more effective, the overall outcomes of many acute vascular pathologies remain unsatisfactory. For instance, an aneurysmal subarachnoid hemorrhage continues to carry a high mortality and morbidity burden. Even with timely aneurysm exclusion, there is a critical need for better strategies in the post-rupture management phase.

Neurosurgery is increasingly embracing a personalized medicine approach. Tailoring treatment strategies to individual patients' anatomy, pathology, biological disease behavior, and personal preferences, while leveraging technical innovations, allows for the formulation of individualized therapeutic plans aimed at achieving optimal outcomes. The integration of artificial intelligence is anticipated to significantly enhance future management strategies [9].

Funding: This research received no external funding.

Conflicts of Interest: The authors declare no conflicts of interest.

References

1. Oya, S. Recent Advancements in the Surgical Treatment of Brain Tumors. *Curr. Oncol.* **2023**, *30*, 8424–8425. [CrossRef] [PubMed]
2. Gerritsen, J.K.W.; Broekman, M.L.D.; De Vleeschouwer, S.; Schucht, P.; Nahed, B.V.; Berger, M.S.; Vincent, A.J.P.E. Safe surgery for glioblastoma: Recent advances and modern challenges. *Neurooncol. Pract.* **2022**, *9*, 364–379. [CrossRef] [PubMed]
3. Andrade, E.J.; Alli, S.; Sindwani, R.; Kshettry, V.R.; Recinos, P.F. Beyond the sella: Expanded endoscopic endonasal approaches for pituitary tumors. *Neurooncol Adv.* **2025**, *7* (Suppl. S1), i29–i39. [CrossRef] [PubMed]
4. Nunna, R.; Tariq, F.; Jummah, F.; Bains, N.; Qureshi, A.I.; Siddiq, F. Advances in the endovascular management of cerebrovascular disease. *Mo Med.* **2024**, *121*, 127–135. [PubMed]
5. Lawton, M.T.; Lang, M.J. The future of open vascular neurosurgery: Perspectives on cavernous malformations, AVMs, and bypasses for complex aneurysms. *J. Neurosurg.* **2019**, *130*, 1409–1416. [CrossRef] [PubMed]
6. Laguardia, S.; Piccioni, A.; Alonso Vera, J.E.; Muqaddas, A.; Garcés, M.; Ambreen, S.; Sharma, S.; Sabzvari, T. A comprehensive review of the role of the latest minimally invasive neurosurgery techniques and outcomes for brain and spinal surgeries. *Cureus* **2025**, *17*, e84682. [CrossRef] [PubMed]
7. Lim-Fat, M.J.; Bennett, J.; Ostrom, Q.; Touat, M.; Franceschi, E.; Schulte, J.; Bindra, R.S.; Fangusaro, J.; Dhall, G.; Nicholson, J.; et al. Central nervous system tumors in adolescents and young adults: A Society for Neuro-Oncology Consensus Review on diagnosis, management, and future directions. *Neuro Oncol.* **2025**, *27*, 13–32. [CrossRef] [PubMed]

8. Baker, M.S., Jr.; Carpenter, K.L.H.; Helmy, A.; Hutchinson, P.J. Multimodality monitoring for the management of severe traumatic brain injury. *Neurosurg. Clin. N. Am.* **2025**, *36*, 343–354. [CrossRef] [PubMed]
9. Tangsrivimol, J.A.; Schonfeld, E.; Zhang, M.; Veeravagu, A.; Smith, T.R.; Härtl, R.; Lawton, M.T.; El-Sherbini, A.H.; Prevedello, D.M.; Glicksberg, B.S.; et al. Artificial intelligence in neurosurgery: A state-of-the-art review from past to future. *Diagnostics* **2023**, *13*, 2429. [CrossRef] [PubMed]

diagnostics

MDPI

Review

Isolated Sagittal Craniosynostosis: A Comprehensive Review

Peter Spazzapan [1] and Tomaz Velnar [1,2,*]

[1] Department of Neurosurgery, University Medical Centre Ljubljana, 1000 Ljubljana, Slovenia; spazzapanpeter@yahoo.it
[2] Alma Mater Europaea ECM, 2000 Maribor, Slovenia
* Correspondence: tvelnar@hotmail.com

Abstract: Sagittal craniosynostosis, a rare but fascinating craniofacial anomaly, presents a unique challenge for both diagnosis and treatment. This condition involves premature fusion of the sagittal suture, which alters the normal growth pattern of the skull and can affect neurological development. Sagittal craniosynostosis is characterised by a pronounced head shape, often referred to as scaphocephaly. Asymmetry of the face and head, protrusion of the fontanel, and increased intracranial pressure are common clinical manifestations. Early recognition of these features is crucial for early intervention, and understanding the aetiology is, therefore, essential. Although the exact cause remains unclear, genetic factors are thought to play an important role. Mutations in genes such as FGFR2 and FGFR3, which disrupt the normal development of the skull, are suspected. Environmental factors and various insults during pregnancy can also contribute to the occurrence of the disease. An accurate diagnosis is crucial for treatment. Imaging studies such as ultrasound, computed tomography, magnetic resonance imaging, and three-dimensional reconstructions play a crucial role in visualising the prematurely fused sagittal suture. Clinicians also rely on a physical examination and medical history to confirm the diagnosis. Early detection allows for quick intervention and better treatment outcomes. The treatment of sagittal craniosynostosis requires a multidisciplinary approach that includes neurosurgery, craniofacial surgery, and paediatric care. Traditional treatment consists of an open reconstruction of the cranial vault, where the fused suture is surgically released to allow normal growth of the skull. However, advances in minimally invasive techniques, such as endoscopic strip craniectomy, are becoming increasingly popular due to their lower morbidity and shorter recovery times. This review aims to provide a comprehensive overview of sagittal craniosynostosis, highlighting the aetiology, clinical presentation, diagnostic methods, and current treatment options.

Keywords: craniosynostosis; scaphocephaly; cranial deformation; surgery; cranial vault remodelling

1. Introduction

The skull of vertebrates consists of the neurocranium, which surrounds and protects the brain, and the viscerocranium, which forms the face. The neurocranium is separated into the following:

1. Membranous neurocranium, which forms through the process of intramembranous ossification and creates the frontal bone, the squamous portion of the temporal bone, the intraparietal portion of the occipital bone, and the parietal bone;
2. Cartilaginous neurocranium, which ossifies via endochondral ossification and gives rise to the ethmoid and sphenoid bones, as well as the petrous and mastoid portions of the temporal bone and the occipital bone.

The skull sutures form at the junctions of the skull bones. Here the bone tissue is gradually deposited; therefore, the cranial sutures act as ossification centres of the skull [1]. The skull sutures allow unrestricted brain growth through progressive bone deposition. Craniosynostosis occurs when the cranial sutures undergo too early ossification and no longer function as ossification centres. In craniosynostosis, the growth of the skull is impaired due to the ossification of one or more cranial sutures, thus giving rise to specific skull deformations. Virchow's law [2] states that if the growth of the skull stops in a direction perpendicular to the ossified suture, the rapidly growing brain finds space for its rapid growth elsewhere, and compensatory growth occurs in a direction parallel to the affected suture and no longer in a perpendicular direction. The clinical picture varies depending on which suture is fused [3].

Craniosynostosis is defined as syndromic or non-syndromic. Of the non-syndromic ones, scaphocephaly, trigonocephaly, and anterior plagiocephaly are the most common. Brachycephaly and posterior plagiocephaly are less common. Syndromic craniosynostoses are more complex conditions, usually involving multiple sutures and usually associated with intracranial hypertension, hydrocephalus, and Chiari malformation. Syndromic forms of craniosynostosis usually present with multiple fused sutures and may include central nervous system, limb, or airway malformations [4].

According to literature data, the incidence is estimated at 1/2100 births, with a male-to-female ratio of 4 to 1. Non-syndromic craniosynostosis accounts for 85 to 95% of all cases, while syndromic cases account for 5 to 15%. In Slovenia, the annual incidence is estimated at 1:1500 births. The prevalence of non-syndromic craniosynostosis is 93%, and that of syndromic craniosynostosis is 7%. The predominance of male children (78.9%) is well known [1,3–5].

In terms of morphological phenotypes, the most common form of craniosynostosis is non-syndromic craniosynostosis (ISS) (40 to 55%) (Figure 1). In second place is the metopic synostosis (15 to 30%), followed by the unilateral and bilateral coronal synostosis (15 to 20%). Lambdoid synostosis is the rarest (0 to 5%). Ossification of two or more sutures is rare and usually occurs in syndromic cases [3]. In Slovenia, ISS accounted for 54.9% of cases, metopic craniosynostosis 25.3%, unilateral coronal craniosynostosis 14%, bilateral coronal craniosynostosis 1.4%, and lambdoid craniosynostosis 1.4%. Multiple suture craniosynostosis occurred in 2.8% of cases [1,5].

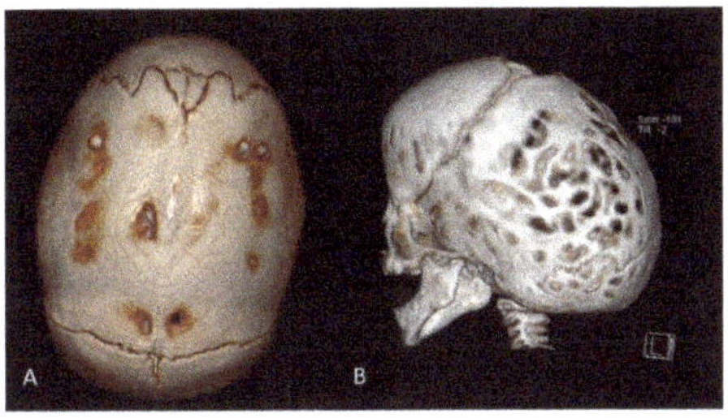

Figure 1. Computed tomography (CT) with 3D reconstructions showing sagittal craniosynostosis (**A**) and subsequent scaphocephalic skull deformity (**B**).

Among the known aetiologies of craniosynostosis, genetic, metabolic, and haematological diseases, mucopolysaccharidosis, and teratogens (valproic acid, retinoic acid) are the most important [3]. The presence of CSF drainage and microcephaly can also be a cause of craniosynostosis, as in both cases, the growth potential of the brain itself is reduced; the cranial sutures are not exposed to the force of the growing brain and, consequently, ossify prematurely. Genetic studies have identified some of the genes involved in the pathogenesis of craniosynostosis. The genes FGFR−1, FGFR−2, FGFR−3, FGFR−4, and TGFBR−2 (associated with Loeys–Dietz syndrome) encode receptors that are involved in the processes of differentiation, proliferation, and migration of cranial suture cells.

The genetic causes of syndromic craniosynostosis also include alterations in the TWIST1, ERF, and EFNB1 genes, which play a specific role in the development of this condition. Understanding the roles of these genes in syndromic craniosynostosis is crucial for diagnosis, genetic counselling, and potentially developing targeted therapies since early identification of mutations in these genes can aid in personalised management and treatment plans for affected individuals [3]. For example, mutations in the TWIST1 gene are associated with Saethre–Chotzen syndrome, one of the syndromes causing craniosynostosis. TWIST1 is involved in the regulation of embryonic development, particularly in the formation of bones and other tissues. Mutations in this gene disrupt normal cranial suture development, leading to premature fusion of the skull bones. ERF (ETS2 repressor factor) is a transcription factor that regulates gene expression by binding to specific DNA sequences. Mutations in ERF have been linked to craniosynostosis, particularly the Muenke syndrome subtype. ERF likely plays a role in controlling the balance of cell proliferation and differentiation during cranial bone development. Disruptions in ERF function can lead to abnormal skull growth and premature fusion of cranial sutures. EFNB1 (Ephrin−B1) is a gene that encodes a cell surface protein involved in cell signaling. Mutations in EFNB1 are associated with craniofrontonasal syndrome, another type of syndromic craniosynostosis. EFNB1 is important for the guidance of migrating neural crest cells during embryonic development, which contribute to the formation of the skull and face. Mutations in EFNB1 disrupt normal cranial bone development, leading to craniosynostosis and other craniofacial abnormalities [1,5].

The diagnosis of craniosynostosis is initially clinical. Depending on the affected suture, characteristic deformations of the cranial vault occur. Other clinical signs are the typical ridge that appears over the ossified suture and the absence of displacement of the two bones adjacent to the suture at palpation. The diagnosis is ultimately confirmed radiologically. Ultrasonography (US) of the head alone confirms the ossification of the suture (Figure 2), and computed tomography (CT) of the head with 3D reconstruction clearly shows the craniosynostosis.

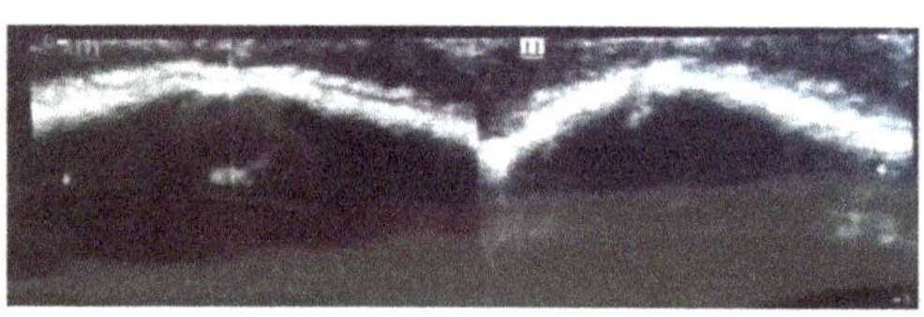

Figure 2. Cranial bone ultrasound confirms the synostosis of the cranial suture, as the hyperechoic bone signal continues uninterrupted, whereas a hypoechoic cranial suture should be identifiable.

These two examinations are particularly important in those rare cases in which craniosynostosis cannot be confirmed with certainty by clinical examination. An ocular fundus examination is indicated to rule out the presence of increased intracranial pressure. More detailed information about the anatomy of the brain can be obtained by magnetic resonance imaging (MRI), although this is rarely indicated in isolated craniosynostosis, as clinically significant brain abnormalities in craniosynostosis are rare and can usually be recognised by ultrasound of the head. Genetic tests are always necessary if an underlying syndromic condition is suspected. In syndromic forms, however, MRI imaging is frequently used to evaluate associated Chiari malformation, syrinx, hydrocephalus, and other CNS malformations [4,5].

The treatment of craniosynostosis is surgical and requires complex remodelling of the deformed parts of the skull [6]. The procedure must eliminate the constricting and deforming tendency that synostosis exerts on the growth of the head. This requires remodelling of the bony structures of the neurocranium and, if necessary, of the viscerocranium. The procedure must be performed not only for cosmetic reasons but, above all, to allow the brain to grow normally. The age at which surgical treatment of craniosynostosis is performed depends on the involved suture, the possible presence of hydrocephalus or Chiari malformation, and the systemic, especially respiratory, condition of the child.

When planning the treatment of a child with craniosynostosis, it is important to consider which suture is affected, the general and neurological condition of the child, and any associated pathologies and malformations. In the vast majority of non-syndromic craniosynostosis, a single procedure is sufficient to reshape the skull. Hydrocephalus or Chiari malformations are very rare in these cases. In syndromic cases, Chiari malformation, raised intracranial pressure, and hydrocephalus are more common [4]. Apneas are also common and occur both due to central reasons (in association with Chiari malformation) and peripherical reasons (in association with maxillary hypoplasia and upper airway stenosis). These are, therefore, complex clinical conditions that need to be corrected by a series of interventions in the correct chronological order. The treatment of such children is time-consuming and multidisciplinary. Surgical treatment of craniosynostosis is complex and not without complications. According to the literature, complications occur in 2 to 8% of cases [7]. The mortality rate in all current series is less than 1%. Possible complications include wound dehiscence, infections, subcutaneous haematomas, dural injuries, and CSF leakage.

The evaluation of the success of craniosynostosis surgery is based on the assessment of the aesthetic and functional outcomes. The aesthetic result is difficult to assess objectively. The most useful methods for this purpose are craniometric measurements, the most important of which is the cranial index (CI), which indicates the ratio of skull width to skull length. In healthy, normocephalic children, the CI is between 76% and 78% [8]. The closer the CI approaches these values after surgery, the more favourable the aesthetic results.

The cognitive outcome is assessed by neuropsychological tests performed throughout the child's development. In children without concomitant hydrocephalus and without raised intracranial pressure, certain neurocognitive problems occur in 30 to 50% of cases despite surgery [9]. These problems are most pronounced in the areas of language acquisition, writing, and reading, although the intelligence quotient (IQ) is usually within normal limits. In this review, we discuss ISS and its management.

2. Isolated Sagittal Craniosynostosis

Scaphocephaly is a skull deformity caused by ISS, i.e., premature, non-syndromic ossification of the sagittal suture. ISS is the most common form of craniosynostosis occurring in clinical practise (incidence 1:5000 births) and accounts for 40 to 60% of all cases [3,10]. It occurs more frequently in boys than in girls. In the neonatal period, it can be easily recognised and diagnosed by a simple clinical examination. It presents with an elongated and narrowed head shape, characterised mainly by frontal and occipital bossing and a narrow bitemporal and biparietal distance (Figure 3). There is no asymmetry of the face, orbits, or brain base in ISS. A thickening of the sagittal suture is often observed, which can be palpated. Radiologically, the thickened suture can be confirmed by a simple X−ray of the head or, more precisely, by CT (Figure 1) or ultrasound (Figure 2).

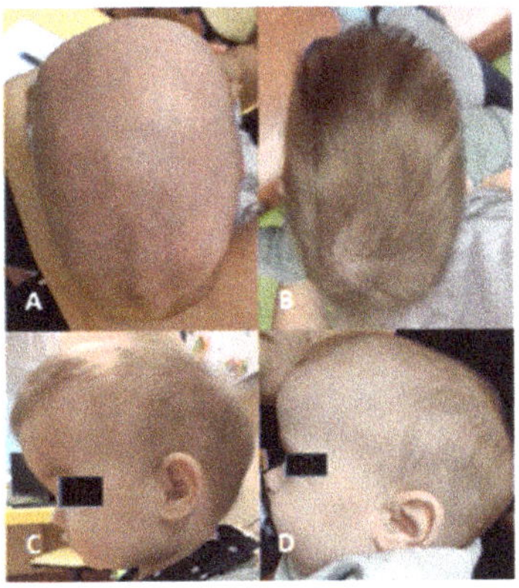

Figure 3. (**A**,**B**) show the scaphocephalic head shape from a bird's eye view, characterised by biparietal constriction and increased anteroposterior circumference. (**C**,**D**) show the lateral view, with prominent frontal convexity and flattening of the vertex.

Although these general data suggest that ISS is a specific, homogeneous, and well-defined pathology, a close examination of each case and a thorough review of the literature may show that this is not the case. In fact, during the routine clinical and radiological examination of a child with ISS, the various anatomical, genetic, and functional abnormalities that can accompany almost every single case of ISS are easily overlooked and not evaluated. When properly recognised, ISS can be considered a much more heterogeneous pathology, which should be evaluated by the multidisciplinary expertise of paediatricians, geneticists, anatomists, neurologists, radiologists, and paediatric neurosurgeons [11].

The sagittal suture does not ossify according to the all-or-nothing principle. Therefore, different morphological forms of scaphocephaly and different clinical presentations may develop depending on the different segments of the sagittal suture involved in the process of craniosynostosis [8,11]:

- Dolichocephaly occurs when the entire sagittal suture is ossified. It is characterised by an elongated and narrow head.
- Leptocephaly occurs when the anterior third of the suture is ossified. It is characterised by a uniform and homogeneous narrowing of the cranial vault, affecting both the parietal and frontal bones.
- Batrocephaly occurs when the middle and anterior third of the sagittal suture are ossified. It is characterised by pronounced occipital bossing.
- Cynocephaly occurs when the middle third of the sagittal suture is ossified. It is characterised by a bony depression that occurs behind the coronal sutures.
- Sphenocephaly is the most common form and occurs when the middle and posterior third of the sagittal suture are ossified. It is mainly characterised by a bossing of the bregma and of the frontal bone. In these cases, from a bird's eye view, the width of the frontal bone is greater than the biparietal width.

The frontal and occipital bossing are clinical features of ISS and represent a compensatory phenomenon due to the limited ability of the skull to grow in a lateral direction, according to Virchow's law. The heterogeneity of the different forms of deformity is, therefore, not only related to the ossification of the sagittal suture per se but, above all, to compensatory mechanisms resulting from the limitation of the normal growth vectors of the skull. It is important to point out that these compensatory processes differ mainly according to the time at which ossification of the sagittal suture takes place in the prenatal period. Thus, early ossification of the suture is associated with a more pronounced scaphocephalic deformity, whereas late ossification of the suture is associated with a less pronounced deformity [12]. These compensatory processes may persist after surgery and may also affect the outcome of surgical treatment, especially if the procedure did not provide sufficient relief or was performed too late.

ISS and the resulting scaphocephaly, with all the morphological forms described above, can be diagnosed at any age. Prenatal diagnosis is quite rare but possible. Prenatal ultrasound measurements in children with ISS are usually within normal limits, although in some cases, a reduced biparietal distance and an increased anteroposterior (fronto-occipital) distance can be observed. Only after birth can the deformity be clearly identified, and the characteristic bony ridge above the sagittal suture can be palpated.

3. Radiology

As we have already written, the clinical picture of ISS is not homogeneous. There are different morphological forms of scaphocephalic deformity, and in each of these forms, specific cranial and intracranial changes occur during development. Although CT and MRI are not usually necessary investigations for surgical treatment planning, many surgeons use CT scans for preoperative planning. Both imaging techniques can be useful for research purposes as they can reveal many intracranial abnormalities or variations, not only in relation to the shape of the cranial sulcus but also in relation to the structure of the brain itself. It is clear that changes in the shape of the cranial sulcus can also affect the deformation and shape of the brain itself [13], which becomes longer in ISS compared to normocephalic children. In addition, other deformities are characteristic of the ISS brain, in particular the narrowing of the occipital lobes, the lengthening of the lateral ventricles, and the lateral widening of the frontal lobes. The thalamus and other deep nuclei are slightly displaced backward compared to the brains of children without craniosynostosis. The subarachnoid spaces are distributed differently in children with ISS than under normal conditions. There may be characteristic subarachnoid accumulations or widening of the subarachnoid spaces in the frontal region (Figure 4) and in the interhemispheric fissure. The lateral ventricles may also be slightly wider than normal, especially in the anterior part of the lateral ventricular bodies. These findings are found in up to two-thirds of children with ISS [11].

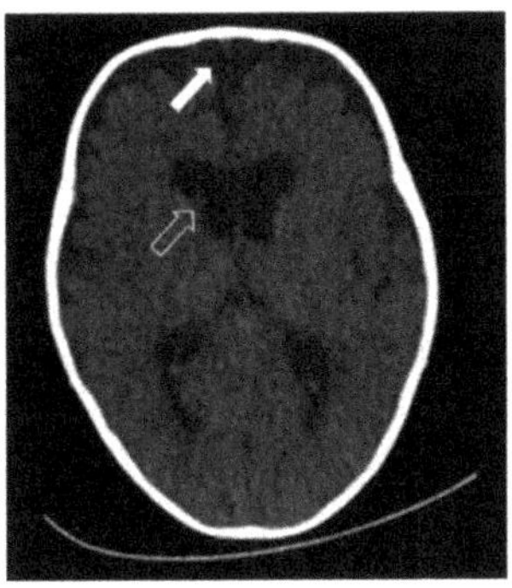

Figure 4. A CT scan of scaphocephaly showed enlarged frontal pericerebral subarachnoid spaces (white arrow) and slightly wider frontal horns of the lateral ventricles (empty arrow).

Two mechanisms have been described that could explain the occurrence of these rearrangements in the intracranial spaces. These are:

1. the above-mentioned passive accumulation of CSF in the subarachnoid spaces as a result of morphological enlargement in the frontal region; and
2. CSF retention as a result of a disturbance in the process of CSF resorption [14].

On the basis of this second theory, the physiopathological process of the development of the bossing of the frontal bone could be at least partially related to the above-mentioned CSF retention. In favour of this hypothesis [14] is the fact that CSF retention is more frequently observed in the frontal subarachnoid cisterns when a bony ridge is seen on CT around the synostotic sagittal suture, surrounding the superior sagittal sinus as a partial or complete bony ring. This is referred to as an Omega sign (Figure 5).

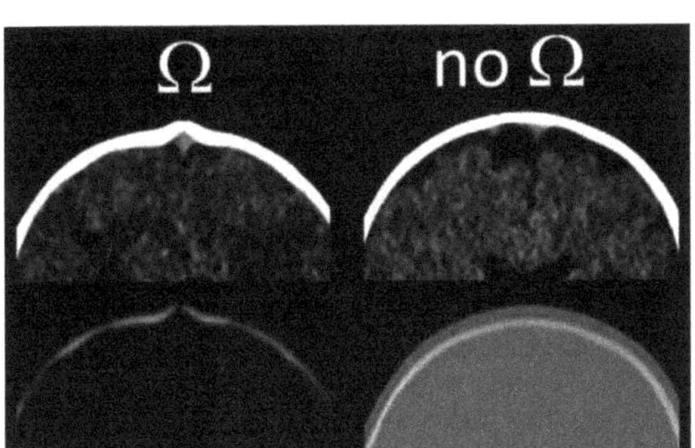

Figure 5. The Omega sign is recognisable on CT scans. It is a bony groove in the area of the synostotic sagittal suture, which hugs the superior sagittal sinus (refer to Ref. [14].)

When this groove is absent and the bony surface overlying the superior sagittal sinus is flat, the CSF accumulations mentioned above are less common. In the past, impaired CSF resorption in children with ISS has also been demonstrated by the technique of infusion into the lumbar subarachnoid space [15,16]. These studies have also shown a decompression of the sagittal sinus after surgery. This improved CSF reabsorption and reduced the extent of subarachnoid CSF collections.

In addition to all these changes, some studies have also described changes in intracranial volume in children with ISS based on CT scans. The data in the literature are rather confusing and often contradictory. In fact, studies using CT scans to assess brain volume have shown that intracranial volume in ISS can remain within normal limits in the first months of life despite the deformity and that it increases with age compared to normocephalic children [17–19]. Other studies [20] have shown partially different results, namely that the intracranial volume in ISS between the third and tenth months of life is lower than in children of the same age without craniosynostosis [20]. These divergent results show that the natural course and process of cranial growth in children with ISS are complex, only partially understood, and unpredictable.

4. Genetics

Although ISS is the most common craniosynostosis, the aetiology of this pathology remains unclear. In recent years, a number of genes have been identified that regulate and control the development and process of progressive, physiological ossification of the sagittal suture. The most important genes involved in this ossification process are FGFR–1–3, TWIST1, RAB23, BMP, EFNB1, TCF12, and PHEX [21]. The diversity of these genes confirms that ISS is also a heterogeneous pathological entity at the molecular level [22].

There is no autosomal inheritability for ISS, and the origin of mutations in the aforementioned genes is multifactorial. In this sense, a second pregnancy will very rarely present with the same condition [21].

Routine genetic testing in children with ISS has limited indications, and it is questionable whether it is clinically appropriate to perform these tests in all children with this diagnosis or only in children in whom a genetic or metabolic defect is suspected. Otherwise, in most cases where an underlying metabolic disease is present (hypophosphatasia, hypophosphatemic rickets, mucolipidosis, mucopolysaccharidosis, osteopetrosis, pseudohypoparathyroidism), this is usually diagnosed before or at the same time as ISS. More rarely, the reverse is the case, where craniosynostosis is recognised and diagnosed first, which serves as a trigger for further diagnoses leading to the final definition of metabolic disease. There is no doubt that systematic genetic testing, routinely performed in the neonatal period, will make an important contribution to the early detection of metabolic diseases in the coming years, including with regard to the diagnosis of ISS [21,22].

5. Intracranial Pressure in ISS

ISS is usually the cause of two different problems:

1. aesthetic deformities and
2. the risk of developing increased intracranial pressure.

The occurrence of increased intracranial pressure with ISS is a complication that is usually due to delayed surgery or poor follow-up of the child after surgery. In rare cases, this complication is attributed to a lack of knowledge about the pathophysiology of ISS itself and limited diagnostic capabilities. Knowledge of the correct management, treatment, and choice of surgical technique is also limited. Opinions still differ in the literature in this regard. Therefore, there are no clear guidelines for the ideal treatment of ISS [23].

The possibility of increased intracranial pressure varies widely, as do the consequences of this condition in children with ISS. In Arnaud's 1995 study, intracranial pressure values measured in the epidural space in the head in 142 patients with ISS at one year of age were not consistent [24]. Values between 3 and 25 mmHg were described. Routine measurement of intracranial pressure in children with ISS is rarely performed, and elevated intracranial pressure is usually diagnosed on the basis of clinical and radiological signs. In this context, it is important to emphasise the importance of diagnosing the condition of papilledema and the resulting potential impairment of visual function. Compared to other forms of craniosynostosis, visual impairment due to papilledema is very rare in ISS, but conversely, in cases where ISS is associated with increased intracranial pressure, papilledema and impaired visual function are common findings. The prevalence of papilledema in ISS is estimated to be approximately 5% [25].

6. Neurocognitive Development in ISS

Increased intracranial pressure not only leads to visual problems but also to a delay in neurocognitive development. As we have seen, the different forms of scaphocephaly can vary depending on the aetiology, morphology of the cranial vault, age at diagnosis, and intracranial findings on imaging of the head. These different conditions can result in different neurocognitive sequelae, which can vary greatly. In this context, the outcomes in terms of learning ability and neurocognitive function may also vary. A number of pathophysiological factors, alone or in combination, may explain the occurrence of neurocognitive problems associated with ISS:

1. increased intracranial pressure [26],
2. deformation of the brain as a result of deformation of the skull [27],
3. problems with the normal development of the brain,
4. compression of the venous sinuses with resulting impairment of venous outflow [14,28].

The scores of the intelligence quotient (IQ) in these children are usually in the average range [27], and there are even studies in which some children with ISS achieved high or very high IQ scores [29,30]. Nevertheless, neurodevelopment is at least partially impaired in children with ISS, and many authors believe that children with ISS are at increased risk of neurodevelopmental disorders, which manifest primarily in the form of learning difficulties in early childhood and adolescence [9,27]. In addition, several studies have shown that the neurocognitive performance of children who have not operated ISS in intelligence tests was in the average range but lower compared to unaffected children. While motor and cognitive development in the first years of life may be in line with expectations, later performance on developmental tests may be lower than expected [31].

Magge et al. described that 50% of children with ISS between the ages of 6 and 16 had learning and reading difficulties, although all of these children had normal IQ scores on intelligence tests [9]. Other authors have also described poorer gross motor skills and significantly lower non-verbal IQ than verbal IQ in children with ISS compared to controls [29,32]. In another study, children operated on ISS performed better on cognitive organisation scales than the control group, whereas they performed significantly worse on working memory and information processing speed scales [33]. Arnaud [24] demonstrated a negative correlation between IQ scores and high ICP values. Of the children with ISS and elevated ICP, 16% showed a developmental delay, while of the children with ISS and normal ICP, 6% showed a developmental delay. Although the difference was not statistically significant, there was a trend suggesting a negative association between ICP and cognitive development, which has been questioned by several other authors in the past [34].

7. The Treatment of ISS

The aim of surgical treatment for sagittal craniosynostosis is to reopen the cranial suture and allow the skull to grow and develop in all directions. This is because the growth of the skull is based on the pressure exerted by the underlying and growing brain, which thus directs and controls the development of the skull. There are differing opinions as to whether the purpose of ISS surgery is purely cosmetic, i.e., aesthetic, or whether it is also necessary to counteract the effects of increased intracranial pressure resulting from the limited capacity of cranial growth and disturbances in physiological CSF circulation [35].

In seeking an answer to these questions, it is worth noting that, unlike most other craniosynostoses, signs of scaphocephaly can also be seen in some cognitively normal adults [11,35]. This is a rare finding but has raised some doubts and questions in the past about the real purpose of surgical treatment, which, based on these facts, should have a predominantly or exclusively aesthetic purpose. Against this background, the early surgical treatment commonly offered to children with ISS cannot be considered absolutely necessary. On the other hand, these doubts are clearly refuted by a number of other studies that clearly show the importance of early surgical treatment. For example, it has been shown that older children diagnosed with ISS after the age of 4 often showed signs of chronically elevated intracranial pressure [11,30].

The two main goals and purposes of surgical treatment are:

1. prevention or treatment of brain dysfunction when clinical signs of increased intracranial pressure are already present,
2. the aesthetic correction of skull deformity.

These two goals are achieved by

1. increasing the volume of the skull,
2. redirecting the vectors of cranial growth,
3. normalising the dynamics of the skull,
4. correcting the aesthetic appearance.

8. Surgical Techniques

Virchow was the first to propose a modern theory of the pathophysiology of craniosynostosis in 1851 [2]. Subsequently, the French surgeon Lannelongue was the first to describe the surgical treatment of craniosynostosis in 1881 [36]. He described the linear craniectomy, in which a bone ligament was removed parallel to the ossified sagittal suture. Later, in 1882, the English surgeon Lane operated on a nine-month-old child who was diagnosed with craniosynostosis in conjunction with microcephaly [37]. He removed the ossified suture from the anterior to the posterior fontanel and performed a bilateral parietal osteotomy so that the osteotomies formed a cross shape. In 1894, Jacobi [38] described a high morbidity and mortality rate in a series of 33 craniosynostosis patients, which even led to craniosynostosis surgery not being performed for the next three decades. Faber and Towne [39] reintroduced surgical treatment for craniosynostosis patients, mainly to prevent visual impairment and blindness. They emphasised the need for surgical intervention in early childhood, between the ages of one and three months. Since then, many surgical techniques have been developed and described for the treatment of ISS. Historically, the first surgical interventions for ISS were limited to the removal of the ossified suture, known as linear suturectomy. Over time, more and more extensive surgical steps were added to this basic procedure, leading to invasive techniques to reshape the entire cranial vault. Despite the more or less invasive individual surgical techniques, the main purpose of open surgery remains the removal of the ossified suture, to which more or less invasive steps are then added to reshape the skull deformity that constitutes the clinical picture of ISS [40–45].

A number of open surgical techniques have been demonstrated and described to actively reshape the convexity of the forehead. All these techniques are based on the removal, displacement, and reimplantation of free bone flaps [41,42,46–50], which allow a more or less pronounced bilateral widening and shortening of the anteroposterior cranial sulcus. In recent decades, this principle has been pursued less through extensive surgical procedures and more through the use of embedding material, usually springs, to reshape the cranial vault. Similarly, endoscopic techniques have gained popularity in the last 10 years and are commonly used for the treatment of ISS. In the endoscopic technique, the endoscope is used to perform a sagittal suturenectomy and short parietal osteotomies. This procedure, therefore, does not aim to radically reshape the entire vault but only to relieve the restrictive effect that ISS has on the growth of the cranial scrotum. Further remodelling of the vault is carried out by a corrective helmet, which is used postoperatively and controls growth based on the physiological growth of the brain and enables remodelling of the skull [51,52].

The aim and objective of all these surgical techniques, both open and endoscopic, are, of course, always the same, namely to allow the brain to develop normally and to achieve an aesthetic state in which it is impossible to see that the child had a skull deformity at any time in the past. The aim is, therefore, to give the child a completely normal appearance. The basic principle of any surgical therapy is to counteract the abnormal longitudinal growth of the skull in favour of transverse growth. There are also different opinions about the ideal age for surgery. The general consensus is that cranial remodelling is more aesthetically successful in children operated on before the age of six months. Neurocognitive studies on operated children have also shown that children operated on before this age have a better outcome than others [30,35,53]. In our institution, for example, we performed a biparietal expansion, namely the Renier H technique (RHT), on 28 consecutive children with ISS between 2015 and 2018. However, at the early postoperative follow-up of these children, we found that the frontal protrusion remained visible and aesthetically disturbing (Figure 6). We then changed the surgical protocol and introduced a more extensive reshaping, which we called total cranial vault reshaping (TCVR), which also included the frontal bone and offered the possibility of a better aesthetic result. In our study [1], the majority of children underwent surgery before the age of 6 months. Such early surgery also allows bone defects and ridges that form in the area of extensive osteotomies to be completely covered and hidden by active overgrowth of bone tissue during the first year of life. If children are operated on later, especially after the first year of life, these bone defects can remain palpable or visible. This is unfavourable, especially if they are located in the forehead area, where they are not covered by the scalp, and thus represent an aesthetic problem [11].

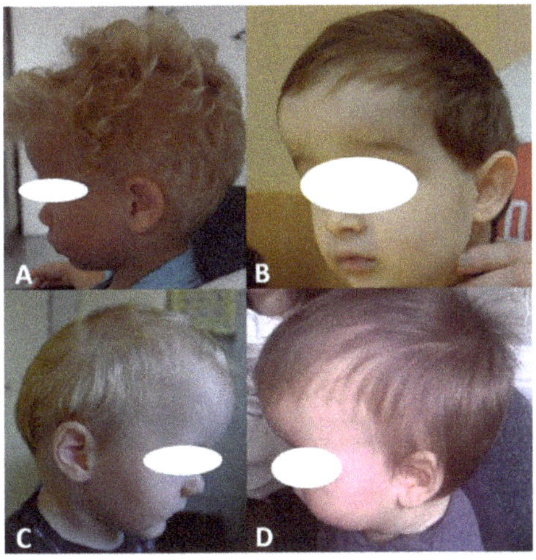

Figure 6. Four cases of children (**A–D**) with marked and persistent frontal bulging at early follow-up after RHT surgery.

Several surgical techniques are described in the literature, but not all of them achieve or fulfil these goals. In scaphocephaly, it is necessary to release the reduction in intracranial space by the synostotic suture and, depending on the surgical technique used, to remodel the entire connective neurocranium to varying degrees. This allows the brain to grow freely in all directions and shape the skull symmetrically. The ideal age for the operation is between three and six months, as the brain still has sufficient growth potential after the operation to give the skull a normocephalic shape. For this reason, no osteosynthetic material is used in these operations that could impair certain growth vectors of the skull in one way or another [11,23].

Despite decades of continuous research, the ideal surgical treatment has not yet been proven, nor has it been proven that one treatment would later show clear advantages over other techniques in the long-term follow-up of these children [23]. Many surgical techniques have been described. The most commonly used are biparietal reshaping with the RHT [54], total vault reshaping, and endoscopic reshaping [35,54–56]. Biparietal remodelling or RHT, is based on the expansion of the parietal part of the skull. Many variations in this procedure have been proposed and described, often named after the shapes of the osteotomies performed during the procedure: Pi technique, T technique, Y technique, inverted Y technique, inverted Pi technique, inverted T technique, double Pi technique, double T technique, and double H technique. Even more invasive and extensive are the techniques for reshaping the entire cranial vault, in which not only osteotomies are created, but the entire vault is gradually reshaped more extensively and more actively (Figure 7). These techniques are based on the removal, displacement, and reimplantation of free bone flaps and are considered to be the most extensive and invasive [54,57–60]. They all go under the common name of remodelling the entire cranial vault. Despite these many well-known open surgical techniques, in recent years, many centres have focused on the introduction of surgical techniques aimed at reducing the morbidity and overall surgical risk of the procedure. To this end, surgical techniques based on small skin incisions have been developed [51,52,56,61] (Figure 8).

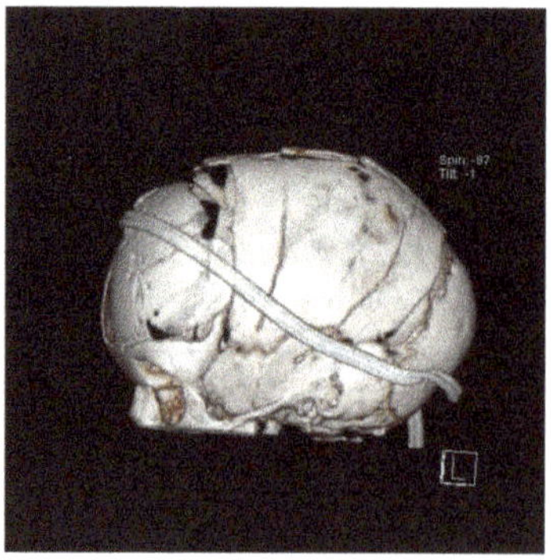

Figure 7. The reshaping of the entire vault involves not only biparietal expansion but also the reshaping of the frontal bone.

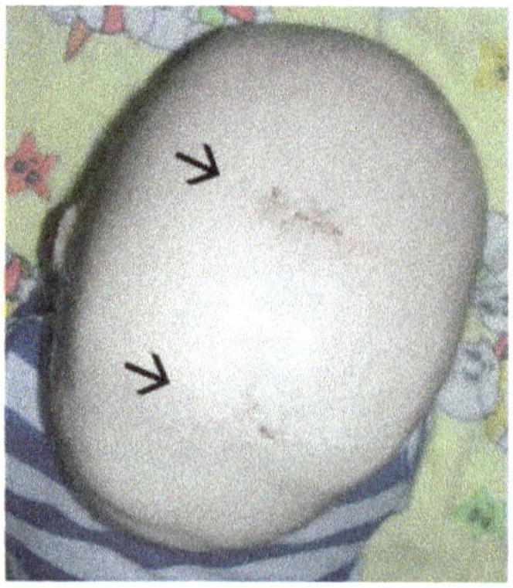

Figure 8. The aim of an endoscopic procedure is to minimise the invasiveness of the surgery itself. The endoscopic approach is performed through two small incisions in the skin (arrows). The synostotic sagittal suture is then removed with the assistance of an endoscope.

These are mainly endoscopic techniques [55] and techniques based on the use of implantable springs (Figure 9) and distractors [51,52,62,63].

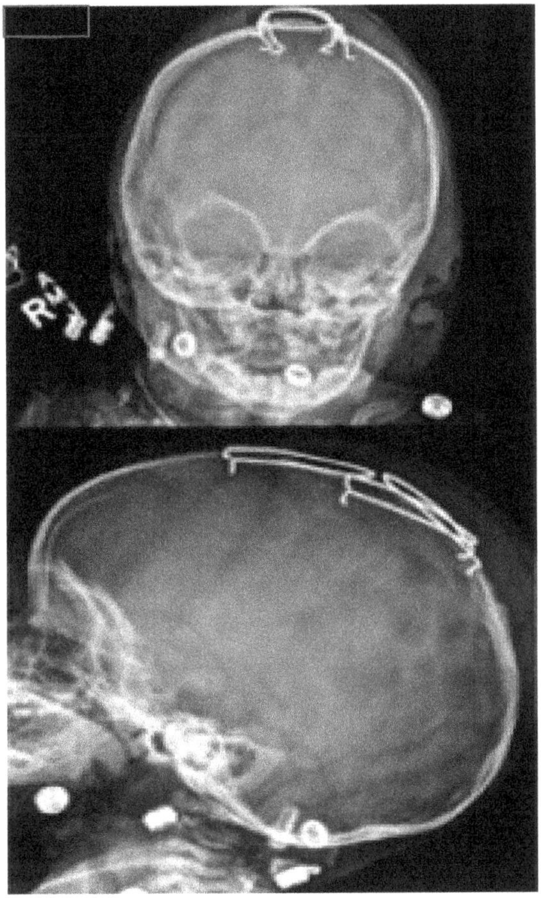

Figure 9. One of the modern surgical methods of ISS treatment involves the insertion of springs into the bone defect created after the suturectomy (refer to Ref. [62]).

Of these less invasive approaches, endoscopic procedures are the most commonly used. They have the advantage of requiring fewer skin incisions and less blood loss and are therefore considered less invasive and more child-friendly [64–70]. Endoscopic techniques are based on the principle of a minimally invasive surgical approach in which the endoscope is used to assist in the creation of a sagittal suturectomy and relieve osteotomies through two small skin incisions. These new osteotomies have the functions of newly surgically formed cranial sutures. Ideally, such procedures are performed on children at a young age, between the first and third months of life. It is important that children wear a corrective helmet for several months after such an operation. It is the wearing of the helmet that determines the final success, not the primary operation itself. Endoscopic treatment is based on the ability of the developing brain to reshape the skull, and the corrective helmet provides adequate support by inhibiting the longitudinal growth vector of the skull and thereby stimulating the lateral growth vector [71,72].

Several studies have shown the efficacy of endoscopic treatment of ISS and comparable results to those after open cranial remodelling [71–73].

The advantages and limitations of each of these individual surgical techniques have been extensively analysed in numerous articles, mainly based on surgical criteria such as:

1. Blood loss during surgery: The amount of blood loss during endoscopic craniosynostosis surgery can vary depending on factors such as the complexity of the case, the patient's medical condition, and the surgical technique employed. It is difficult to provide exact quantities as they can differ widely, especially between individual cases. Endoscopic craniosynostosis surgery is typically associated with minimal blood loss compared to traditional open procedures. In many cases, blood loss may be limited to a few millilitres to tens of millilitres.
2. The need for blood transfusions: The need for blood transfusions during endoscopic craniosynostosis surgery varies depending on several factors, including the patient's age, medical condition, the complexity of the surgery, and the amount of blood loss experienced during the procedure. Paediatric patients have lower blood volumes compared to adults. As a result, even a small amount of blood loss relative to body size can have a more significant impact and may necessitate a blood transfusion. Despite efforts to minimise blood loss, some degree of bleeding can occur during surgery. Patients with pre-existing anaemia or lower-than-normal haemoglobin levels may be at higher risk of requiring blood transfusions during surgery, particularly if significant intraoperative bleeding occurs. Endoscopy is, therefore, a suitable surgical technique for this group of patients.
3. The duration of the operation: The duration of endoscopic craniosynostosis surgery can vary depending on several factors, including the complexity of the case, the specific techniques employed, the number of sutures involved, and the surgeon's experience. Generally, endoscopic craniosynostosis surgery tends to be shorter in duration compared to traditional open cranial vault reconstruction. The duration of endoscopic surgery typically ranges from 1 to 4 h, depending on various factors, including the number of involved sutures, the experience of surgeons, and surgical technique, among others.
4. The length of hospitalisation.

9. Clinical Outcome of the Surgical Treatment

It must be said that long-term results, both aesthetic and functional, are rarely demonstrated in most studies. Therefore, despite the relatively large number of studies, we do not have the data to draw firm conclusions about the long-term effectiveness of certain surgical techniques. As far as the aesthetic outcome is concerned, the conclusions of these studies are mainly based on postoperative measurements of the CI (ratio of skull width to skull length), which is not a perfect indicator of the morphology of the cranial body. At the same time, the results of the various studies are very heterogeneous, as children with different initial stages of deformity, different ages, and different surgical techniques were included in the studies. In any case, all studies describe an improvement in CI after surgery, and it is generally recognised that the lateral, biparietal head circumference increases after the surgery while the anteroposterior head circumference decreases to a lesser extent [74].

Different surgical techniques may have different effects on the final morphological appearance of the skull. In his study, Panchal compared linear suturectomy (without postoperative wearing of a helmet) with whole skull remodelling and described a more significant improvement in CI after whole skull remodelling compared to suturectomy one year after surgery. However, the long-term outcome was not analysed in this study, so no definitive conclusions could be drawn [75].

Although the aesthetic outcome is usually only assessed on the basis of a subjective evaluation, and these results should, therefore, be treated with caution, the literature shows that the aesthetic outcome is rated as good or very good in most cases. Only a few children show a poor aesthetic result and the need for a second operation. In this context, it should be noted that surgical treatment can also lead to more or less large bony defects in the vaulted skull, which occasionally require subsequent surgical coverage or cranioplasty.

10. ISS Relapse and Secondary Craniosynostosis of a Different Suture

Regardless of the surgical technique used, ISS recurrence is one of the rare but important causes of poor long-term aesthetic outcomes. In a series of 79 children who underwent linear suturectomy [76], four children required reoperation due to the recurrence of craniosynostosis and the occurrence of increased intracranial pressure. In the second series, which included 181 children operated for ISS, eleven children had to be reoperated due to proven recurrent synostosis [54,57–60]. Clinical and radiological evidence of increased intracranial pressure was found in six cases [74]. It should certainly be noted that in some of these children, sagittal craniosynostosis was part of the syndromic disease and that the predisposition for the occurrence of increased intracranial pressure was, therefore, increased in these children. This shows, among other things, the importance of the fact that even in apparently simple forms of ISS, there may be an underlying syndromic disease that is not yet recognised in the early neonatal period. On the other hand, these results indicate that the risk of increased intracranial pressure is always present, even in children with non-syndromic ISS. A strict follow-up after surgical treatment permits the early recognition of a persistent scaphocephalic deformation. An ophthalmologic diagnosis of papilledema and a radiological confirmation of a recurrent synostosis are the criteria on which the diagnosis of a recurrent ISS is based [74,75].

Other studies have also confirmed the risk of postoperative increased intracranial pressure and have shown that secondary craniosynostosis of another previously opened cranial suture may occur after surgery. Postoperative synostosis of the coronal suture is the most common in this context and can occur in up to 10% of children after removal of the sagittal suture if both coronal sutures were not also removed at the time of surgery [77]. Secondary synostosis of the coronary or lambdoid sutures may also occur after remodelling of the entire cranial vault, according to the literature [78]. Finally, this condition may also occur in some children who have not undergone surgery for ISS at all [77,79].

11. The Effect of Treatment on Neurocognitive Outcome

With appropriate and successful surgical treatment of ISS, the likelihood of neurocognitive impairment in children is very low and has been reported to be up to 9% in a mild form [3]. However, as we have already seen, the narrower shape of the cranial vault can result in the growing brain not having enough space for normal physiological development, which can lead to clinical signs of increased intracranial pressure, i.e., visual disturbances due to papilledema, headaches, and neurocognitive delays [80].

The impact of surgery on long-term neurocognitive functional outcomes is not clearly known, although surgery for scaphocephaly has been performed for several decades. The results in the literature are contradictory, and, most importantly, most studies have significant methodological limitations so that no realistic and long-term conclusions can be drawn. Different studies have compared different initial levels of deformity, different ages at the time of surgery, different surgical techniques, and different ages at clinical outcome assessment. All these factors, especially age at surgery, surgical technique, type of anaesthesia, and duration of surgery, can influence the final clinical outcome in one way or another. Neuroanaesthesia may also pose a risk for further cognitive delays. Taking all these limitations into account, we can conclude that most studies agree that children with ISS can develop long-term neurocognitive problems, particularly with regard to language development, despite surgical treatment. In a population of 18-year-olds operated on before the age of 30 weeks using a linear sagittal suture technique, a delay in language development was demonstrated [81]. Similar language problems were also demonstrated in another study [30] in which language development was delayed in 28 of the 76 children operated on. It has also been shown that children's motor functions generally improve after surgery and that these improvements persist over time [32].

Age at surgery is obviously important and has an impact on postoperative status and neurocognitive improvement. Several studies have shown that children operated on in the first year or first six months of life have better outcomes than children operated on later or those operated on at a later age for objective reasons (poor general condition or late referral to a surgical facility). Indeed, children may be referred for surgery because of a late diagnosis of ISS at the time of hospitalisation due to a general neurocognitive delay [1,30,32].

In the study by Hashim [35], the long-term neuropsychological outcome of children operated on for ISS was compared by age at surgery and by the surgical technique used. He compared linear suturectomy (without postoperative wearing of a helmet) with open total cranial vault remodelling. Neuropsychological tests were performed on 70 children (age range 5.75–24.42 years—mean age 10.04 years). The study included measures of IQ, verbal ability, reading ability, and reading comprehension. The worst results were found in the children for whom the intervention was carried out after the age of 12 months. However, in the two groups of children operated on before six months of age, linear suturectomy was associated with worse outcomes (i.e., it was not possible to expand and remodel the cranial vault sufficiently) than the remodelling of the entire vault. This showed that the surgical technique also has an impact on the final neurocognitive outcome and that the functional outcome varies depending on the surgical technique used and the age at surgery. Considering all these data, it is worth considering that the choice of surgical technique has an impact not only on the aesthetic but also on the functional outcome of children with ISS [35].

12. Conclusions

ISS continues to be a fascinating field of research that combines genetics, radiology, embryology, and clinical medicine. Advances in diagnostic methods and surgical techniques continue to improve our understanding and patient outcomes. The long-term outcomes of intervention for ISS are multifaceted and include not only the physical aspects of skull morphology but also cognitive development and psychosocial well-being. Early intervention has been associated with better neurocognitive outcomes, emphasising the importance of timely diagnosis and treatment. The importance of interdisciplinary collaboration in the comprehensive management of ISS and the need for continued research to further unravel the complexity of this anomaly cannot be overemphasised.

Author Contributions: Conceptualisation, P.S. and T.V.; resources, T.V.; data curation, P.S.; writing—original draft preparation, P.S. and T.V.; project administration, T.V.; funding acquisition, T.V. All authors have read and agreed to the published version of the manuscript.

Funding: This research received no external funding.

Institutional Review Board Statement: Not applicable.

Informed Consent Statement: Written informed consent has been obtained from the patients' parents to publish this paper.

Data Availability Statement: Not applicable.

Conflicts of Interest: The authors declare no conflicts of interest.

References

1. Spazzapan, P.; Kočar, M.; Eberlinc, A.; Velnar, T. Kraniofacialne rekonstrukcije pri otrocih s kraniosinostozo. *Slov. Pediatr.* **2021**, *28*, 67–77. [CrossRef]
2. Virchow, R. Uber den Cretinismus, namentlich in Franken, und uber pathologische Schadelformen. *Verh. Phys. Med. Ges. Wurzbg.* **1851**, *2*, 230.
3. Kajdic, N.; Spazzapan, P.; Velnar, T. Craniosynostosis—Recognition, clinical characteristics, and treatment. *Bosn. J. Basic. Med. Sci.* **2018**, *18*, 110–116. [CrossRef]
4. Cinalli, G.; Sainte-Rose, C.; Kollar, E.M.; Zerah, M.; Brunelle, F.; Chumas, P.; Arnaud, E.; Marchac, D.; Pierre-Kahn, A.; Renier, D. Hydrocephalus and craniosynostosis. *J. Neurosurg.* **1998**, *88*, 209–214. [CrossRef]
5. Spazzapan, P.; Kocar, M.; Eberlinc, A.; Haber, B.; Velnar, T. Craniofacial reconstructions in children with craniosynostosis. *J. Integr. Neurosci.* **2022**, *21*, 106. [CrossRef] [PubMed]

6. Arnaud, E.; Paternoster, G.; James, S.; Morisseau-Durand, M.P.; Couloigner, V.; Diner, P.; Tomat, C.; Viot-Blanc, V.; Fauroux, B.; Cormier-Daire, V.; et al. Stratégie craniofaciale pour les faciocraniosténoses [Craniofacial strategy for syndromic craniosynostosis]. *Ann. Chir. Plast. Esthétique* **2016**, *61*, 408–419. [CrossRef]
7. Esparza, J.; Hinojosa, J.; García-Recuero, I.; Romance, A.; Pascual, B.; de Aragón, A.M. Surgical treatment of isolated and syndromic craniosynostosis. Results and complications in 283 consecutive cases. *Neurocirugia* **2008**, *19*, 509–529. [CrossRef]
8. Ruiz-Correa, S.; Sze, R.W.; Starr, J.R.; Lin, H.T.; Speltz, M.L.; Cunningham, M.L.; Hing, A.V. New scaphocephaly severity indices of sagittal craniosynostosis: A comparative study with cranial index quantifications. *Cleft Palate-Craniofacial J.* **2006**, *43*, 211–221. [CrossRef] [PubMed]
9. Magge, S.N.; Westerveld, M.; Pruzinsky, T.; Persing, J.A. Long-term neuropsychological effects of sagittal craniosynostosis on child development. *J. Craniofacial Surg.* **2002**, *13*, 99–104. [CrossRef]
10. Di Rocco, F.; Zerah, M. Introduction au rapport sur les craniosténoses. *Neurochirurgie* **2019**, *65*, 195. [CrossRef] [PubMed]
11. Di Rocco, F.; Gleizal, A.; Szathmari, A.; Beuriat, P.A.; Paulus, C.; Mottolese, C. Sagittal suture craniosynostosis or craniosynostoses? The heterogeneity of the most common premature fusion of the cranial sutures. *Neurochirurgie* **2019**, *65*, 232–238. [CrossRef]
12. Calandrelli, R.; Pilato, F.; Massimi, L.; Panfili, M.; Colosimo, C. A systematic quantitative morpho-volumetric analysis in infants with sagittal craniosynostosis and relationship with the severity of scaphocephalic deformity. *Radiol. Med.* **2020**, *125*, 585–594. [CrossRef]
13. Aldridge, K.; Kane, A.A.; Marsh, J.L.; Yan, P.; Govier, D.; Richtsmeier, J.T. Relationship of brain and skull in pre- and postoperative sagittal synostosis. *J. Anat.* **2005**, *206*, 373–385. [CrossRef]
14. Usami, K.; Nicolini, F.; Arnaud, E.; Di Rocco, F. Cerebrospinal fluid collections in sagittal suture synostosis. *Childs Nerv. Syst.* **2016**, *32*, 519–525. [CrossRef]
15. Caldarelli, M.; Di Rocco, C.; Rossi, G.F. Lumbar subarachnoid infusion test in pediatric neurosurgery. *Dev. Med. Child. Neurol.* **1979**, *21*, 71–82. [CrossRef]
16. Di Rocco, C.; Caldarelli, M.; Mangiola, A.; Milani, A. The lumbar infusion test in infants. *Childs Nerv. Syst.* **1988**, *4*, 16–21. [CrossRef] [PubMed]
17. Heller, J.B.; Heller, M.M.; Knoll, B. Intracranial volume and cephalic index outcome. *Plast. Reconstr. Surg.* **2008**, *121*, 187–195. [CrossRef] [PubMed]
18. Posnick, J.C.; Armstrong, D.; Bite, U. Metopic and sagittal synostosis: Intracranial volume measurements prior to and after cranio-orbital reshaping in childhood. *Plast. Reconstr. Surg.* **1995**, *96*, 299–309. [CrossRef] [PubMed]
19. Posnick, J.C.; Lin, K.Y.; Chen, P.; Armstrong, D. Sagittal synostosis: Quantitative assessment of presenting deformity and surgical results based on CT scans. *Plast. Reconstr. Surg.* **1993**, *92*, 1015–1024. [CrossRef] [PubMed]
20. Seeberger, R.; Hoffmann, J.; Freudlsperger, C.; Berger, M.; Bodem, J.; Horn, D.; Engel, M. Intracranial volume (ICV) in isolated sagittal craniosynostosis measured by 3D photocephalometry: A new perspective on a controversial issue. *J. Cranio-Maxillofac. Surg.* **2016**, *44*, 626–631. [CrossRef] [PubMed]
21. Chauhan, B.K.; Hoover, J.M.; Scanga, H.; Medsinge, A.; Arnold, G.L.; Nischal, K.K. Isolated Sagittal Synostosis in a Boy with Craniofrontonasal Dysplasia and a Novel EFNB1 Mutation. *Plast. Reconstr. Surg. Glob. Open* **2015**, *3*, e427. [CrossRef] [PubMed]
22. Rothenbuhler, A.; Fadel, N.; Debza, Y.; Bacchetta, J.; Diallo, M.T.; Adamsbaum, C.; Linglart, A.; Di Rocco, F. High Incidence of Cranial Synostosis and Chiari I Malformation in Children With X-Linked Hypophosphatemic Rickets (XLHR). *J. Bone Miner. Res.* **2019**, *34*, 490–496. [CrossRef] [PubMed]
23. Lee, B.S.; Hwang, L.S.; Doumit, G.D.; Wooley, J.; Papay, F.A.; Luciano, M.G.; Recinos, V.M. Management options of non-syndromic sagittal craniosynostosis. *J. Clin. Neurosci.* **2017**, *39*, 28–34. [CrossRef]
24. Arnaud, E.; Renier, D.; Marchac, D. Prognosis for mental function in scaphocephaly. *J. Neurosurg.* **1995**, *83*, 476–479. [CrossRef] [PubMed]
25. Florisson, J.M.; van Veelen, M.L.; Bannink, N.; van Adrichem, L.N.; van der Meulen, J.J.; Bartels, M.C.; Mathijssen, I.M. Papilledema in isolated single-suture craniosynostosis: Prevalence and predictive factors. *J. Craniofacial Surg.* **2010**, *21*, 20–24. [CrossRef]
26. Renier, D.; Sainte-Rose, C.; Marchac, D.; Hirsch, J.F. Intracranial pressure in craniostenosis. *J. Neurosurg.* **1982**, *57*, 370–377. [CrossRef]
27. Speltz, M.L.; Collett, B.R.; Wallace, E.R.; Starr, J.R.; Cradock, M.M.; Buono, L.; Cunningham, M.; Kapp-Simon, K. Intellectual and academic functioning of school-age children with single-suture craniosynostosis. *Pediatrics* **2015**, *135*, e615–e623. [CrossRef]
28. Massimi, L.; Caldarelli, M.; Tamburrini, G.; Paternoster, G.; Di Rocco, C. Isolated sagittal synostosis: Definition, classification and surgical indications. *Childs Nerv. Syst.* **2012**, *28*, 1311–1317. [CrossRef]
29. Bellew, M.; Chumas, P. Long-term developmental follow-up in children with nonsyndromic craniosynostosis. *J. Neurosurg. Pediatr.* **2015**, *16*, 445–451. [CrossRef]
30. Shipster, C.; Hearst, D.; Somerville, A.; Stackhouse, J.; Hayward, R.; Wade, A. Speech, language, and cognitive development in children with isolated sagittal synostosis. *Dev. Med. Child. Neurol.* **2003**, *45*, 34–43. [CrossRef]
31. Da Costa, A.C.; Anderson, V.A.; Savarirayan, R.; Wrennall, J.A.; Chong, D.K.; Holmes, A.D.; Greensmith, A.L.; Meara, J.G. Neurodevelopmental functioning of infants with untreated single-suture craniosynostosis during early infancy. *Childs Nerv. Syst.* **2012**, *28*, 869–877. [CrossRef]

32. Bellew, M.; Liddington, M.; Chumas, P.; Russell, J. Preoperative and postoperative developmental attainment in patients with sagittal synostosis: 5-year followup. *J. Neurosurg. Pediatr.* **2011**, *7*, 121–126. [CrossRef]
33. Kljajić, M.; Maltese, G.; Tarnow, P.; Sand, P.; Kölby, L. The cognitive profile of children with nonsyndromic craniosynostosis. *Plast. Reconstr. Surg.* **2019**, *143*, 1037–1052. [CrossRef] [PubMed]
34. Gewalli, F.; Guimarães-Ferreira, J.P.; Sahlin, P.; Emanuelsson, I.; Horneman, G.; Stephensen, H.; Lauritzen, C.G. Mental development after modified pi procedure: Dynamic cranioplasty for sagittal synostosis. *Ann. Plast. Surg.* **2001**, *46*, 415–420. [CrossRef] [PubMed]
35. Hashim, P.W.; Patel, A.; Yang, J.F.; Travieso, R.; Terner, J.; Losee, J.E.; Pollack, I.; Jane, J., Sr.; Jane, J., Jr.; Kanev, P.; et al. The effects of whole-vault cranioplasty versus strip craniectomy on long-term neuropsychological outcomes in sagittal craniosynostosis. *Plast. Reconstr. Surg.* **2014**, *134*, 491–501. [CrossRef] [PubMed]
36. Lannelongue, M. De la craniectomie dans la microcéphalie. *Compt. Rend. Seances Acad. Sci.* **1890**, *110*, 1382–1385.
37. Lane, L.C. Pioneer craniectomy for relief of mental imbecility due to premature sutural closure and microcephalus. *JAMA* **1892**, *18*, 49–59. [CrossRef]
38. Jacobi, A. Non nocere. *Med. Rec.* **1894**, *45*, 609.
39. Faber, H.K.; Towne, E.B. Early craniectomy as a preventive measure in oxycephaly and allied conditions. With special reference to the prevention of blindness. *Am. J. Med. Sci.* **1927**, *173*, 701–711. [CrossRef]
40. Hunter, A.G.W.; Rudo, N.L. Craniosynostosis I. Sagittal synostosis: Its genetics and associated clinical findings in 214 patients who lacked involvement of the coronal suture(s). *Teratology* **1976**, *14*, 185–193. [CrossRef] [PubMed]
41. Albright, A.L.; Towbin, R.B.; Schultz, B.L. Long term outcome after sagittal synostosis operations. *Pediatr. Neurosurg.* **1996**, *25*, 78–82. [CrossRef]
42. Greene, C.S., Jr.; Winston, K.R. Treatment of scaphocephaly with sagittal craniectomy and biparietal morcellation. *Neurosurgery* **1988**, *23*, 196–202. [CrossRef]
43. Epstein, N.; Epstein, F.; Newman, G. Total vertex craniectomy for the treatment of scaphocephaly. *Childs Brain* **1982**, *9*, 309–316. [CrossRef]
44. Jane, J.A.; Edgerton, M.T.; Futrell, J.W.; Park, T.S. Immediate correction of sagittal synostosis. *J. Neurosurg.* **1978**, *49*, 705–710. [CrossRef] [PubMed]
45. Marchac, D.; Renier, D. *Craniofacial Surgery for Craniosynostosis*; Little Brown: Boston, MA, USA, 1982; pp. 87–92.
46. Amm, C.A.; Denny, A.D. Correction of sagittal synostosis using foreshortening and lateral expansion of the cranium activated by gravity: Surgical technique and postoperative evolution. *Plast. Reconstr. Surg.* **2005**, *116*, 723–735. [CrossRef] [PubMed]
47. Berry-Candelario, J.; Ridgway, E.D.; Grondin, R.T.; Rogers, G.F.; Proctor, M.R. Endoscope-assisted strip craniectomy and postoperative helmet therapy for treatment of craniosynostosis. *Neurosurg. Focus* **2011**, *31*, E5. [CrossRef] [PubMed]
48. Boop, F.A.; Chadduck, W.M.; Shewmake, K.; Teo, C. Outcome analysis of 85 patients undergoing the pi procedure for correction of sagittal synostosis. *J. Neurosurg.* **1996**, *85*, 50–55. [CrossRef] [PubMed]
49. Renier, D.; Lajeunie, E.; Arnaud, E.; Marchac, D. Management of craniosynostoses. *Childs Nerv. Syst.* **2000**, *16*, 645–658. [CrossRef]
50. Tullous, M.W.; Henry, M.N.; Wang, P.T.H.; Vollmer, D.G.; Auber, A.E.; Mancuso, P.A. Multiple-revolution spiral osteotomy for cranial reconstruction. *J. Neurosurg.* **2001**, *94*, 671–678. [CrossRef] [PubMed]
51. Van Veelen, M.L.; Mathijssen, I.M. Spring-assisted correction of sagittal suture synostosis. *Childs Nerv. Syst.* **2012**, *28*, 1347–1351. [CrossRef] [PubMed]
52. David, L.R.; Plikaitis, C.M.; Couture, D. Outcome analysis of our first 75 spring-assisted surgeries for scaphocephaly. *J. Craniofacial Surg.* **2010**, *21*, 3–9. [CrossRef]
53. Kolar, J.C.; Salter, E.M.; Weinberg, S.M. Preoperative craniofacial dysmorphology in isolated sagittal synostosis: A comprehensive anthropometric evaluation. *J. Craniofacial Surg.* **2010**, *21*, 1404–1410. [CrossRef]
54. Di Rocco, F.; Knoll, B.I.; Arnaud, E.; Blanot, S.; Meyer, P.; Cuttarree, H.; Sainte-Rose, C.; Marchac, D. Scaphocephaly correction with retrocoronal and prelambdoid craniotomies (Renier's "H" technique). *Childs Nerv. Syst.* **2012**, *28*, 1327–1332. [CrossRef]
55. Jimenez, D.F.; Barone, C.M.; Rogers, J.N. *Endoscopic Wide Vertex Craniectomy in Controversies in Pediatric Neurosurgery*; Jallo, G.I., Kothbauer, K.F., Pradilla, G., Eds.; Thieme: New York, NY, USA, 2010.
56. Jugović, D.; Spazzapan, P. Endoskopsko zdravljenje skafocefalije: Prikaz primera in nove operacijske tehnike. *Zdr. Vestn.* **2015**, *84*, 642–648. [CrossRef]
57. Di Rocco, F.; Ben Gbulie, U.; Meyer, P.; Arnaud, E. Current techniques and protocols in the surgical management of scaphocephaly in young infants. *J. Craniofacial Surg.* **2014**, *25*, 39–41. [CrossRef]
58. Jane, J.A.; Francel, P.C. *The Evolution of Treatment for Sagittal Synostosis: A Personal Record in Craniofacial Anomalies: Growth and Development from a Surgical Perspective*; Goodrich, J.T., Hall, C.D., Eds.; Thieme: New York, NY, USA, 1995.
59. Kiehna, E.N.; Jane, J.A. *Early Strip Craniectomy in Controversies in Pediatric Neurosurgery*; Jallo, G.I., Kothbauer, K.F., Pradilla, G., Eds.; Thieme: New York, NY, USA, 2010.
60. Mori, K.; Sakamoto, T.; Nakai, K. *The Surgical Management of Scaphocephaly in Craniofacial Anomalies: Growth and Development from a Surgical Perspective*; Goodrich, J.T., Hall, C.D., Eds.; Thieme: New York, NY, USA, 1995.
61. Di Rocco, C. How to decrease the impact of surgical scar in the correction of sagittal synostosis. *Childs Nerv. Syst.* **2003**, *19*, 42–45. [CrossRef]

62. Arko, L., 4th; Swanson, J.W.; Fierst, T.M.; Henn, R.E.; Chang, D.; Storm, P.B.; Bartlett, S.P.; Taylor, J.A.; Heuer, G.G. Spring-mediated sagittal craniosynostosis treatment at the Children's Hospital of Philadelphia: Technical notes and literature review. *Neurosurg. Focus* **2015**, *38*, E7. [CrossRef] [PubMed]
63. Lauritzen, C.G.; Davis, C.; Ivarsson, A.; Sanger, C.; Hewitt, T.D. The evolving role of springs in craniofacial surgery: The first 100 clinical cases. *Plast. Reconstr. Surg.* **2008**, *121*, 545–554. [CrossRef] [PubMed]
64. Fearon, J.A.; McLaughlin, E.B.; Kolar, J.C. Sagittal craniosynostosis: Surgical outcomes and long-term growth. *Plast. Reconstr. Surg.* **2006**, *117*, 532–541. [CrossRef] [PubMed]
65. Goobie, S.M.; Meier, P.M.; Pereira, L.M.; McGowan, F.X.; Prescilla, R.P.; Scharp, L.A. Efficacy of tranexamic acid in pediatric craniosynostosis surgery: A double-blind, placebo-controlled trial. *Anesthesiology* **2011**, *114*, 862–871. [CrossRef] [PubMed]
66. Jimenez, D.F.; Barone, C.M. Endoscopic craniectomy for early surgical correction of sagittal craniosynostosis. *J. Neurosurg.* **1998**, *88*, 77–81. [CrossRef]
67. Jimenez, D.F.; Barone, C.M. Endoscopic technique for sagittal synostosis. *Childs Nerv. Syst.* **2012**, *28*, 1333–1339. [CrossRef]
68. Shah, M.N.; Kane, A.A.; Petersen, J.D.; Woo, A.S.; Naidoo, S.D.; Smyth, M.D. Endoscopically assisted versus open repair of sagittal craniosynostosis: The St. Louis Children's Hospital experience. *J. Neurosurg. Pediatr.* **2011**, *8*, 165–170. [CrossRef] [PubMed]
69. Thomas, G.P.L.; Johnson, D.; Byren, J.C.; Judge, A.D.; Jayamohan, J.; Magdum, S.A. The incidence of raised intracranial pressure in nonsyndromic sagittal craniosynostosis following primary surgery. *J. Neurosurg. Pediatr.* **2015**, *15*, 350–360. [CrossRef] [PubMed]
70. Thompson, D.R.; Zurakowski, D.; Haberkern, C.M.; Stricker, P.A.; Meier, P.M.; Bannister, C.; Benzon, H.; Binstock, W.; Bosenberg, A.; Brzenski, A.; et al. Endoscopic Versus Open Repair for Craniosynostosis in Infants Using Propensity Score Matching to Compare Outcomes: A Multicenter Study from the Pediatric Craniofacial Collaborative Group. *Anesth. Analg.* **2018**, *126*, 968–975. [CrossRef] [PubMed]
71. Hinojosa, J.; Esparza, J.; Muñoz, M.J. Endoscopic-assisted osteotomies for the treatment of craniosynostosis. *Childs Nerv. Syst.* **2007**, *23*, 1421–1430. [CrossRef] [PubMed]
72. Murad, G.J.; Clayman, M.; Seagle, M.B.; White, S.; Perkins, L.A.; Pincus, D.W. Endoscopic-assisted repair of craniosynostosis. *Neurosurg. Focus* **2005**, *19*, E6. [CrossRef] [PubMed]
73. Isaac, K.V.; Meara, J.G.; Proctor, M.R. Analysis of clinical outcomes for treatment of sagittal craniosynostosis: A comparison of endoscopic suturectomy and cranial vault remodeling. *J. Neurosurg. Pediatr.* **2018**, *22*, 467–474. [CrossRef] [PubMed]
74. Collmann, H.; Solomon, B.D.; Schweitzer, T.; Kress, W.; Muenke, M. Nonsyndromic craniosynostoses in Craniosynostoses: Molecular genetics, principles of diagnosis and treatment. In *Monographs in Human Genetics*; Muenke, M., Kress, W., Collmann, H., Solomon, B.D., Eds.; Karger: Basel, Switzerland, 2011; Volume 19, pp. 165–176.
75. Panchal, J.; Marsh, J.L.; Park, T.S.; Kaufman, B.; Pilgram, T.; Huang, S.H. Sagittal craniosynostosis outcome assessment for two methods and timings of intervention. *Plast. Reconstr. Surg.* **1999**, *103*, 1574–1584. [CrossRef]
76. Van Veelen, M.L.; Eelkman Rooda, O.H.; de Jong, T.; Dammers, R.; van Adrichem, L.N.; Mathijssen, I.M. Results of early surgery for sagittal suture synostosis:long-term follow-up and the occurrence of raised intracranial pressure. *Childs Nerv. Syst.* **2013**, *29*, 997–1005. [CrossRef]
77. Arnaud, E.; Capon-Degardin, N.; Michienzi, J.; Di Rocco, F.; Renier, D. Scaphocephaly part II: Secondary coronal synostosis after scaphocephalic surgical correction. *J. Craniofacial Surg.* **2009**, *20* (Suppl. S2), 1843–1850. [CrossRef] [PubMed]
78. Seruya, M.; Tan, S.Y.; Wray, A.C.; Penington, A.J.; Greensmith, A.L.; Holmes, A.D. Total cranial vault remodeling for isolated sagittal synostosis: Part I. Postoperative cranial suture patency. *Plast. Reconstr. Surg.* **2013**, *132*, 602–610. [CrossRef] [PubMed]
79. Yarbrough, C.K.; Smyth, M.D.; Holekamp, T.F.; Ranalli, N.J.; Huang, A.H.; Patel, K.B. Delayed synostoses of uninvolved sutures after surgical treatment of nonsyndromic craniosynostosis. *J. Craniofacial Surg.* **2014**, *25*, 119–123. [CrossRef] [PubMed]
80. Gault, D.T.; Renier, D.; Marchac, D.; Jones, B.M. Intracranial pressure and intracranial volume in children with craniosynostosis. *Plast. Reconstr. Surg.* **1992**, *90*, 377–381. [CrossRef] [PubMed]
81. Virtanen, R.; Korhonen, T.; Fagerholm, J.; Viljanto, J. Neurocognitive sequelae of scaphocephaly. *Pediatrics* **1999**, *103*, 791–795. [CrossRef]

diagnostics MDPI

Article

Results of Surgical Treatment of Occult Spinal Dysraphisms—A Single Centre Experience

Peter Spazzapan [1], Tomaz Velnar [1,2,*], Nina Perosa [2], Andrej Porcnik [2] and Borut Prestor [2]

[1] Unit of Paediatric Neurosurgery, University Medical Centre Ljubljana, 1000 Ljubljana, Slovenia; spazzapanpeter@yahoo.it
[2] Department of Neurosurgery, University Medical Centre Ljubljana, 1000 Ljubljana, Slovenia; nina.vrbnjak@gmail.com (N.P.); andrej.porcnik@kclj.si (A.P.); borut.prestor@kclj.si (B.P.)
* Correspondence: tvelnar@hotmail.com

Abstract: Occult spinal dysraphisms (OSDs) are caused by various defects in the embryogenesis of the spinal cord and represent an obstacle to the ascent of the conus, which allows the conus to pass from the lower levels of the spinal canal to the final position between L1 and L2 during normal foetal life. When an OSD tethers the spinal cord at the lower levels, it can lead to neurological symptoms, better known as tethered cord syndrome. Surgical treatment of OSD is primarily aimed at untethering the spinal cord. In asymptomatic patients, this can protect against the long-term development of neurological deficits. In symptomatic patients, this can halt or limit the progression of existing symptoms. The aim of this study is to examine all paediatric and adult patients diagnosed with OSD and treated in the Department of Neurosurgery at the University Medical Centre Ljubljana during the 5-year period of 2016–2021. All patients diagnosed with OSD during this period were included in the study. Patient characteristics, treatment modalities and outcomes were studied with the aim of describing the differences between the paediatric and adult population and defining the rationality of treating these pathological conditions. We included in the study 52 patients with 64 occult dysraphic lesions. Adults (>18 years old) represented 15/52 (28.8%) of all patients, while 37/52 (71.8%) were children. The most common OSDs were conus lipomas, followed by dermal sinus tracts, filum terminale lipomas and split cord malformations. Surgical treatment was performed in 35/52 (67.3%) cases, while conservative management was chosen in 17/52 (32.6%) cases. The preoperative presence of symptoms was statistically higher in adults than in children ($p = 0.0098$). Surgery on complex spinal cord lipomas was statistically related to a higher rate of postoperative neurological complications ($p = 0.0002$). The treatment of OSD is complex and must be based on knowledge of the developmental anomalies of the spine and spinal cord. Successful surgical treatment relies on microsurgical techniques and the use of neuromonitoring. Successful treatment can prevent or limit the occurrence of neurological problems.

Keywords: dysraphisms; tethered cord; sphincter dysfunction; paresis; pain; orthopaedic deformation

1. Introduction

Occult spinal dysraphisms (OSDs) are malformations of the spinal axis of the nervous system, caused by disorders at different stages of the embryogenesis of the nervous system. Depending on the developmental stage at which the defect occurs, they are categorised as gastrulation defects, primary neurulation defects and secondary neurulation defects, which are described as follows:

- Gastrulation defects: Gastrulation is the process by which the epiblast gives rise to the trilaminar disc (ectoderm, mesoderm and endoderm). Defects at this stage can lead to the development of diastematomyelia (split cord malformation—SCM) and neurenteric cysts.

- Primary neurulation defects: Primary neurulation is the process of neural tube closure. A defect at this stage can lead to the development of a myelomeningocele (MMC) (open spinal dysraphism, not discussed in this article), dermal sinus tract, limited dorsal myeloschisis (LDM) and conus lipoma.
- Secondary neurulation defects: Secondary neurulation is the process of formation of the most caudal part of the nervous system (conus, cauda equina and filum terminale). Defects at this stage lead to the development of lipomas of the filum terminale (LFTs), Currarino syndrome, caudal regression syndrome and myelocystocele.

One of the key moments in the development of the spinal cord and cauda equina is the ascent of the conus, i.e., the process by which the conus ascends from the low, sacral levels to the final L1–L2 position, during the last months of gestation. All forms of OSD can interfere with this process to some degree, by impeding the ascent of the conus or spinal cord, which remains tethered in the lower levels of the spinal canal. This condition is called tethered spinal cord. A tethered spinal cord may be asymptomatic in early childhood. Later, during growth, some children may develop tethered cord syndrome, which is characterised by orthopaedic deformities, paresis, muscle atrophy, paraesthesia, pain and sphincter dysfunction. Asymptomatic children with tethering of the spinal cord have a varying risk of becoming symptomatic in the first 10 years of life, depending on the type of OSD. For conus lipomas, which are one of the most common forms of OSD, this risk is estimated at 40–43% [1–3]. Some children with OSD may already show symptoms in the neonatal period, though cutaneous stigmata in the lumbosacral region remain the most common cause that induce further investigations and lead to the diagnosis of OSD [1,2]. In all cases of OSD, it must be assessed whether it is appropriate to surgically untether the spinal cord to prevent the onset of symptoms and to prevent the progression of pre-existing neurological deficits.

In this study we analysed the preoperative, operative and postoperative data of a series of consecutive patients treated in a single centre for OSD. The aim was to compare the preoperative data between adults and children and define the operative risks of different types of OSDs.

2. Materials and Methods

In this paper, we retrospectively review all preoperative and postoperative data of patients treated with newly diagnosed OSD in the Department of Neurosurgery at the University Medical Centre Ljubljana between 2016 and 2021.

We collected data on the demographic, clinical and radiological characteristics of the patients. Lipomas of the spinal cord were classified, based on the definition of Pang [3], as dorsal (located on the dorsal side of the placode and above the conus, which is spared), transitional (located on the dorsal side of the placode, but at the level of the conus, which is affected) and chaotic (located on the ventral and dorsal side of the conus, which is embedded in the fatty tissue). The treatment was divided into conservative or surgical and the outcome of treatment was classified on the basis of new postoperative neurological deficits. To compare the differences between paediatric and adult patients we used a Student's t-test for two independent means. We further analysed the operative risks for those subtypes of OSD related to the highest surgical challenges and risks, namely the transitional and chaotic conus lipomas. The statistical results were significant, at $p < 0.05$.

3. Results

Between 2016 and 2021, 52 patients were diagnosed with some form of OSD. Table 1 summarises the demographic, clinical and radiological aspects of the patients (Table 1). Adults (>18 years old) represented 15/52 (28.8%) of all patients, while 37/52 (71.8%) were children. Of paediatric diagnoses, 21/37 (56.7%) were made within the first 3 months of life. Cutaneous stigmata (haemangioma, subcutaneous lipoma or dermal pit) were present in 44/52 (84.6%) patients; they were recognized in 34/37 (91.8%) paediatric patients and in 10/15 (66.6%) adult patients.

Table 1. Demographic characteristics of the patients included in the case series.

	Total	Children	Adults
Total number of patients	52	37/52 (71.8%)	15/52 (28.8%)
Total number of OSDs	64	49/64 (76.5%)	15/64 (23.4%)
Cutaneous stigmata	44/52 (84.6%)	34/37 (91.8%)	10/15 (66.6%)
Conus lipoma	22/64 (34.3%)	17/22 (77.2%)	5/22 (22.7%)
Dorsal	13/22 (59%)	12/13 (92.3%)	1/13 (7.6%)
Transitional	7/22 (31.8%)	3/7 (42.8%)	4/7 (57.1%)
Chaotic	2/22 (9%)	2/2 (100%)	0
Dermal tract	13/64 (20.3%)	12/13 (83.3%)	1/13 (7.6%)
LFT	12/64 (18.7%)	10/12 (83.3%)	2/12 (16.6%)
SCM	5/64 (7.8%)	4/5 (80%)	1/5 (20%)
Conus agenesis	3/64 (4.6%)	3/3 (100%)	0
LDM	2/64 (3.1%)	2/2 (100%)	0
Dermoid cyst	2/64 (3.1%)	2/2 (100%)	0
Presacral meningocele	2/64 (3.1%)	0	2/2 (100%)
Neurenteric cyst	1/64 (1.5%)	0	1/1 (100%)
Epithelialized MMC	1/64 (1.5%)	0	1/1 (%)
Meningocele	1/64 (1.5%)	1/1 (100%)	0

In 13/52 (25%) cases there were two different dysraphic lesions. Two patients had three different dysraphic lesions (Figure 1). In total, there were 64 dysraphic lesions (Table 1): 22/64 (34.3%) conus lipomas (transitional in 13/22 (59%) cases, dorsal in 7/22 (31.8%) cases and chaotic in 2/22 (9%) cases); 13/64 (20.3%) dermal tracts; 12/64 (18.7%) LFTs; 5/64 (7.8%) SCMs; 3/64 (4.6%) agenesis of the conus as part of caudal regression syndrome; 2/64 (3.1%) LDM; 2/64 (3.1%) dermoid cysts; 2/64 (3.1%) presacral meningoceles as part of Currarino syndrome; 1/64 (1.5%) neurenteric cyst; 1/64 (1.5%) epithelialized MMC; and 1/64 (1.5%) meningocele.

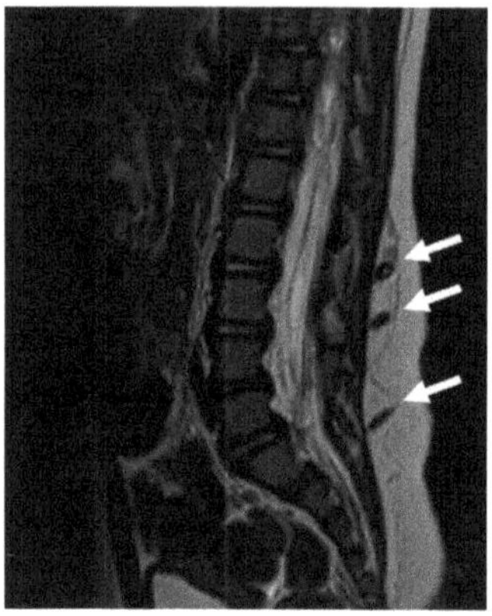

Figure 1. MR scan of a paediatric patient with three concomitant dermal tracts (white arrows). The conus is located at a physiological level L1.

The only case of epithelialized MMC (Figure 2) was included in the OSD series because the patient presented in adulthood and the placode was completely covered with intact skin. The spinal cord was untethered from the overlying fibrous epithelialized tissue, and the dural sac was reconstructed using the same techniques and principles of untethering for spinal cord lipomas.

In 8/52 (15.3%) cases, the conus was at the physiological level of L1, while, in all other cases, the spinal cord was tethered at lower levels. The VACTERL association (combination of spinal defects, anal atresia, cardiac defects, tracheoesophageal fistula, renal anomalies and orthopaedic deformities of the lower limbs) was present in 2/52 (3.8%) cases. Genetic syndromes were present as follows: Currarino syndrome in 3/52 (5.7%) cases (Figure 3), caudal regression syndrome in 3/52 (5.7%) cases (Figure 4) and sacral syndrome, Down syndrome and PNET hamartoma syndrome each in 1/52 (1.9%) cases. A Chiari malformation was present in 4/52 (7.6%) cases (Chiari 2 in two cases with an underlying MMC). The two cases in which the primary underlying malformation was an open neural tube defect, namely an MMC, had also associated hydrocephalus, which were treated by means of a ventriculoperitoneal shunt. Overall, 17/52 (32.6%) patients were not treated surgically, and 35/52 (67.3%) patients were treated with a neurosurgical procedure (Table 2).

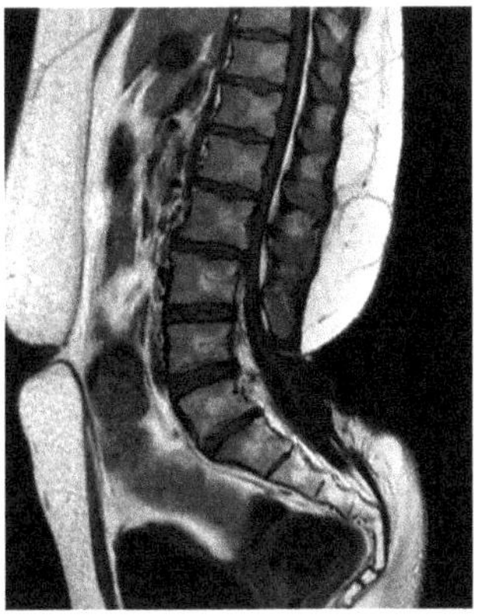

Figure 2. MR scan of an adult patient who presented with an epithelized MMC tethering the spinal cord. The spinal cord was untethered and the dural sac reconstructed by means of a wide dural sac.

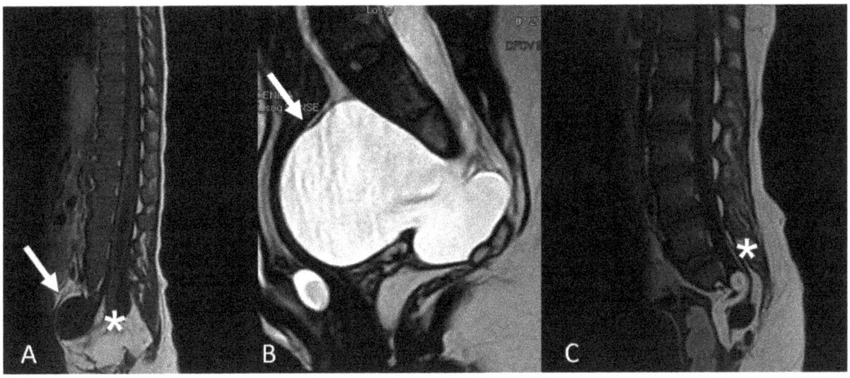

Figure 3. Two patients with Currarino syndrome, characterised by a presacral mass, which is most often represented by a meningocele (**A**,**B**) (white arrows). The spinal cord can be tethered by a conus lipoma (**A**) or by a LFT (**C**) (asterisks).

The reasons for not undergoing surgery were as follows: rejection of the risks of surgery or an older age of the patient (the preventive potential of surgical untethering is lower in adults than in children) [1–3]. In three cases with caudal regression syndrome, no surgery was indicated, as magnetic resonance imaging (MRI) showed only agenesis of the conus without spinal cord tethering.

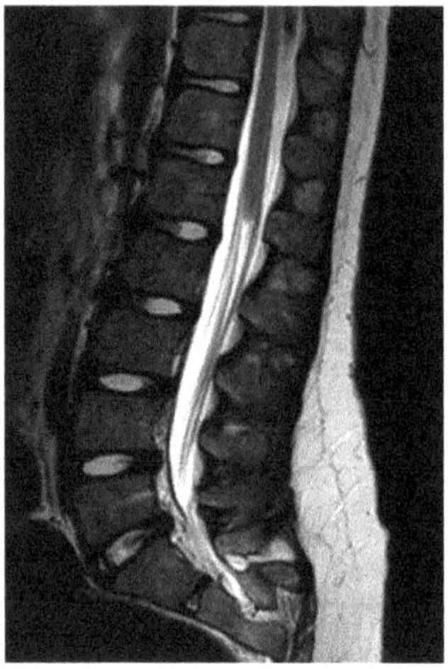

Figure 4. A case of caudal regression syndrome, where the conus, cauda equina and filum terminale are not developed, due to an absent process of secondary neurulation.

Table 2. Treatment strategies for the treatment of OSD and complications after surgical treatment.

	Total Number of Patients	Children	Adults
Conservative treatment	17/52 (32.6%)	10/17 (58.8%)	7/17 (41.1%)
Surgical treatment	35/52 (67.3%)	29/35 (82.8%)	6/35 (17.1%)
Transient sphincter dysfunction	2/35 (5.7%)	2/2 (100%)	0
Permanent sphincter dysfunction	1/35 (2.8%)	1/1 (100%)	0
Segmental sensory loss	3/35 (8.5%)	3/3 (100%)	0

In the preoperative neurological status, we observed the following (Table 3): spinal deformities in 5/37 (13.5%) paediatric cases and in 3/15 (20%) adult cases ($p = 0.566$); urological problems in 7/37 (18.9%) paediatric cases and 5/15 (33.3%) adult cases ($p = 0.272$); orthopaedic deformities in 9/37 (24.3%) paediatric cases and 8/15 (53.3%) adult cases ($p = 0.044$); lower limb paresis in 8/37 (21.6%) paediatric cases and 7/15 (46.6%) adult cases ($p = 0.073$); pain in 5/37 (13.5%) paediatric cases and 11/15 (73.3%) adult cases ($p = 0.0001$); and paraesthesia in 10/37 (27%) paediatric cases and 10/15 (66.6%) adult cases ($p = 0.007$). Overall, the statistical analysis confirmed a statistically significant difference in the presence of symptoms between children and adults ($p = 0.0098$).

Syringomyelia was present in 12/37 (32.4%) paediatric cases and in none of the adult cases. In four paediatric cases (three caudal regression syndromes and one MMC), the primary spinal cord malformation, rather than the spinal cord tethering, was the direct cause of the neurological deficits. In the group of symptomatic children, no subtype of dysraphism was predominant (three LFTs, four conus lipomas, two SCMs and three caudal regression syndromes).

Neurosurgical untethering of the spinal cord was performed in 35/52 (67.3%) cases. Postoperative transient sphincter dysfunction occurred in 2/35 (5.7%) cases and permanent sphincter dysfunction occurred in 1/35 (2.8%) case. In 3/35 (8.5%) cases, a permanent loss of sensation was observed in some isolated dermatomes of the lower limbs after the untethering. All of these complications occurred after transitional conus lipoma surgery. Wound infection occurred in 2/35 (5.7%) cases, while we observed cerebrospinal fluid (CSF) leakage in 3/35 (8.5%) cases. A second operation was not necessary in any case. Taking into account the complexity of surgical treatment of transitional and chaotic lipomas, we observed that 4/9 (44.4%) of these surgeries were complicated by a permanent neurological deficit, compared to the 0% rate of permanent neurological deficits of the other 26 OSD surgical procedures ($p = 0.0002$).

Table 3. Preoperative signs and symptoms of the tethered cord syndrome recorded in adult and paediatric patients of our series.

	Total	Children	Adults	*t*-Test
Spinal deformities	8/52 (15.3%)	5/37 (13.5%)	3/15 (20%)	$p = 0.566$
Urological problems	12/52 (23%)	7/37 (18.9%)	5/15 (33.3%)	$p = 0.272$
Orthopaedic deformities	17/52 (32.6%)	9/37 (24.3%)	8/15 (53.3%)	$p = 0.044$
Lower limb paresis	15/52 (28.8%)	8/37 (21.6%)	7/15 (46.6%)	$p = 0.073$
Pain	16/52 (30.7%)	5/37 (13.5%)	11/15 (73.3%)	$p = 0.0001$
Paraesthesia	20/52 (38.4%)	10/37 (27%)	10/15 (66.6%)	$p = 0.007$

4. Discussion

OSDs are developmental anomalies of the spinal neural axis that can cause tethered cord syndrome. In the last trimester of pregnancy, when the nervous system is already developed, the physiological process of the ascent of the conus takes place. Due to the asymmetry between the development and growth of the vertebrae and the spinal cord, the conus ascents from its original low position to the physiological level of L1–L2. In the vast majority of cases, OSD interferes with this process and tether the spinal cord at a low level. In the long term, this leads to ischemia, compression and myelodysplasia of the spinal cord, which can result in tethered cord syndrome, characterized by spinal and orthopaedic deformities, urological problems, paresis, paraesthesia and pain in the lower limbs.

OSDs are caused by a variety of early embryological neurodevelopmental defects. The most appropriate classification of dysraphisms is, therefore, based on knowledge of the developmental stages of embryonic development.

4.1. Defects in the Gastrulation Stage

Gastrulation occurs between days 14 and 16 of gestational age and leads to the development of the trilaminar embryonic disc, which consists of the endoderm, mesoderm and ectoderm. The ectoderm is the most important from the point of view of neurosurgical pathology.

1. Diastematomyelia—Split cord malformation (SCM):

SCM is characterised by a split, double spinal cord. It is caused by a defect in the phase of cellular migration from the epiblast to the primitive cord, a process that normally leads to cellular integration and the formation of the notochord. If integration does not occur, two notochords are formed, triggering the formation of two hemicords [4]. A distinction is made between SCM1, in which there is a bone spur between the two halves of the spinal cord, and SCM2, in which the two hemicords are separated by a fibrous membrane. SCM1 is characterised by two dural sacs, while the dural sac in SCM2 is a single one. Both forms hinder the normal ascent of the conus and the spinal cord. For this reason, it is necessary to remove the bone or membrane separating the two hemicords and create a single dural sac. In our series, SCM1 was present in three cases and SCM2 in two cases. Two patients with SCM1 were treated surgically (Figure 5), and one patient with SCM1 rejected surgical treatment. Both patients with SCM2 are asymptomatic and are under strict follow-up with annual electromyographic and urodynamic tests.

2. Neurenteric cyst:

Between days 18 and 20 of gestation, the yolk sac and amniotic cavity are temporarily connected by the neurenteric canal of Kovalevsky, which remains open for 3–4 days and closes with the closure of the primitive streak, leaving the notochord behind [5]. If this channel does not close, this leads to a permanent connection between the ectodermal (neural) and endodermal structures. This form of OSD is called a neurenteric cyst, which manifests as a tumour in the spinal canal (Figure 6). The cyst is surrounded by a characteristic enteric epithelium and can compress the spinal cord, leading to neurological deficits. A neurenteric cyst is always located on the ventral or lateral side of the spinal cord, never on the dorsal side. It is often associated with bony abnormalities of the spine and is never located under the S2 neurotome, as the nervous system distal to this level develops through a separate process called secondary neurulation. The neurenteric cyst occurred in only one case in our series: it became symptomatic in adulthood due to compression of the spinal cord and was not associated with a definite bony abnormality of the spine. A neurenteric cyst must be removed microsurgically. Any associated bony malformations or deformities of the spine should be treated separately, if necessary, with spondylodesis. In our series, one adult patient presented with a neurenteric cyst at the level of C2–3, which was successfully removed through a posterior approach.

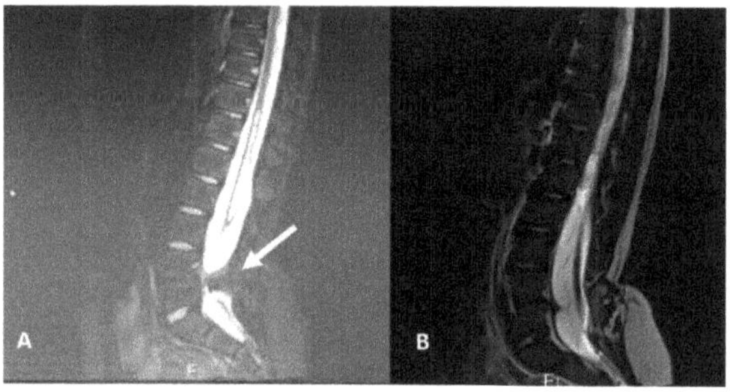

Figure 5. A preoperative (**A**) scan of a SCM1 with a bone spur separating two dural sacs and two hemicords (white arrow). The postoperative image (**B**) shows the removal of the bone spur and the reconstruction of a single dural sac.

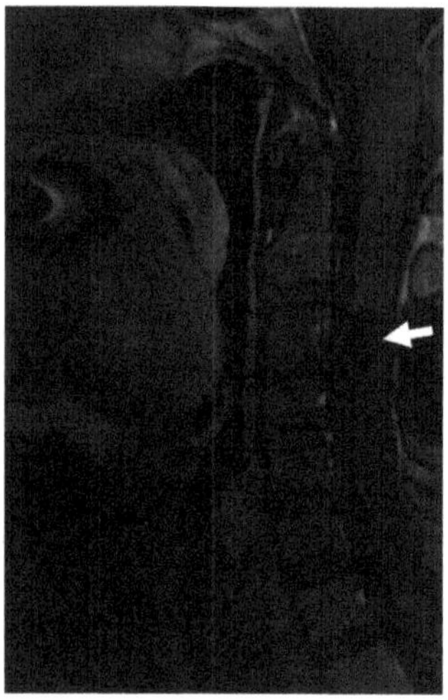

Figure 6. A neurenteric cyst located on the ventral side of the cervical spinal cord (white arrow). The patient presented in adulthood due to neurological symptoms related to the compression of the spinal cord.

4.2. Defects in the Primary Neurulation Stage

Primary neurulation is a process that occurs between days 17 and 23 of gestational age, in which two neural crests within the ectoderm elevate and fuse to form the neural tube. Primary neurulation also includes the process of disjunction: this is the moment when the closed neural tube (neuroectoderm) separates from the overlying cutaneous ectoderm. From this moment on, the closed neural tube will be surrounded by cells of mesodermal origin.

The most common and dramatic defect that occurs at this stage of embryonic development is MMC, which results from incomplete closure of the neural tube. MMC is an open spinal dysraphism, in which the open neural tube is directly exposed to the outside. MMC is a malformation that affects the entire nervous system and leads to a Chiari 2 malformation, hydrocephalus and many other malformations of the central nervous system (polymicrogyria, agenesis of the vermis, agenesis of the corpus callosum, etc.). Since it is an open neural tube defect, it will not be discussed here.

The other forms of OSD that occur at the stage of primary neurulation are related to defects in the process of disjunction, which may be either incomplete or premature.

1. Dermal tract and limited dorsal myeloschisis (LDM):

A dermal tract develops when the disjunction process is incomplete [6]. A dermal tract is a thin fibrous band that connects the skin (dermal ectoderm) to the central nervous system (neuroectoderm). The tract usually runs through the dysraphic dorsal elements of the spinal column and through the dura and attaches to the spinal cord or another intradural neural element. The dermal tract is often associated with an intradural inclusion cyst (dermoid or epidermoid) (Figure 7), which may compress the surrounding neural structures.

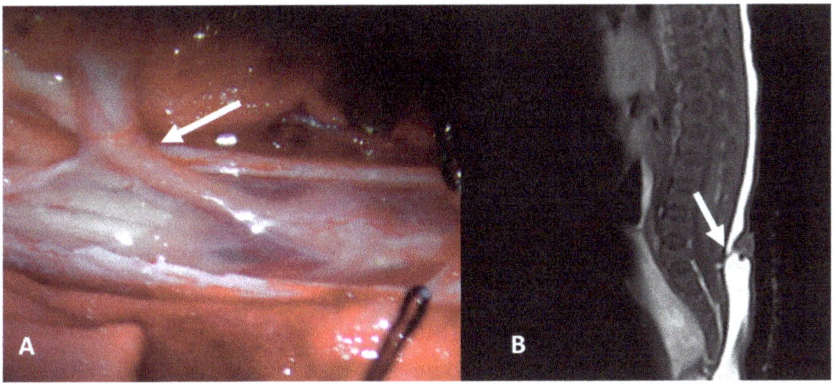

Figure 7. Intraoperative view (**A**) and MR scan (**B**) of a child with a lumbosacral dermal tract (white arrow) and an intradural dermoid cyst. The tract must be removed completely, as close as possible to the spinal cord.

If the histological composition of the fibrous tract is predominantly neural rather than fibrous, it is better defined as LDM (Figure 8) [7]. When there is communication between the CSF and the subcutaneous compartment through the neural tract, the LDM can take on a cystic morphology. In these cases, the skin overlying the subcutaneous cyst can be very thin, so these cases may be difficult to distinguish from MMC, especially on prenatal ultrasounds. Undoubtedly, the neurological and general prognosis is much worse in MMC than in LDM.

Dermal tracts were a fairly common finding in our series, accounting for 20.3% of all OSD. LDM was a rather rare diagnosis, at 3.1% of all OSD. Surgical removal of the dermal tract or LDM is necessary to relieve the spinal cord and prevent possible infection associated with the abnormal dermal and epidermal tissue. The aim of surgery should be to completely remove the dermal tract or LDM, as close to the spinal cord as possible, without causing neurological deficits. Neurophysiological monitoring is essential for these and all other OSD operations.

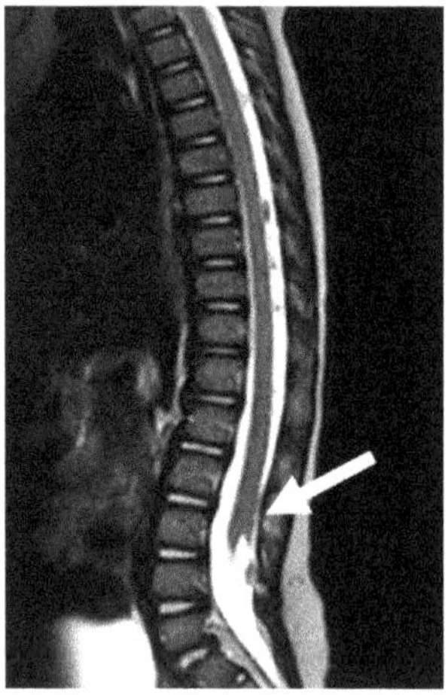

Figure 8. LDM is formed by neural tissue that is tethered toward the extraspinal mesodermal tissues. Note the deformed dorsal aspect of the spinal cord at the level of the dysraphic lesion (white arrow), which can be located at any level of the spinal cord.

2. Lipoma of the conus:

Premature disjunction leads to the formation of spinal cord lipomas. If the neuroectoderm separates from the cutaneous ectoderm too early, when the neural tube has not yet closed, this leads to infiltration of the still open neural tube by mesodermal tissue. The neural tube can therefore not close, and the placode (the exposed neural plate) is infiltrated by subcutaneous fatty tissue (Figure 9). This more or less thick lipomatous stalk can migrate from the subcutaneous tissue through the dysraphic bone and the dura into the intradural space. Lipomas of the spinal cord can be of the dorsal type (located on the dorsal side of the spinal cord and cranial to the still recognisable conus), of the transitional type (located on the dorsal side of the spinal cord and at the level of the no longer recognisable conus) or of the chaotic type (located on the dorsal and ventral side of the spinal cord, with an unrecognisable conus). Surgery for spinal cord lipomas, especially of the transitional and chaotic type, is complex and risky. Without surgery, 40–43% of these children develop tethered cord syndrome within 10 years [1,2,8,9]. At the same time, partial resection is also not recommended, as the results of subtotal removal are even worse than those of conservative treatment (follow-up with electromyography and urodynamic examinations), with 46% of these children developing tethered cord syndrome [8,9]. It is therefore necessary to completely remove the fatty tissue, undertake neurulation of the placode and create a wide dural sac with extensive duraplasty. Intraoperatively, it is often difficult to recognize the border between fatty and neural tissue, which is why neurophysiological monitoring is an absolute priority in these procedures. Using this technique, the risk of new neurological deficits is reduced to 0.8% over 10 years [8]. It is important to note that the risk of neurological deficits and the long-term prognosis vary, according to the type of lipoma and the position of the conus. Transitional lipomas with a low-lying conus are at high risk, compared to dorsal lipomas where the conus may be located at L1, L2 or L3 level. The higher risk carried by transitional and chaotic lipomas was confirmed also by our results: adult patients, in whom neurological deficits were statistically significantly more frequent than in children ($p = 0.0098$), also had a higher incidence of transitional and chaotic lipomas at diagnosis compared to children (57.1% vs. 44.4%). In our series, 15/22 (68.1%) conus lipomas were surgically treated (Figure 10). Our results confirm that conus lipoma surgery is safe, although the complexity of treatment of transitional and chaotic lipomas was evident, since permanent neurological deficits (one neurogenic bladder and three dermatomal sensorial deficits) were present exclusively in four of nine (44.4%) patients who had a transitional or chaotic lipoma ($p = 0.0002$).

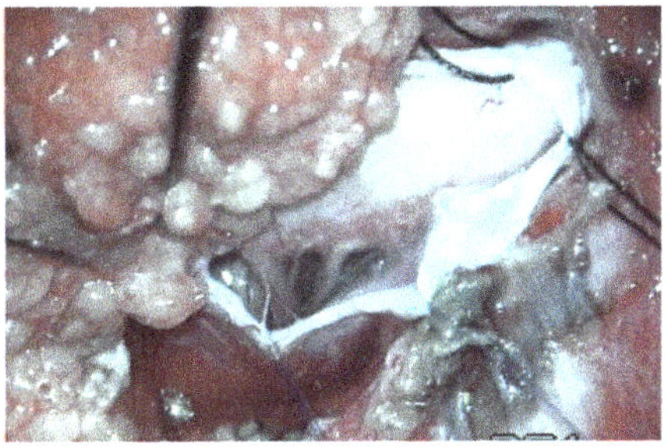

Figure 9. Intraoperative picture of a transitional conus lipoma, attached to the neural placode. The adipose tissue must be completely removed to guarantee a long-term protective effect against neurological deterioration.

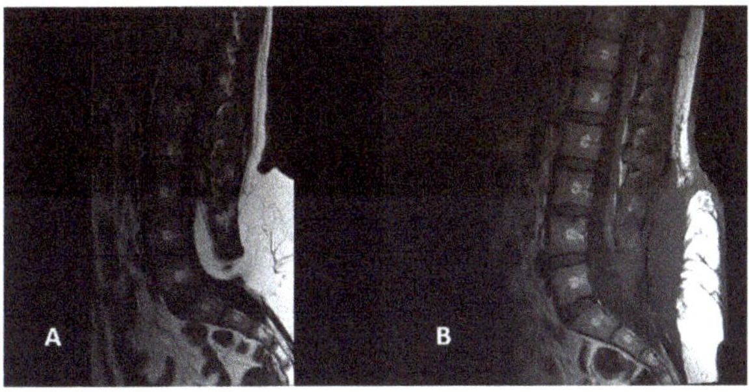

Figure 10. Preoperative (**A**) and postoperative (**B**) MR image of a completely removed transitional conus lipoma.

4.3. Defects in the Secondary Neurulation Stage

While the central nervous system, cranial to the S2 neurotome, is formed by the process of primary neurulation, a completely different process called secondary neurulation occurs caudal to this level. Around the 25th to 27th day of gestational age, a caudal cellular mass, consisting of undifferentiated pluripotent cells, forms in the caudal part of the embryo. These cells undergo an extraordinary proliferation phase, followed by a phase of apoptotic decline and regression of the caudal cell mass. This process gives rise to the conus, the filum terminale and the cauda equina. These tissues then connect to the caudal part of the neural tube that was formed by primary neurulation. The process of secondary neurulation is closely linked to the development of the cloaca. Failures at this stage can therefore lead to complex syndromes in which the nervous, urogenital and digestive organs are affected simultaneously.

1. Lipomas of the filum terminale:

Inadequate apoptosis and regression of the caudal cell mass can lead to a thickened, "fatty" filum terminale. On MRI, the LFT appears as a thick, hyperintensive tract on T1 images (Figure 11). The surgical procedure for untethering is relatively simple: the LFT must be exposed distal to the conus and cut under neurophysiological monitoring. As the risks associated with this procedure are very low, it is worth performing it as early as possible, i.e., in the first months of life [10], in order to protect the child from the onset of symptoms of tethered cord syndrome. In our series, LFTs represented 12/64 (18.7%) of all OSDs and were surgically sectioned in all cases.

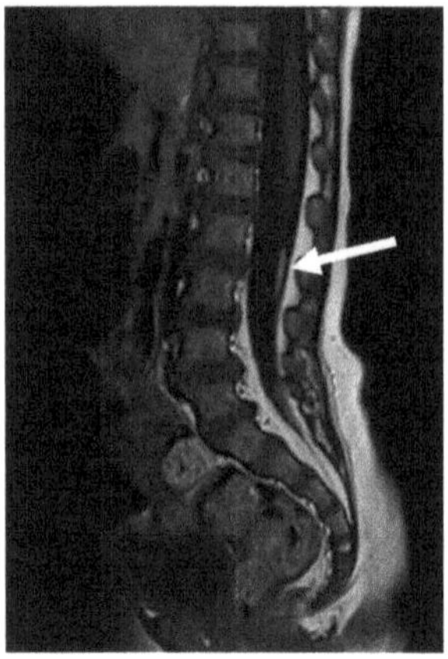

Figure 11. MR appearance of a lipoma of the filum terminale (white arrow), also known as "thickened filum" or "fatty filum".

2. Currarino syndrome:

Currarino syndrome is characterised by a triad: anal malformation, presacral mass and dysgenesis (or agenesis) of the sacrum. In the case of an associated LFT or conus lipoma, a tethered cord may be present [11]. The presacral mass is, in most cases, a meningocele (Figure 3), but can also represent a teratoma [10]. In the absence of a tethered cord, a conservative approach may be considered if the radiological diagnosis of a presacral meningocele is clear and there is no suspicion of a presacral teratoma.

3. Caudal regression syndrome:

If the process of secondary neurulation does not occur at all, there is complete agenesis of the conus and nerve roots caudal to the S2 level (Figure 4). These patients may have more or less impaired lower limb function, but some can walk normally. Sphincter function is completely absent, as the innervation of these segments is completely undeveloped. Surgical treatment is not indicated in these patients since the conus is absent, but not tethered.

4. Myelocystocele:

Myelocystocele is a cystic malformation that occurs within the developing conus and other neural structures that arise through the process of secondary neurulation. These lesions appear as large cystic formations in the sacral and perineal region. The aim of surgical treatment is to reconstruct the caudal segments of the spinal canal, the dural sac and the anatomy of the pelvic floor itself, which is always severely affected.

4.4. Indication for Treatment

OSD are malformations that are specific to the neurosurgical field and for which a neurosurgical opinion should always be sought. Any form of OSD can lead to spinal cord tethering and is therefore a risk factor for progressive neurological symptoms. In this context, the neurosurgeon must always assess whether it is possible to release the spinal cord tethering by surgery. When determining the indication for an operation, the risks of the procedure itself must always be taken into account, in particular the possibility of neurological impairment as a result of the surgical procedure itself.

In most cases, the diagnosis is made in early childhood on the basis of cutaneous stigmata, and the children are usually neurologically intact at birth. If the imaging diagnosis reveals a simple form of OSD, e.g., an LFT, the beneficial effect of surgery is significantly greater compared to a conservative approach. The diagnosis of a transitional or chaotic conus lipoma raises more difficult questions about potential neurological complications associated with surgery, which may be unacceptable to many parents. However, it is becoming increasingly clear in the literature that it is better to operate on the child than to observe them [1,2,8].

In the adult population, the diagnosis of OSD is usually made on the basis of signs and symptoms of neurological deterioration rather than skin manifestations. This can be clearly seen in Table 3, where symptoms of tethered cord syndrome are much more common in adult patients than in children ($p = 0.0098$). Among the symptoms of tethered cord syndrome, pain ($p = 0.0001$) and paraesthesia in the lower limbs ($p = 0.007$) showed the greatest and significant differences between the paediatric and adult populations. Most cases, both paediatric and adult, present with sphincter dysfunction or paresis of the lower limbs. As neurological problems are usually irreversible once they have occurred, it is generally assumed that the protective effect of surgery is less pronounced in adults than in children [1,8]. Nevertheless, certain problems, particularly pain, paresis and paraesthesia, can disappear or at least be alleviated after successful surgical treatment. In particular, it is possible to halt progressive neurological deterioration with surgical treatment and thus prevent further neurological deficits [3].

Based on our results, we have to ask ourselves whether a 44.4% prevalence of permanent neurological deficits after the surgery of complex (transitional and chaotic) conus lipomas is an acceptable fact for parents, compared to a 40–43% chance of having neurological deficits due to the natural history of these lesions [3]. We must underline that more than half of these neurological deficits were represented by isolated dermatomal loss of sensorial function, which, despite being troublesome for the patients, still remains compatible with normal life, normal gait pattern and normal urological function. Statistical models are increasingly in favour of surgery [8], but robust and convincing results can only be based on long-term follow-ups and the long surgical learning curve required for the surgical treatment of the most complex forms of lipomas and, in general, OSD.

5. Conclusions

The treatment of OSD requires proper knowledge of the defects that occur during embryological development and can lead to complex malformations. Surgical treatment is always indicated if the OSD constricts the spinal cord below the L1 level and if the malformation itself has a compressive effect on the surrounding nerve tissue. If spinal cord tethering is detected radiologically, it is advisable to perform the untethering as early as possible, to avoid neurological damage caused by spinal cord tension. In our series, the preoperative presence of symptoms was statistically higher in adults than in children ($p = 0.0098$). Surgery of complex spinal cord lipomas was statistically related to a higher rate of postoperative neurological complications ($p = 0.0002$). Such procedures should be carried out in facilities that have the relevant experience and where neurophysiological monitoring is available at all times. After the untethering procedure, children should be monitored throughout their lives, as tethered cord syndrome may recur due to scarring, other associated dysraphic lesions or the incomplete removal of the primary OSD.

Author Contributions: All authors contributed equally. P.S. and N.P. analysed the data; P.S., B.P., A.P. and T.V. wrote the paper. All authors have read and agreed to the published version of the manuscript.

Funding: This research received no external funding.

Institutional Review Board Statement: The study was conducted in accordance with the Declaration of Helsinki, and approved by the Department of Neurosurgery, University Medical Centre Ljubljana, Slovenia. Ethical approval number: 4/2023, January 2023.

Informed Consent Statement: Not applicable.

Data Availability Statement: No new data were created or analyzed in this study. Data sharing is not applicable to this article.

Conflicts of Interest: The authors declare no conflicts of interest.

References

1. Kulkarni, H.V.; Pierre-Kahn, A.; Zerah, M. Conservative management of asymptomatic spinal lipomas of the conus. *Neurosurgery* **2004**, *54*, 868–875. [CrossRef] [PubMed]
2. Wykes, V.; Desai, D.; Thompson, D.N. Asymptomatic lumbosacral lipomas—A natural history study. *Child's Nerv. Syst.* **2012**, *28*, 1731–1739. [CrossRef] [PubMed]
3. Pang, D.; Zovickian, J.; Wong, S.T.; Hou, Y.J.; Moes, G.S. Surgical treatment of complex spinal cord lipomas. *Child's Nerv. Syst.* **2013**, *29*, 1485–1513. [CrossRef] [PubMed]
4. Beuriat, P.A.; Di Rocco, F.; Szathmari, A.; Mottolese, C. Management of split cord malformation in children: The Lyon experience. *Child's Nerv. Syst.* **2018**, *34*, 883–891. [CrossRef] [PubMed]
5. Baek, W.K.; Lachkar, S.; Iwanaga, J.; Oskouian, R.J.; Loukas, M.; Oakes, W.J.; Tubbs, R.S. Comprehensive Review of Spinal Neurenteric Cysts with a Focus on Histopathological Findings. *Cureus* **2018**, *10*, 3379. [CrossRef] [PubMed]
6. Tisdall, M.M.; Hayward, R.D.; Thompson, D.N. Congenital spinal dermal tract: How accurate is clinical and radiological evaluation? *J. Neurosurg. Pediatr.* **2015**, *15*, 651–656. [CrossRef] [PubMed]
7. Pang, D.; Zovickian, J.; Oviedo, A.; Moes, G.S. Limited dorsal myeloschisis: A distinctive clinicopathological entity. *Neurosurgery* **2010**, *67*, 1555–1579. [CrossRef] [PubMed]
8. Pierre-Kahn, A.; Zerah, M.; Renier, D.; Cinalli, G.; Sainte-Rose, C.; Lellouch-Tubiana, A.; Brunelle, F.; Le Merrer, M.; Giudicelli, Y.; Pichon, J.; et al. Congenital lumbosacral lipomas. *Child's Nerv. Syst.* **1997**, *13*, 298–334. [CrossRef] [PubMed]
9. Pierre-Kahn, A.; Lacombe, J.; Pichon, J.; Giudicelli, Y.; Renier, D.; Sainte-Rosse, C.; Perrigot, M.; Hirsch, J.-F. Intraspinal lipomas with spina bifida: Prognosis and treatment in 73 cases. *J. Neurosurg.* **1986**, *65*, 756–761. [CrossRef] [PubMed]
10. Usami, K.; Lallemant, P.; Roujeau, T.; James, S.; Beccaria, K.; Levy, R.; Di Rocco, F.; Sainte-Rose, C.; Zerah, M. Spinal lipoma of the filum terminale: Review of 174 consecutive patients. *Child's Nerv. Syst.* **2016**, *32*, 1265–1272. [CrossRef]
11. Cearns, M.D.; Hettige, S.; De Coppi, P.; Thompson, D.N.P. Currarino syndrome: Repair of the dysraphic anomalies and resection of the presacral mass in a combined neurosurgical and general surgical approach. *J. Neurosurg. Pediatr.* **2018**, *22*, 584–590. [CrossRef] [PubMed]

diagnostics

MDPI

Article

The Impact of Surgical Telementoring on Reducing the Complication Rate in Endoscopic Endonasal Surgery of the Skull Base

Janez Ravnik [1,*], Hojka Rowbottom [1], Carl H. Snyderman [2], Paul A. Gardner [3], Tomaž Šmigoc [1], Matic Glavan [4], Urška Kšela [5], Nenad Kljaić [6] and Boštjan Lanišnik [4]

1 Department of Neurosurgery, Maribor University Medical Centre, 2000 Maribor, Slovenia; tomaz.smigoc@ukc-mb.si (T.Š.)
2 Departments of Otolaryngology and Neurological Surgery, University of Pittsburgh School of Medicine, Pittsburgh, PA 15213, USA
3 Department of Neurological Surgery, University of Pittsburgh School of Medicine, Pittsburgh, PA 15213, USA
4 Department of Otorhinolaryngology, Head and Neck Surgery, Maribor University Medical Centre, 2000 Maribor, Slovenia
5 Department of Endocrinology and Diabetology, Maribor University Medical Centre, 2000 Maribor, Slovenia
6 Department of Ophthalmology, Maribor University Medical Centre, 2000 Maribor, Slovenia; nenad.kljaic@ukc-mb.si
* Correspondence: janez.ravnik@ukc-mb.si

Abstract: Background: Pituitary adenomas represent the most common pituitary disorder, with an estimated prevalence as high as 20%, and they can manifest with hormone hypersecretion or deficiency, neurological symptoms from mass effect, or incidental findings on imaging. Transsphenoidal surgery, performed either microscopically or endoscopically, allows for a better extent of resection while minimising the associated risk in comparison to the transcranial approach. Endoscopy allows for better visualisation and improvement in tumour resection with an improved working angle and less nasal morbidity, making it likely to become the preferred surgical treatment for pituitary neoplasms. The learning curve can be aided by telementoring. Methods: We retrospectively analysed the clinical records of 94 patients who underwent an endoscopic endonasal resection of a pituitary neoplasm between the years 2011 and 2023 at Maribor University Medical Centre in Slovenia. Remote surgical telementoring over 3 years assisted with the learning curve. Results: The proportion of complication-free patients significantly increased over the observed period (60% vs. 79%). A gradual but insignificant increase in the percentage of patients with improved endocrine function was observed. Patients' vision improved significantly over the observed period. By gaining experience, the extent of gross total tumour resection increased insignificantly (67% vs. 79%). Conclusions: Telementoring for the endoscopic endonasal approach to pituitary neoplasms enables low-volume centres to achieve efficiency, decreasing rates of postoperative complications and increasing the extent of tumour resection.

Keywords: pituitary neoplasms; telementoring; endoscopic endonasal approach; outcomes

1. Introduction

Over the last three decades, the endoscopic endonasal approach (EEA) has become the predominant approach for surgical treatment of different skull base pathologies, and is currently recognised as the standard for most pituitary adenomas [1–3]. EEA enables surgery in parasellar regions and sagittal and coronal plane corridors to the central skull base [1,4]. Microscopic transsphenoidal surgery had long been considered the "gold standard" in the surgical treatment of pituitary neoplasms, and at the beginning, the endoscope was used solely as an assisting tool to explore the sellar cavity for residual tumour tissue, but due to its wide panoramic, up-close visualisation, and recent developments of endoscopic instrumentation and techniques, EEA has gained popularity [4,5].

EEA is associated with a steep learning curve, which is necessary to increase the effectiveness of EEA and decrease the length of surgery [6–8]. A great deal of learning takes place in the operating theatre; however, sufficient time has to be spent in a dissection laboratory to acquire enough anatomical knowledge [1,9]. Additionally, EEA requires the adoption of new technology and instrumentation with a transition from three-dimensional to two-dimensional visualisation; however, newer three-dimensional endoscope technology has been developed to improve visualisation and understanding of the anatomy, which mirrors the view offered by a traditional microscope [1,10].

Telementoring, whereby an expert employs telecommunication technology to guide a less experienced learner from a remote location, provides a unique solution to increase quality and enhance access to surgical care in low-volume medical centres [11,12].

Collaboration between a neurosurgeon and an ear, nose, and throat (ENT) surgeon is crucial for successful patient management in the operating theatre, as well as outside [1,2]. The development of a skull base team that is efficient in performing EEA is a demanding task, even more-so in a low-volume centre; thus, telementoring by an experienced centre represents a possible solution to establish proficiency in EEA when on-site mentoring cannot be established [1,9,11].

The collaboration between neurosurgeons and ENT surgeons in endoscopic endonasal surgery at the Maribor University Medical Center (MUMC) in Slovenia started in 2009. The Maribor surgeons (JR and BL) were the first to establish a skull base team at this centre. In 2010, they attended the endoscopic skull base surgery course at the University of Pittsburgh Medical Center (UPMC), followed by a visit to the skull base centre at UPMC for an additional two weeks. A collaboration was established with the co-authors (CS and PG). The MUMC surgeons repeated their visit to the UPMC course and skull base department four years later. The collaboration between the four surgeons continued with regular consultations and an annual endoscopic skull base surgery course with lectures and hands-on cadaver dissections conducted in Maribor attended by the two surgeons from UPMC. The telementoring programme started in 2013 and finished in 2015.

Throughout the telementoring programme and thereafter, several adaptations and improvements were made. The extent of safe resection gradually improved and extended endonasal approaches for skull base pathology were introduced. Regarding pituitary tumours, a great effort was required to improve endocrinological results for non-secretory and secretory adenomas. The main goal was to preserve the endocrinological function of the remaining pituitary gland with the gross total resection of the pituitary adenoma. Important progress was achieved with skull base reconstruction with the introduction of the nasoseptal flap [13]. A multidisciplinary team comprising a neurosurgeon, otolaryngologist-head and neck surgeon (OHNS), endocrinologist, and ophthalmologist was established to provide better patient care with greater continuity of care and less duplication of services.

This article analyses the results and complications after successfully applying a three-year telementoring programme by evaluating the extent of surgery, endocrinological results, and rate of complications after pituitary tumour surgery.

2. Material and Methods

2.1. Study Design and Patient Data

2.1.1. Study Design

We conducted a retrospective analysis of patients who underwent endoscopic endonasal transsphenoidal surgery performed at the MUMC between January 2011 and December 2023. A total of 94 patients were identified, of whom 93 regularly attended postoperative follow-up appointments. Patients included in the study analysis had to be older than 18 years. The observed timeframe was divided into 4 periods: from 2011 to 2014, 2015 to 2017, 2018 to 2020, and 2021 to 2023. For statistical comparison, the four groups of patients were further united into early (year 2011–2017) and late (year 2018–2023) periods.

During the telementoring programme, which started in 2013 and finished in 2015, 10 endoscopic endonasal surgeries of the skull base were mentored preoperatively and during the key part of the procedure. The telementoring programme required consent and a liability waiver from both groups, and the main team was solely responsible for the surgery and the outcome. Surgical instrumentation was standardised, and surgical techniques were adopted from the UPMC Center for Cranial Base Surgery. An educational programme was completed at the courses organised by the University of Pittsburgh Center for Cranial Base Surgery.

Prior to the start of telementoring, the technological needs and capabilities of both institutions were determined, and real-time two-way video and audio streaming was established using existing technology (Polycom Video Conferencing Equipment, Karl Storz Image 1 and Aida Video System, Tuttlingen, Germany). The surgical plan was laid out before surgery, and imaging was reviewed by both groups. Operative times were adjusted so that the key period of telementoring was in the range of 5:30–8:30 EST. Telementoring started and continued during the critical phases of the surgery, resection and reconstruction. Following each procedure, an evaluation form was used to document the interventions and rates of experience. Postoperative radiographs were shared via e-mail [1].

2.1.2. Patient Data and Institutional Review Board

The local ethics committee of the MUMC reviewed and approved our study. Patient data were collected via the online medical record system, and the imaging examination data were collected via the local PACS system. The following data were collected from the electronic medical record: year of surgery, gender, age, length of hospitalisation, type of pituitary neoplasm and its location, exact cell type, postoperative complications, extent of resection, rehospitalisation after surgery for pituitary neoplasm, hypopituitarism before surgery, tumour hormonal activity, tumour size, hormonal syndrome before surgery, neurologic symptoms/signs before surgery, residual tumour tissue seen on control MRI 6 months after surgery, tumour recurrence after surgery and treatment, endocrine function before and after surgery, vision before and after surgery, and presence of hypopituitarism after surgery. Statistical data analysis was performed using the Statistical Package for Social Sciences (IBM SPSS Statistics for Windows, Version 29.0.2.0, Armonk, NY, USA). A Pearson Chi-Square test and Fisher's exact test for 2 × 2 tables were used for the statistical comparison of the groups' frequencies. p value < 0.05 was considered statistically significant.

2.1.3. Clinical Management

Each patient with a sellar pathology was presented to the multidisciplinary team, which examined the MRI imaging, the results of the endocrinologic tests, and the results of the neuro-ophthalmic examination. Patients with visual deficits, growing neoplasms, and uncontrollable hormonal deficits were identified as suitable candidates for surgery. The operative procedure, purpose, and risks were explained to every patient who chose operative treatment or conservative management. Most patients were hospitalised at the University Department of Otorhinolaryngology, Head and Neck Surgery, and a few at the Department of Neurosurgery. The surgeries were performed in a dedicated endoscopic operating room enabling a four-handed endoscopic technique. Image guidance was used in all cases. The telementoring link was established and tested prior to the surgery. Each surgery started with the preparation of the nasoseptal flap, usually on the right side. A one-sided corridor was created, and bilateral sphenoidotomy was performed. At this stage, telementoring started. The most common intervention from the overseeing team was increased exposure at the level of the rostrum and medial opticocarotid recesses (medial OCR) to improve suprasellar exposure. Particular care was taken to identify both carotid and optic protuberances. The sellar floor was removed in the usual fashion. At this point, the performing surgeons were usually advised to remove more bone in all directions to reach optic and carotid protuberances and gain sufficient access to the intrasellar pathology.

The resection phase was also subject to telementoring, with tips on tumour resection in the suprasellar region. The performing surgeons were instructed to carefully inspect the boundaries of the tumour, and they were assisted in properly identifying tumour borders and the remnant of the pituitary gland. Special care was taken not to damage the healthy pituitary tissue. The removal of the tumour tissue with two aspirators (one with a neuronavagated tip) was extremely useful. Reconstruction was monitored only in the first intradural phase. After ensuring watertight intradural reconstruction, the defect was covered with a nasoseptal flap. After surgery, patients were transferred to the intensive unit within the Department of Otorhinolaryngology while awake. Packing was removed between the 3rd and 5th postoperative day.

After discharge, they were examined by an endocrinologist 3 months following surgery, where endocrinologic tests were repeated and hormonal replacement therapy was adjusted. After surgery, all patients had the following follow-up appointments: 3 months after surgery, they were re-examined by an endocrinologist; and 6 months after surgery, a control MRI was performed, which was examined by two independent neuroradiologists to assess the extent of tumour resection, and they were later examined by a neurosurgeon and an ophthalmologist. Patients with no radiologic and/or endocrinologic signs of tumour recurrence were followed-up with an annual MRI and regular appointments with an endocrinologist, neurosurgeon, and ophthalmologist. Patients with a recurrence of sellar pathology were either further treated or monitored.

3. Results

From 2011 to 2023, 94 patients underwent endoscopic endonasal surgery for a sellar pathology, and from that sample, 49 (52.1%) were women. The mean age of the included patients was 58 years (range 20–82 years, SD = 14).

Table 1 demonstrates the number and proportion of operated patients per observed period. During the telementoring programme (2013–2015), ten endoscopic endonasal surgeries of the skull base were performed, and clinical follow-up was provided with postoperative imaging diagnostics shared by e-mail between the consultants with intense communication. No technical difficulties were encountered during the telementoring programme with a good and stable audio-visual connection. The general results of the telementoring programme were described in the previous publication [1].

Table 1. Number and percentage of patients operated per period.

		Number	Percentage
Period	2011–2014	15	16.0%
	2015–2017	21	22.3%
	2018–2020	24	25.5%
	2021–2023	34	36.2%
	Total	94	100.0%

The operations performed from 2011 to 2012 were conducted with no help of telementoring from an experienced centre, and surgeries after 2015, when the telementoring period finished, comprised discussions amongst surgeons; however, these were not live during surgery, but were either prior to or after the operations.

Adenomas represented the most common pituitary neoplasm in the observed group, with null cell adenomas diagnosed in 45.7% of the observed population, plurihormonal adenomas present in 31.9%, and monohormonal adenomas in 13.8% of patients.

The majority of tumours were in the intrasellar and suprasellar regions. Most patients were diagnosed with macroadenomas, and more than half had hypopituitarism before surgery. The hormonal activity of the pituitary neoplasm was present in 20.2% of cases, and from those, more than half (55.6%) were diagnosed with a growth-hormone-secreting adenoma, followed by prolactinomas in 38.9%, adrenocorticotropic hormone-secreting tumours in 11.1%, and thyroid-stimulating hormone secretion in 5.6% of cases, as illustrated in Table 2.

Table 2. Sellar pathology in the observed group of patients.

		Number	Percentage
Neoplasm type	Adenoma	86	91.5%
	Craniopharyngioma	2	2.1%
	Schwannoma	1	1.1%
	Metastasis	3	3.2%
	Rathke cleft cyst	1	1.1%
	Lymphocytic hypophysitis	1	1.1%
	Total	94	100.0%
Neoplasm location	Intrasellar region	16	17.0%
	Intrasellar and suprasellar region	72	76.6%
	Intrasellar, suprasellar and parasellar region	4	4.3%
	Intrasellar and parasellar region	2	2.1%
	Total	94	100.0%
Hypopituitarism prior surgery	No deficit	39	41.5%
	Hypopituitarism	55	58.5%
	Total	94	100.0%
Hormonal activity	No	75	79.8%
	Yes	19	20.2%
	Total	94	100.0%
Size	Microadenoma	2	2.1%
	Macroadenoma	92	97.9%
	Total	94	100.0%

Around a quarter (25.5%) were diagnosed with a hormonal syndrome before surgery, with hyperprolactinemia being the most common one, followed by acromegaly, and 84% had neurological symptoms and deficits, with vision impairments being the most common ones, as illustrated in Table 3.

Table 3. Preoperative signs and symptoms.

		Number	Percentage
Cushing syndrome	No	90	95.7%
	Yes	4	4.3%
	Total	94	100.0%
Hyperprolactinemia	No	82	87.2%
	Yes	12	12.8%
	Total	94	100.0%
Hyperthyroidism	No	93	98.9%
	Yes	1	1.1%
	Total	94	100.0%
Acromegaly	No	84	89.4%
	Yes	10	10.6%
	Total	94	100.0%
Vision deficits	No	28	29.8%
	Yes	66	70.2%
	Total	94	100.0%
Apoplexy	No	81	86.2%
	Yes	13	13.8%
	Total	94	100.0%
Seizures	No	93	98.9%
	Yes	1	1.1%
	Total	94	100.0%
Headaches	No	60	63.8%
	Yes	34	36.2%
	Total	94	100%

There was one death in our series of patients, as demonstrated in Table 4 and Figure 1. The cause of death was a respiratory infection unrelated to the surgical procedure. Over the observed period, the percentage of complication-free patients after surgery gradually increased, as is demonstrated in Table 4. Diabetes insipidus was transient in all cases. In the early period (from 2011 to 2017), 19 patients were complication-free, whereas in the late period (from 2018 to 2023), 45 were complication-free. The difference in the overall number of complications is statistically significant between the early and late period ($p = 0.022$, Fisher's Exact Test). However, the difference between the two periods (early vs. late) for each individual complication was not statistically significant ($p > 0.05$, Fisher's Exact Test).

Table 4. Occurrence of postoperative complications per observed period.

		Period							
		2011–2014		2015–2017		2018–2020		2021–2023	
		Number	Percentage	Number	Percentage	Number	Percentage	Number	Percentage
Syndrome of inappropriate antidiuretic hormone secretion	No	14	93.3%	21	100.0%	24	100.0%	31	91.2%
	Yes	1	6.7%	0	0.0%	0	0.0%	3	8.8%
	Total	15	100.0%	21	100.0%	24	100.0%	34	100.0%
Diabetes insipidus	No	12	80.0%	15	71.4%	20	83.3%	31	91.2%
	Yes	3	20.0%	6	28.6%	4	16.7%	3	8.8%
	Total	15	100.0%	21	100.0%	24	100.0%	34	100.0%
Cerebrospinal fluid leak	No	15	100.0%	17	81.0%	23	95.8%	33	97.1%
	Yes	0	0.0%	4	19.0%	1	4.2%	1	2.9%
	Total	15	100.0%	21	100.0%	24	100.0%	34	100.0%
Meningitis	No	15	100.0%	19	90.5%	23	95.8%	34	100.0%
	Yes	0	0.0%	2	9.5%	1	4.2%	0	0.0%
	Total	15	100.0%	21	100.0%	24	100.0%	34	100.0%
Haemorrhage	No	12	80.0%	19	90.5%	22	91.7%	34	100.0%
	Yes	3	20.0%	2	9.5%	2	8.3%	0	0.0%
	Total	15	100.0%	21	100.0%	24	100.0%	34	100.0%
Death	No	15	100.0%	21	100.0%	23	95.8%	34	100.0%
	Yes	0	0.0%	0	0.0%	1	4.2%	0	0.0%
	Total	15	100.0%	21	100.0%	24	100.0%	34	100.0%
Other complications	No	15	100.0%	20	95.2%	23	95.8%	34	100.0%
	Yes	0	0.0%	1	4.8%	1	4.2%	0	0.0%
	Total	15	100.0%	21	100.0%	24	100.0%	34	100.0%

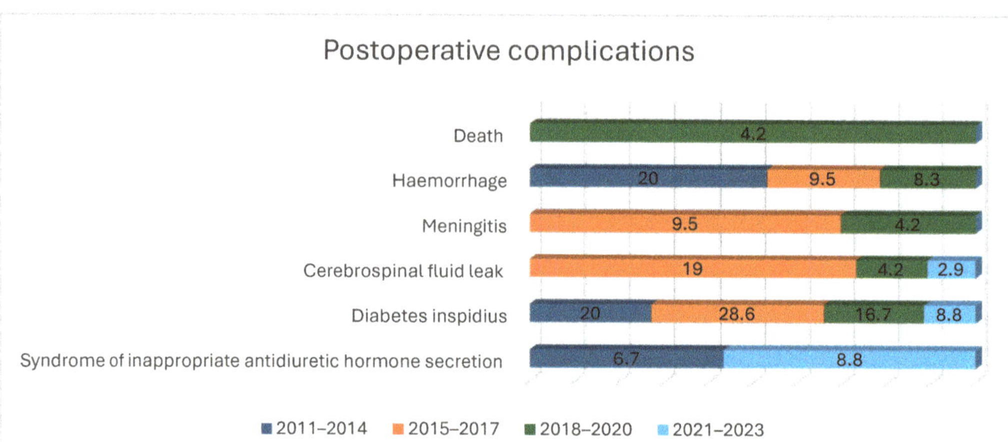

Figure 1. Postoperative complications per observed period.

A gradual increase in improved endocrine function after surgery, which was determined by the reduction in hormonal replacement therapy or its discontinuation, was observed, as well as an improvement in patients' vision after surgery, as is shown in Table 5 and Figure 2. When comparing postoperative endocrine function and postoperative hypopituitarism, there were no statistically significant differences between the early (2011–2017) and late period (2018–2023) ($p > 0.05$, Fisher's Exact Test). However, patients' eyesight improved significantly ($p = 0.013$, Fisher's Exact Test) in the late period.

Table 5. Postoperative endocrine function and eyesight per observed period.

		Period							
		2011–2014		2015–2017		2018–2020		2021–2023	
		Number	Percentage	Number	Percentage	Number	Percentage	Number	Percentage
Endocrine function	Better	1	6.7%	3	14.3%	2	8.3%	6	17.6%
	Same	11	73.3%	16	76.2%	15	62.5%	24	70.6%
	Worse	3	20.0%	2	9.5%	7	29.2%	4	11.8%
	Total	15	100.0%	21	100.0%	24	100.0%	34	100.0%
Eyesight	Better	4	26.7%	6	28.6%	11	45.8%	22	64.7%
	Same	11	73.3%	15	71.4%	13	54.2%	11	32.4%
	Worse	0	0.0%	0	0.0%	0	0.0%	1	2.9%
	Total	15	100.0%	21	100.0%	24	100.0%	34	100.0%
Hypopituitarism after surgery	No	2	13.3%	7	33.3%	5	20.8%	16	47.1%
	Yes	13	86.7%	14	66.7%	19	79.2%	18	52.9%
	Total	15	100.0%	21	100.0%	24	100.0%	34	100.0%

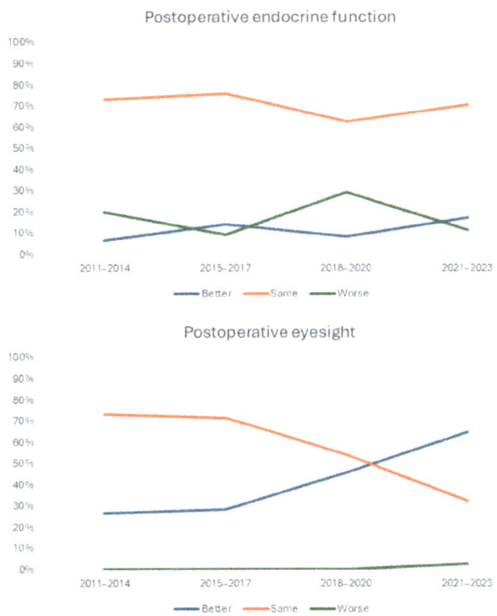

Figure 2. Postoperative endocrine function and eyesight per observed period.

The extent of neoplasm resection, which was ascertained using MRI 6 months after surgery, progressively increased from 66.7% in the first period to 79.4% in the last period, as illustrated in Table 6 and Figure 3; however, a chi-square test of independence showed that the difference was not statistically significant (X^2 (3, N = 94) = 3.788, $p = 0.285$).

Table 6. Extent of tumour resection per observed period.

		Period							
		2011–2014		2015–2017		2018–2020		2021–2023	
		Number	Percentage	Number	Percentage	Number	Percentage	Number	Percentage
Extent of tumour resection	Gross total resection	10	66.7%	15	71.4%	12	50.0%	27	79.4%
	Subtotal resection	2	13.3%	6	28.6%	10	41.7%	6	17.6%
	Partial resection	1	6.7%	0	0.0%	2	8.3%	1	2.9%
	Biopsy	2	13.3%	0	0.0%	0	0.0%	0	0.0%
	Total	15	100.0%	21	100.0%	24	100.0%	34	100.0%

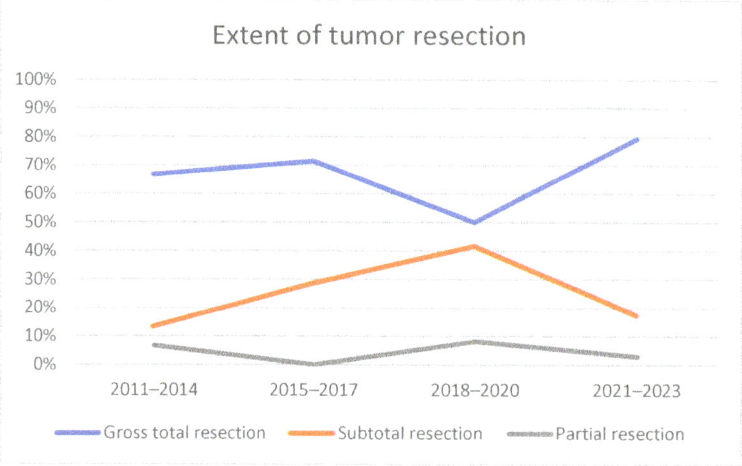

Figure 3. Extent of tumour resection per observed period.

The proportion of patients who required rehospitalisation after EEA gradually decreased. After being discharged, four patients (26.7%) were rehospitalised in the first period; one was diagnosed with a nasal septal abscess and was discharged after 4 days; the second patient was diagnosed with diabetes insipidus and was discharged after 5 days; and two patients had suboptimal hydrocortisone therapy and were both discharged after 2 days. In the second period, one patient (4.8%) had to be rehospitalised for an additional 40 days, as they developed a cerebrospinal fluid leak and meningitis. In the third period, one patient (4.2%) was re-admitted for 12 days for additional tumour resection after the control MRI; there were no postoperative complications.

Out of 94 patients, 11 had recurrences of the following: Rathke cleft cysts and adenoma that required no revision surgery each recurred in 1 patient; a craniopharyngioma that required additional surgery was present in 1 patient; and 8 patients had adenomas that regrew and required revision surgery. EEA was utilised in all cases of revision surgery.

The senior surgeons at Maribor operated on 22 patients before becoming proficient enough to operate without telementoring from surgeons at UPMC. Pituitary tumours present the ideal first step in the endoscopic learning curve based on their location in the centre of the skull base outside the subarachnoid space and with the natural corridor provided by the sphenoid sinus in line with the nasal cavity [14].

4. Discussion

This study demonstrates a successful implementation of EEA for pituitary neoplasms in a low-volume centre, such as MUMC, with an emphasis on the combined efforts of a newly established skull base team and their collaboration with an experienced skull base centre. The number of patients gradually increased over the observed period, with 34 patients having been operated on in the last 3 year period from 2021 to 2023 in comparison to only 15 in the first 4 year period from 2011 to 2014. The major reason for the rise in patient numbers was an increased referrals of patients from other hospitals to our institution. The steady increase in the number of patients operated on each year for pituitary tumours with the addition of other endoscopic endonasal procedures ensured a safe and efficient EEA in a low-volume centre.

This study has potential limitations. Despite a gradual increase in the number of operated patients, the number of patients included in the study was relatively small, since MUMC is a midsize hospital in a country with a population of approximately 2 million. Additionally, in this study, we included patients with different sellar pathologies, which share distinctive behaviours and characteristics; however, the main aim of our work was to demonstrate the acquirement of the surgical technique and the learning curve of the newly established skull base team with the help of telementoring from an experienced centre. Furthermore, the follow-up period for patients operated on in the last period (2021–2023) was considerably shorter than for those in the first period (2011–2014); hence, the comparison of long-term effects of treatment could not be performed.

Pituitary adenomas, benign neoplasms that comprise up to 15% of all intracranial masses, represent the most common pituitary disorder, with an estimated prevalence as high as 20% based on autopsy and radiologic studies, with the majority having no clinical significance [14–18]. Neoplasms can manifest with syndromes of hormone hypersecretion or deficiency, neurological symptoms from a mass effect of the expanding gland, or they can be an incidental finding on imaging performed for unrelated issues [19–21]. In our observed patient population, the neurological signs and symptoms were the most common, present in more than 80% of cases. Treatment aims to reduce hormone hypersecretion, remove the mass effect, and correct hormone deficiency [22–24]. Nonfunctioning asymptomatic microadenomas do not require immediate treatment; however, patients require careful monitoring with regular control MRIs [25,26].

Transsphenoidal surgery for the resection of pituitary neoplasms can be performed either microscopically or endoscopically, and has been proven to achieve a better extent of resection while minimising the associated risks in comparison to the transcranial approach; thus, it represents the first-line treatment for the vast majority of pituitary adenomas [14,27,28]. Microscopic transsphenoidal surgery used to be the gold standard for pituitary tumour removal; however, poor visualisation due to the deep location of adenomas, combined with a narrow surgical space, presented a major obstacle [4]. Endoscopy, with its panoramic view, has led to better visualisation and, thus, improvements in the extent of tumour resection; it also provides an improved working angle and less nasal morbidity [28–30]. The growing acceptance of endoscopic transsphenoidal surgery for pituitary adenomas amongst surgeons is making it highly likely to become the first line of approach for pituitary neoplasm in the future [27,31–33]. Currently, at the MUMC, with the establishment of a proficient skull base team, EEA represents the main surgical modality in the treatment of pituitary pathologies.

EEA allows for surgery in the parasellar regions, namely planum/tuberculum sellae, cavernous sinus, and clivus, where larger and more complex adenomas invade, as the endoscope can be introduced through narrow corridors to reach deep spaces, and with angled lenses, it provides enhanced vision to achieve what is commonly known as "looking around the corners" [4,14].

Endocrinologic outcomes after endoscopic adenoma removal have been comparable, and in some cases even superior, to those after microsurgical tumour removal [34]. A systematic review by Strychowsky demonstrated that EEA for pituitary neoplasms is associated with less mean blood loss, shorter hospitalisation and operative time, fewer nasal complications, and an increase in the proportion of gross total tumour resection with decreasing incidence of postoperative diabetes insipidus [35].

The learning curve for EEA to the pituitary tumour is steep and is often associated with an increase in complications, as the surgeon is faced with unfamiliar anatomy and new technologies, as well as new surgical skills [9,28]. The ideal number of cases to achieve proficiency is not established and depends on the surgeon's prior experiences and skills, the composition of the practice, and the frequency of surgeries [36]. Based on limited published data, it is recommended that a team should perform 30 to 50 pituitary surgeries together to gain proficiency prior to taking on more difficult surgical cases, namely EEA to vascular malformations and highly vascular tumours [9]. The surgeons at MUMC performed 22 operations before becoming accomplished; however, they had previous experience with other endonasal endoscopic procedures that they could build on. Due to its steep learning curve, mentorship is vital for mastering the EEA; however, centralisation of care in high-income countries can restrict access to surgical training outside of metropolitan hubs. Telementoring can help face these challenges, as it can be used effectively in a variety of settings [12,37,38]. Studies have shown that there was no significant difference in outcomes for trainees who received telementoring or on-site mentoring [11]. The advent of augmented and virtual reality utilised for telementoring could further increase autonomy for trainee surgeons [39–41]. The main disadvantages to a wider implementation of telementoring are costs, technical limitations, reliable internet connection, and cyber security [11,12]. The potential drawbacks of telementoring must be addressed before the programme starts. Both groups involved must be familiar with surgical hands-on capabilities and dexterity, and mutual trust is paramount for success. There is also a question of liability that must be cleared up before the surgery. In our case, the domestic team at MUMC was solely responsible for the management of patients as well as potential complications. A team must have a surgical plan laid out before the surgery, as well as a backup plan in case of problems with audio-visual connection. Despite some potential limitations, the benefits of telementoring outweigh them if the programme starts under careful consideration and in a collaborative environment.

The primary goal of most pituitary surgeries is gross total resection. In a study conducted by Dehdashti, gross total resection of macroadenomas was achieved in 96% of cases [35]. Similarly, Wang and colleagues managed to achieve a gross total resection in 92% of cases, whereas total resection was achieved in 76% of cases of giant adenomas [24]. Yu and colleagues cited a gross total resection of pituitary adenomas to be achieved in 60–73% of all cases, which was higher than expected based on a systematic review conducted by Komotar, where gross total resection was achieved in 47.2% of cases [30,42–44]. In our patient series, the proportion of cases of GTR increased from 66.7% in the first observed period up to almost 80% (79.4%) in the last period; however, the difference was not statistically significant when comparing the extent of resection in the early period (2011–2017) and the late one (2018–2023). In the first period, subtotal and partial resections were present more often than in other periods, as the primary focus was avoiding postoperative complications rather than the extent of resection. Wang and colleagues managed to achieve the GTR of macroadenomas in the majority of cases by using intraoperative MRI and neuronavigation during surgery for assessing residual tumour tissue and determining further safe tumour resection, second transcranial surgery, radiotherapy, or radiosurgery [30]. The usefulness of intraoperative MRIs is controversial, with some studies reporting a higher rate of gross total resection, but others showing no difference [45,46].

Patients with nonfunctioning pituitary adenomas most often present with signs and symptoms of hypopituitarism, headaches, hemianopsia, progressive loss of vision, and diplopia [30,45,47–52]. Headaches are present in 16% to 70% of cases, and are mainly localised in the frontal and occipital regions [45,53,54]; in our patients series, 36.2% presented with headaches. Visual impairments, most often bitemporal visual deficits due to midchiasmal compression, are present in larger adenomas, whereas diplopia is rare [3,55,56]. Amongst our patient group, 70.2% had visual deficits. Additionally, nonfunctioning pituitary adenomas, especially macroadenomas, can cause hypopituitarism with at least one hormone deficiency [57,58]. The patients in our study were mainly diagnosed with macroadenomas (97.9%), and 58.5% had hypopituitarism before surgery. Asymptomatic nonfunctioning adenomas are not recommended for surgical treatment, except for young patients. In cases of incomplete tumour resection with no obvious symptoms, patients are recommended for further observation rather than second surgery, which is required in cases of tumour regrowth [30,59]. Following surgery for nonfunctioning adenomas, visual impairments often improve, whereas data regarding hypopituitarism is inconsistent [60,61]. In our case series, the proportion of patients whose vision improved after pituitary tumour removal increased over the observed period from 26.7% in the first period to 64.7% by the last period. When comparing patients' postoperative vision between the early period (2011–2017) and the late one, there was a statistically significant improvement. An improvement in postoperative endocrine function was also observed over the period; in the first period, 6.7% experienced endocrine function improvement, whereas by the last period, that proportion increased to 17.6%; however, it was not statistically significant.

In a study conducted by Alexopoulou, 80% of patients with nonfunctioning adenomas had at least one pituitary axis deficiency, and following surgery, that proportion dropped to 61%, with the improvement mostly present in cases of adenomas affecting the LH/FSH and TSH axis [62]. Hypopituitarism was present in 58.5% of cases before surgery and 68.1% after surgery in our series; however, over the observed period, we managed to reduce the percentage of cases with hypopituitarism following surgery from 86.7% in the first period to 52.9% in the last. With experience, distinguishing the normal pituitary gland from the tumour tissue was easier.

Tumour size is recognised as a preoperative predictor of new pituitary deficiency, with surgery of larger neoplasms more often leading to a new hormone deficiency [60]. The function of the hypothalamic-pituitary axis continues to change postoperatively, even without radiotherapy [60]. Surgery for prolactinomas is suggested when patients are intolerant to the side effects of medications or they are ineffective, and in cases of pituitary apoplexy [30,63].

Complications after endoscopic surgery for pituitary adenomas occur in the range from 3.4% to 36.1% with a 1% mortality [18,30,45,64–66]. In our patient series, the percentage of complications following surgery gradually decreased over the observed period from 40% in the first period to 20.6% in the final period. The most often encountered postoperative complications are diabetes insipidus, anterior lobe dysfunction, and cerebrospinal fluid leak [30]. In our study, 16% developed diabetes insipidus after surgery, which was transient in all cases, cerebrospinal fluid leak was present in 6.4%, and intracranial haemorrhages that required revision surgery occurred in 7.4%.

Most cases of cerebrospinal fluid leak stop spontaneously during surgery; however, their incidence is higher in cases of macroadenomas, and a tear in the diaphragm or arachnoid membrane has to be appropriately reconstructed at the end of the procedure [18,64,67,68]. The risk of cerebrospinal fluid leak after EEA is increased in larger adenomas with suprasellar extension, intraoperative leakage, repeat surgery, and high body mass index [69,70]. The rate of cerebrospinal fluid leak after transsphenoidal surgery for pituitary adenomas is approximately 5%, with no significant difference between the endoscopic and microscopic approach [14,71,72]. Over the observed period, the percentage of patients who required rehospitalisation after surgery also decreased from 26.7% in the first period to 2.9% in the fourth period. By effectively reconstructing the sellar floor and utilising the multilayer techniques and nasoseptal grafts, we managed to decrease the complication rates following EEA for pituitary tumours.

No clear evidence is available on the timing, frequency, and duration of postoperative endocrine, radiologic, and ophthalmologic assessments, with most studies suggesting postoperative endocrine evaluation 4 to 8 weeks after surgery and others suggesting 2 to 6 months postoperatively [45,73]. MRI imaging performed immediately after surgery can be misleading due to debris, blood, and packing material; therefore, it is usually performed 3 to 6 months after the operation, when most postoperative changes cease [45,52,74]. In our study, the control MRI was performed 6 months after surgery. The interval for further MRI follow-up is decided upon residual tumour size and its distance to the optic chiasm [45]. Postoperatively, 68% of patients with preoperative visual impairment experience an overall improvement and approximately 5% deteriorate, with longer duration of visual field deficits and severity of visual symptoms being linked to worse postoperative visual outcomes [56,75–77]. Overall, in our study group, 2.9% of patients experienced a decline in their postoperative vision. It has been suggested that a visual examination be performed 3 months after surgery and then from every 4 to 6 months until stabilisation of the visual function, since visual defects tend to progressively improve, especially in the first year following surgery [78,79]. Nonfunctioning pituitary adenomas have regrowth rates between 15% and 66% when treated with surgery or 2% to 28% when combining surgery with radiotherapy; therefore, long-term follow-up is recommended [80,81]. Tumour recurrence was present in 11.7% of cases in our study, with a majority (81.8%) being adenomas, and most recurrences (81.8%) were treated using a second operation, and a minority were monitored using regular control MRI (18.2%).

The recurrence rate peaks between 1 and 5 years after surgery and declines after 10 years; hence, 10 or more years of postoperative imagining surveillance is indicated, with some suggesting lifelong monitoring of patients after surgery for pituitary adenoma, especially in cases of tumour remnants [45,81]. Radiosurgery was utilised in 3.2% of cases in our study with no further recurrence; one was a case of adenoma and two were metastases.

A grading system based on predicting factors, such as tumour invasion seen on MRI, immunohistochemical profile, mitotic index, and Ki-67 and p53 positivity, has been recently suggested to identify patients with a high risk of recurrence of progression [82]. Combining surgery and radiotherapy has been more effective than surgery alone in tumour recurrence prevention; however, radiotherapy can cause significant side effects, namely radiation-induced optic neuropathy, hypopituitarism, and secondary brain tumours; thus, it is reserved for cases of incomplete resection of adenomas with high proliferative activity or in cases of recurrence after repeated operations [83,84].

5. Conclusions

EEA represents a safe and effective modality for the treatment of pituitary adenomas where GTR is vital. Telementoring from an experienced centre enables less-experienced surgeons to establish a proficient skull base team with improving results, and it represents a cost-effective model for the global education of surgeons.

Author Contributions: Conceptualization, J.R., C.H.S., P.A.G. and B.L.; Methodology, J.R., H.R., T.Š. and B.L.; Formal analysis, J.R., H.R., T.Š. and B.L.; Resources, J.R.; Writing—original draft, J.R., H.R., T.Š. and B.L.; Writing—review & editing, J.R., H.R., T.Š., M.G., U.K., N.K. and B.L.; Supervision, J.R., C.H.S., P.A.G., T.Š. and B.L. All authors have read and agreed to the published version of the manuscript.

Funding: This research received no external funding.

Institutional Review Board Statement: The study was conducted in accordance with the Declaration of Helsinki, and approved by the Medical Ethics Commission of the Maribor University Medical Centre (protocol code UKC-MB-KME-31/24 on the 4 July 2024).

Informed Consent Statement: Patient consent was waived due to the retrospective nature and complete anonymity of the research.

Data Availability Statement: The original contributions presented in the study are included in the article, further inquiries can be directed to the corresponding author.

Conflicts of Interest: The authors declare no conflict of interest.

References

1. Snyderman, C.H.; Gardner, P.A.; Lanisnik, B.; Ravnik, J. Surgical telementoring: A new model for surgical training. *Laryngoscope* **2016**, *126*, 1334–1338. [CrossRef]
2. Van Furth, W.R.; De Vries, F.; Lobatto, D.J.; Kleijwegt, M.C.; Schutte, P.J.; Pereira, A.M.; Biermasz, N.R.; Verstegen, M.J. Endoscopic Surgery for Pituitary Tumors. *Endocrinol. Metab. Clin.* **2020**, *49*, 487–503. [CrossRef] [PubMed]

3. Molitch, M.E. Diagnosis and Treatment of Pituitary Adenomas: A Review. *JAMA* **2017**, *317*, 516. [CrossRef]
4. Byun, Y.H.; Kang, H.; Kim, Y.H. Advances in Pituitary Surgery. *Endocrinol. Metab.* **2022**, *37*, 608–616. [CrossRef]
5. Nishioka, H. Recent Evolution of Endoscopic Endonasal Surgery for Treatment of Pituitary Adenomas. *Neurol. Med.-Chir.* **2017**, *57*, 151–158. [CrossRef] [PubMed]
6. Singh, H.; Essayed, W.I.; Cohen-Gadol, A.; Zada, G.; Schwartz, T.H. Resection of pituitary tumors: Endoscopic versus microscopic. *J. Neurooncol.* **2016**, *130*, 309–317. [CrossRef] [PubMed]
7. Kenan, K.; İhsan, A.; Dilek, O.; Burak, C.; Gurkan, K.; Savas, C. The learning curve in endoscopic pituitary surgery and our experience. *Neurosurg. Rev.* **2006**, *29*, 298–305. [CrossRef] [PubMed]
8. Laws, E.R.; Barkhoudarian, G. The Transition from Microscopic to Endoscopic Transsphenoidal Surgery: The Experience at Brigham and Women's Hospital. *World Neurosurg.* **2014**, *82*, S152–S154. [CrossRef]
9. Snyderman, C.; Kassam, A.; Carrau, R.; Mintz, A.; Gardner, P.; Prevedello, D.M. Acquisition of Surgical Skills for Endonasal Skull Base Surgery: A Training Program. *Laryngoscope* **2007**, *17*, 699–705. [CrossRef]
10. Vasudevan, K.; Saad, H.; Oyesiku, M.N. The Role of Three-Dimensional Endoscopy in Pituitary Adenoma Surgery. *Neurosurg. Clin. N. Am.* **2019**, *30*, 421–432. [CrossRef]
11. Erridge, S.; Yeung, D.K.T.; Patel, H.R.H.; Purkayastha, S. Telementoring of Surgeons: A Systematic Review. *Surg. Innov.* **2019**, *26*, 95–111. [CrossRef] [PubMed]
12. Schlachta, C.M.; Nguyen, N.T.; Ponsky, T.; Dunkin, B. Project 6 Summit: SAGES telementoring initiative. *Surg. Endosc.* **2016**, *30*, 3665–3672. [CrossRef] [PubMed]
13. Hadad, G.; Bassagasteguy, L.; Carrau, R.L.; Mataza, J.C.; Kassam, A.; Snyderman, C.H.; Mintz, A. A Novel Reconstructive Technique After Endoscopic Expanded Endonasal Approaches: Vascular Pedicle Nasoseptal Flap. *Laryngoscope* **2006**, *116*, 1882–1886. [CrossRef]
14. Guinto, G.; Guinto-Nishimura, G.Y.; Sangrador-Deitos, M.V.; Uribe-Pacheco, R.; Soto-Martinez, R.; Gallardo, D.; Guinto, P.; Vargas, A.; Aréchiga, N. Current and Future Perspectives of Microscopic and Endoscopic Transsphenoidal Surgery for Pituitary Adenomas: A Narrative Review. *Arch. Med. Res.* **2023**, *54*, 102872. [CrossRef]
15. Famini, P.; Maya, M.M.; Melmed, S. Pituitary Magnetic Resonance Imaging for Sellar and Parasellar Masses: Ten-Year Experience in 2598 Patients. *J. Clin. Endocrinol. Metab.* **2011**, *96*, 1633–1641. [CrossRef] [PubMed]
16. Fernandez, A.; Karavitaki, N.; Wass, J.A.H. Prevalence of pituitary adenomas: A community-based, cross-sectional study in Banbury (Oxfordshire, UK). *Clin. Endocrinol.* **2010**, *72*, 377–382. [CrossRef]
17. Ezzat, S.; Asa, S.L.; Couldwell, W.T.; Barr, C.E.; Dodge, W.E.; Vance, M.L.; McCutcheon, I.E. The prevalence of pituitary adenomas: A systematic review. *Cancer* **2004**, *101*, 613–619. [CrossRef]
18. Wang, M.; Cai, Y.; Jiang, Y.; Peng, Y. Risk factors impacting intra- and postoperative cerebrospinal fluid rhinorrhea on the endoscopic treatment of pituitary adenomas: A retrospective study of 250 patients. *Medicine* **2021**, *100*, e27781. [CrossRef]
19. Lake, M.G.; Krook, L.S.; Cruz, S.V. Pituitary Adenomas: An Overview. *Am. Fam. Physician* **2013**, *88*, 319–327.
20. Lubomirsky, B.; Jenner, Z.B.; Jude, M.B.; Shahlaie, K.; Assadsangabi, R.; Ivanovic, V. Sellar, suprasellar, and parasellar masses: Imaging features and neurosurgical approaches. *Neuroradiol. J.* **2022**, *35*, 269–283. [CrossRef]
21. Sitoci-Ficici, K.H.; Sippl, C.; Prajsnar, A.; Saffour, S.; Linsler, S. Sellar metastasis: A rare intraoperative finding—Surgical treatment, strategies and outcome. *Clin. Neurol. Neurosurg.* **2024**, *241*, 108280. [CrossRef]
22. Melmed, S.; Casanueva, F.F.; Hoffman, A.R.; Kleinberg, D.L.; Montori, V.M.; Schlechte, J.A.; Wass, J.A.H. Diagnosis and Treatment of Hyperprolactinemia: An Endocrine Society Clinical Practice Guideline. *J. Clin. Endocrinol. Metab.* **2011**, *96*, 273–288. [CrossRef]
23. Webster, J.; Piscitelli, G.; Polli, A.; Ferrari, C.I.; Ismail, I.; Scanlon, M.F. A comparison of cabergoline and bromocriptine in the treatment of hyperprolactinemic amenorrhea. Cabergoline Comparative Study Group. *N. Engl. J. Med.* **1994**, *331*, 904–909. [CrossRef] [PubMed]
24. Biller, B.M.K.; Grossman, A.B.; Stewart, P.M.; Melmed, S.; Bertagna, X.; Bertherat, J.; Buchfelder, M.; Colao, A.; Hermus, A.R.; Hofland, L.J.; et al. Treatment of Adrenocorticotropin-Dependent Cushing's Syndrome: A Consensus Statement. *J. Clin. Endocrinol. Metab.* **2008**, *93*, 2454–2462. [CrossRef] [PubMed]
25. Freda, P.U.; Beckers, A.M.; Katznelson, L.; Molitch, M.E.; Montori, V.M.; Post, K.D.; Vance, M.L. Pituitary Incidentaloma: An Endocrine Society Clinical Practice Guideline. *J. Clin. Endocrinol. Metab.* **2011**, *96*, 894–904. [CrossRef] [PubMed]
26. Fernández-Balsells, M.M.; Murad, M.H.; Barwise, A.; Gallegos-Orozco, J.F.; Paul, A.; Lane, M.A.; Lampropulos, J.F.; Natividad, I.; Perestelo-Pérez, L.; de León-Lovatón, P.G.P.; et al. Natural History of Nonfunctioning Pituitary Adenomas and Incidentalomas: A Systematic Review and Metaanalysis. *J. Clin. Endocrinol. Metab.* **2011**, *96*, 905–912. [CrossRef]
27. Ordóñez-Rubiano, E.G.; Capacho-Delgado, Y.A.; Jacomussi-Alzate, L.; Galvis-Oñate, K.A.; Pérez-Chadid, D.; Tamara-Prieto, J.A.; Fabio-Restrepo, H.; Pinzón, M.; Patiño-Gómez, J.G. Dando forma a la curva desde el abordaje transesfenoidal microscópico al endonasal endoscópico para la región selar. *Cir. Cir.* **2024**, *92*, 11497. [CrossRef]
28. Wong, C.E.; Chen, P.W.; Hsu, H.J.; Cheng, S.Y.; Fan, C.C.; Chen, Y.C.; Chiu, Y.-P.; Lee, J.-S.; Liang, S.-F. Collaborative Human–Computer Vision Operative Video Analysis Algorithm for Analyzing Surgical Fluency and Surgical Interruptions in Endonasal Endoscopic Pituitary Surgery: Cohort Study. *J. Med. Internet Res.* **2024**, *26*, e56127. [CrossRef]
29. Jho, H.D. Endoscopic transsphenoidal surgery. *J. Neurooncol.* **2001**, *54*, 187–195. [CrossRef]
30. Wang, F.; Zhou, T.; Wei, S.; Meng, X.; Zhang, J.; Hou, Y.; Sun, G. Endoscopic endonasal transsphenoidal surgery of 1,166 pituitary adenomas. *Surg. Endosc.* **2015**, *29*, 1270–1280. [CrossRef]

31. Khalafallah, A.M.; Liang, A.L.; Jimenez, A.E.; Rowan, N.R.; Oyesiku, N.M.; Mamelak, A.N.; Mukherjee, D. Trends in endoscopic and microscopic transsphenoidal surgery: A survey of the international society of pituitary surgeons between 2010 and 2020. *Pituitary* **2020**, *23*, 526–533. [CrossRef] [PubMed]
32. de Divitiis, E. Endoscopic transsphenoidal surgery: Stone-in-the-pond effect. *Neurosurgery* **2006**, *59*, 512–520. [CrossRef]
33. Emanuelli, E.; Zanotti, C.; Munari, S.; Baldovin, M.; Schiavo, G.; Denaro, L. Sellar and parasellar lesions: Multidisciplinary management. *Acta Otorhinolaryngol. Ital.* **2021**, *41* (Suppl. 1), S30–S41. [CrossRef] [PubMed]
34. D'Haens, J.; Van Rompaey, K.; Stadnik, T.; Haentjens, P.; Poppe, K.; Velkeniers, B. Fully endoscopic transsphenoidal surgery for functioning pituitary adenomas: A retrospective comparison with traditional transsphenoidal microsurgery in the same institution. *Surg. Neurol.* **2009**, *72*, 336–340. [CrossRef] [PubMed]
35. Strychowsky, J.; Nayan, S.; Reddy, K.; Farrokhyar, F.; Sommer, D. Purely endoscopic transsphenoidal surgery versus traditional microsurgery for resection of pituitary adenomas: Systematic review. *J. Otolaryngol.-Head Neck Surg.* **2011**, *40*, 175–185. [PubMed]
36. Dagash, H.; Chowdhury, M.; Pierro, A. When can I be proficient in laparoscopic surgery? A systematic review of the evidence. *J. Pediatr. Surg.* **2003**, *38*, 720–724. [CrossRef]
37. Birkmeyer, J.D.; Lucas, F.L. Hospital Volume and Surgical Mortality in the United States. *N. Engl. J. Med.* **2002**, *346*, 1128–1137. [CrossRef]
38. Shively, E.H.; Shively, A.A. Threats to rural surgery. *Am. J. Surg.* **2005**, *190*, 200–205. [CrossRef]
39. Jarc, A.M.; Stanley, A.A.; Clifford, T.; Gill, I.S.; Hung, A.J. Proctors exploit three-dimensional ghost tools during clinical-like training scenarios: A preliminary study. *World J. Urol.* **2017**, *35*, 957–965. [CrossRef]
40. Vera, A.M.; Russo, M.; Mohsin, A.; Tsuda, S. Augmented reality telementoring (ART) platform: A randomized controlled trial to assess the efficacy of a new surgical education technology. *Surg. Endosc.* **2014**, *28*, 3467–3472. [CrossRef]
41. Schlachta, C.M.; Lefebvre, K.L.; Sorsdahl, A.K.; Jayaraman, S. Mentoring and telementoring leads to effective incorporation of laparoscopic colon surgery. *Surg. Endosc.* **2010**, *24*, 841–844. [CrossRef] [PubMed]
42. Dehdashti, A.R.; Ganna, A.; Karabatsou, K.; Gentili, F. Pure endoscopic endonasal approach for pituitary adenomas: Early surgical results in 200 patients and comparison with previous microsurgical series. *Neurosurgery* **2008**, *62*, 1006–1015; discussion 1015-7. [PubMed]
43. Komotar, R.J.; Starke, R.M.; Raper, D.M.S.; Anand, V.K.; Schwartz, T.H. Endoscopic endonasal compared with microscopic transsphenoidal and open transcranial resection of giant pituitary adenomas. *Pituitary* **2012**, *15*, 150–159. [CrossRef] [PubMed]
44. Yu, S.; Du, Q.; Yao, S.; Zhang, K.; Wang, J.; Zhu, Z.; Jiang, X. Outcomes of endoscopic and microscopic transsphenoidal surgery on non-functioning pituitary adenomas: A systematic review and meta-analysis. *J. Cell. Mol. Med.* **2018**, *22*, 2023–2027. [CrossRef]
45. Esposito, D.; Olsson, D.S.; Ragnarsson, O.; Buchfelder, M.; Skoglund, T.; Johannsson, G. Non-functioning pituitary adenomas: Indications for pituitary surgery and post-surgical management. *Pituitary* **2019**, *22*, 422–434. [CrossRef]
46. Berkmann, S.; Schlaffer, S.; Nimsky, C.; Fahlbusch, R.; Buchfelder, M. Intraoperative high-field MRI for transsphenoidal reoperations of nonfunctioning pituitary adenoma. *J. Neurosurg.* **2014**, *121*, 1166–1175. [CrossRef]
47. Daly, A.F.; Rixhon, M.; Adam, C.; Dempegioti, A.; Tichomirowa, M.A.; Beckers, A. High Prevalence of Pituitary Adenomas: A Cross-Sectional Study in the Province of Liège, Belgium. *J. Clin. Endocrinol. Metab.* **2006**, *91*, 4769–4775. [CrossRef]
48. Gruppetta, M.; Mercieca, C.; Vassallo, J. Prevalence and incidence of pituitary adenomas: A population based study in Malta. *Pituitary* **2013**, *16*, 545–553. [CrossRef]
49. Raappana, A.; Koivukangas, J.; Ebeling, T.; Pirilä, T. Incidence of Pituitary Adenomas in Northern Finland in 1992–2007. *J. Clin. Endocrinol. Metab.* **2010**, *95*, 4268–4275. [CrossRef]
50. Ntali, G.; Wass, J.A. Epidemiology, clinical presentation and diagnosis of non-functioning pituitary adenomas. *Pituitary* **2018**, *21*, 111–118. [CrossRef]
51. Olsson, D.S.; Hammarstrand, C.; Bryngelsson, I.L.; Nilsson, A.G.; Andersson, E.; Johannsson, G.; Ragnarsson, O. Incidence of malignant tumours in patients with a non-functioning pituitary adenoma. *Endocr. Relat. Cancer* **2017**, *24*, 227–235. [CrossRef] [PubMed]
52. Chen, L.; White, W.L.; Spetzler, R.F.; Xu, B. A prospective study of nonfunctioning pituitary adenomas: Presentation, management, and clinical outcome. *J. Neurooncol.* **2011**, *102*, 129–138. [CrossRef]
53. Arafah, B.M.; Prunty, D.; Ybarra, J.; Hlavin, M.L.; Selman, W.R. The Dominant Role of Increased Intrasellar Pressure in the Pathogenesis of Hypopituitarism, Hyperprolactinemia, and Headaches in Patients with Pituitary Adenomas. *J. Clin. Endocrinol. Metab.* **2000**, *85*, 1789–1793. [PubMed]
54. Schankin, C.J.; Reifferscheid, A.K.; Krumbholz, M.; Linn, J.; Rachinger, W.; Langer, S.; Sostak, P.; Arzberger, T.; Kretzschmar, H.; Straube, A. Headache in patients with pituitary adenoma: Clinical and paraclinical findings. *Cephalalgia* **2012**, *32*, 1198–1207. [CrossRef]
55. Lee, I.H.; Miller, N.R.; Zan, E.; Tavares, F.; Blitz, A.M.; Sung, H.; Yousem, D.M.; Boland, M.V. Visual Defects in Patients With Pituitary Adenomas: The Myth of Bitemporal Hemianopsia. *Am. J. Roentgenol.* **2015**, *205*, W512–W518. [CrossRef]
56. Muskens, I.S.; Zamanipoor Najafabadi, A.H.; Briceno, V.; Lamba, N.; Senders, J.T.; Van Furth, W.R.; Verstegen, M.J.T.; Smith, T.R.S.; Mekary, R.A.; Eenhorst, C.A.E.; et al. Visual outcomes after endoscopic endonasal pituitary adenoma resection: A systematic review and meta-analysis. *Pituitary* **2017**, *20*, 539–552. [CrossRef] [PubMed]
57. Raverot, G.; Assié, G.; Cotton, F.; Cogne, M.; Boulin, A.; Dherbomez, M.; Bonneville, J.F.; Massart, C. Biological and radiological exploration and management of non-functioning pituitary adenoma. *Ann. Endocrinol.* **2015**, *76*, 201–209. [CrossRef]

58. Drange, M.R.; Fram, N.R.; Herman-Bonert, V.; Melmed, S. Pituitary Tumor Registry: A Novel Clinical Resource. *J. Clin. Endocrinol. Metab.* **2000**, *85*, 168–174. [CrossRef]
59. Anagnostis, P.; Adamidou, P.; Polyzos, S.A.; Efstathiadou, Z.; Panagiotou, A.; Kita, M. Non-Functioning Pituitary Adenomas: A Single Center Experience. *Exp. Clin. Endocrinol. Diabetes* **2011**, *119*, 314–319. [CrossRef]
60. Al-Shamkhi, N.; Berinder, K.; Borg, H.; Burman, P.; Dahlqvist, P.; Höybye, C.; Olsson, D.S.; Ragnarsson, O.; Ekman, B.; Engström, B.E. Pituitary function before and after surgery for nonfunctioning pituitary adenomas—Data from the Swedish Pituitary Register. *Eur. J. Endocrinol.* **2023**, *189*, 217–224. [CrossRef]
61. Webb, S.M.; Rigla, M.; Gner, A.W.; Oliver, B.; Bartumeus, F. Recovery of Hypopituitarism after Neurosurgical Treatment of Pituitary Adenomas. *J. Clin. Endocrinol. Metab.* **1999**, *84*, 3696–3700. [CrossRef] [PubMed]
62. Alexopoulou, O.; Everard, V.; Etoa, M.; Fomekong, E.; Gaillard, S.; Parker, F.; Raftopoulos, C.; Chanson, P.; Maiter, D. Outcome of pituitary hormone deficits after surgical treatment of nonfunctioning pituitary macroadenomas. *Endocrine* **2021**, *73*, 166–176. [CrossRef]
63. Tatsi, C.; Stratakis, C.A. Aggressive pituitary tumors in the young and elderly. *Rev. Endocr. Metab. Disord.* **2020**, *21*, 213–223. [CrossRef]
64. Berker, M.; Hazer, D.B.; Yücel, T.; Gürlek, A.; Cila, A.; Aldur, M.; Önerci, M. Complications of endoscopic surgery of the pituitary adenomas: Analysis of 570 patients and review of the literature. *Pituitary* **2012**, *15*, 288–300. [CrossRef]
65. Gondim, J.A.; Almeida, J.P.C.; Albuquerque, L.A.F.; Schops, M.; Gomes, E.; Ferraz, T.; Sobreira, W.; Kretzmann, M.T. Endoscopic endonasal approach for pituitary adenoma: Surgical complications in 301 patients. *Pituitary* **2011**, *14*, 174–183. [CrossRef] [PubMed]
66. Zada, G.; Cavallo, L.M.; Esposito, F.; Fernandez-Jimenez, J.C.; Tasiou, A.; De Angelis, M.; Cafiero, T.; Cappabianca, P.; Laws, E.R. Transsphenoidal surgery in patients with acromegaly: Operative strategies for overcoming technically challenging anatomical variations. *Neurosurg. Focus* **2010**, *29*, E8. [CrossRef]
67. Rotenberg, B.; Tam, S.; Ryu, W.H.; Duggal, N. Microscopic versus endoscopic pituitary surgery: A systematic review. *Laryngoscope* **2010**, *120*, 1292–1297. [CrossRef] [PubMed]
68. Ding, Z.; Lu, X.; Wang, Q.; Qian, X.; Lu, H.; Xu, R.; Zhu, A. Endoscopic endonasal surgery of Rathke's cleft cysts–preoperative imaging evaluation, personalized removal and multilevel sellar floor reconstruction. *Clin. Neurol. Neurosurg.* **2024**, *236*, 108111. [CrossRef]
69. Dlouhy, B.J.; Madhavan, K.; Clinger, J.D.; Reddy, A.; Dawson, J.D.; O'Brien, E.K.; Chang, E.; Graham, S.M.; Greenlee, J.D. Elevated body mass index and risk of postoperative CSF leak following transsphenoidal surgery: Clinical article. *J. Neurosurg.* **2012**, *116*, 1311–1317. [CrossRef]
70. Zhang, C.; Ding, X.; Lu, Y.; Hu, L.; Hu, G. Cerebrospinal fluid rhinorrhoea following transsphenoidal surgery for pituitary adenoma: Experience in a Chinese centre. *Acta Otorhinolaryngol. Ital.* **2017**, *37*, 303–307. [CrossRef]
71. Starke, R.M.; Raper, D.M.S.; Payne, S.C.; Vance, M.L.; Oldfield, E.H.; Jane, J.A. Endoscopic vs Microsurgical Transsphenoidal Surgery for Acromegaly: Outcomes in a Concurrent Series of Patients Using Modern Criteria For Remission. *J. Clin. Endocrinol. Metab.* **2013**, *98*, 3190–3198. [CrossRef]
72. Dai, W.; Zhuang, Z.; Ling, H.; Yang, Y.; Hang, C. Systematic review and network meta-analysis assess the comparative efficacy and safety of transsphenoidal surgery for pituitary tumor. *Neurosurg. Rev.* **2021**, *44*, 515–527. [CrossRef] [PubMed]
73. Ziu, M.; Dunn, I.F.; Hess, C.; Fleseriu, M.; Bodach, M.E.; Tumialan, L.M.; Oyesiku, N.M.; Patel, K.S.; Wang, R.; Carter, B.S.; et al. Congress of Neurological Surgeons Systematic Review and Evidence-Based Guideline on Posttreatment Follow-up Evaluation of Patients With Nonfunctioning Pituitary Adenomas. *Neurosurgery* **2016**, *79*, E541–E543. [CrossRef] [PubMed]
74. Dekkers, O.M.; Karavitaki, N.; Pereira, A.M. The epidemiology of aggressive pituitary tumors (and its challenges). *Rev. Endocr. Metab. Disord.* **2020**, *21*, 209–212. [CrossRef] [PubMed]
75. Barzaghi, L.R.; Medone, M.; Losa, M.; Bianchi, S.; Giovanelli, M.; Mortini, P. Prognostic factors of visual field improvement after trans-sphenoidal approach for pituitary macroadenomas: Review of the literature and analysis by quantitative method. *Neurosurg. Rev.* **2012**, *35*, 369–379. [CrossRef]
76. Gnanalingham, K.K. The time course of visual field recovery following transphenoidal surgery for pituitary adenomas: Predictive factors for a good outcome. *J. Neurol. Neurosurg. Psychiatry* **2005**, *76*, 415–419. [CrossRef]
77. Marcus, M.; Vitale, S.; Calvert, P.C.; Miller, N.R. Visual parameters in patients with pituitary adenoma before and after transsphenoidal surgery. *Aust. N. Z. J. Ophthalmol.* **1991**, *19*, 111–118. [CrossRef]
78. Dekkers, O.M.; De Keizer, R.J.W.; Roelfsema, F.; Vd Klaauw, A.A.; Honkoop, P.J.; Van Dulken, H.; Smit, J.W.A.; Romijn, J.A.; Pereira, A.M. Progressive improvement of impaired visual acuity during the first year after transsphenoidal surgery for non-functioning pituitary macroadenoma. *Pituitary* **2007**, *10*, 61–65. [CrossRef]
79. Abouaf, L.; Vighetto, A.; Lebas, M. Neuro-ophthalmologic exploration in non-functioning pituitary adenoma. *Ann. Endocrinol.* **2015**, *76*, 210–219. [CrossRef]
80. Roelfsema, F.; Biermasz, N.R.; Pereira, A.M. Clinical factors involved in the recurrence of pituitary adenomas after surgical remission: A structured review and meta-analysis. *Pituitary* **2012**, *15*, 71–83. [CrossRef]
81. Tampourlou, M.; Ntali, G.; Ahmed, S.; Arlt, W.; Ayuk, J.; Byrne, J.V.; Chavda, S.; Cudlip, S.; Gittoes, N.; Grossman, A.; et al. Outcome of Nonfunctioning Pituitary Adenomas That Regrow After Primary Treatment: A Study From Two Large UK Centers. *J. Clin. Endocrinol. Metab.* **2017**, *102*, 1889–1897. [CrossRef] [PubMed]

82. Raverot, G.; Dantony, E.; Beauvy, J.; Vasiljevic, A.; Mikolasek, S.; Borson-Chazot, F.; Jouanneau, E.; Roy, P.; Trouillas, J. Risk of Recurrence in Pituitary Neuroendocrine Tumors: A Prospective Study Using a Five-Tiered Classification. *J. Clin. Endocrinol. Metab.* **2017**, *102*, 3368–3374. [CrossRef] [PubMed]
83. Loeffler, J.S.; Shih, H.A. Radiation Therapy in the Management of Pituitary Adenomas. *J. Clin. Endocrinol. Metab.* **2011**, *96*, 1992–2003. [CrossRef] [PubMed]
84. Minniti, G.; Jaffrain-Rea, M.L.; Osti, M.; Cantore, G.; Enrici, R.M. Radiotherapy for nonfunctioning pituitary adenomas: From conventional to modern stereotactic radiation techniques. *Neurosurg. Rev.* **2007**, *30*, 167–176. [CrossRef] [PubMed]

diagnostics

MDPI

Article

Hypopituitarism, Diabetes Insipidus, and Syndrome of Inappropriate Antidiuretic Hormone Secretion after Pituitary Macroadenoma Surgery with Indocyanine Green Dye

Tomislav Felbabić [1,2,*], Tomaž Velnar [1,2] and Tomaž Kocjan [2,3]

1 Department of Neurosurgery, University Medical Centre Ljubljana, 1000 Ljubljana, Slovenia; tvelnar@hotmail.com
2 Faculty of Medicine, University of Ljubljana, 1000 Ljubljana, Slovenia
3 Department of Endocrinology, Diabetes and Metabolic Diseases, University Medical Centre Ljubljana, 1000 Ljubljana, Slovenia
* Correspondence: tomislav.felbabic@kclj.si

Abstract: (1) Background: Pituitary adenomas are benign tumors comprising about 18% of all intracranial tumors, and they often require surgical intervention. Differentiating pituitary tissue from adenoma during surgery is crucial to minimize complications. We hypothesized that using ICG dye would reduce the hormonal complication rates. (2) Methods: A prospective randomized study (February 2019–October 2023) included 34 patients with non-functional macroadenomas of the pituitary gland randomly assigned to receive intraoperative ICG or be in the control group. All underwent endoscopic endonasal transsphenoidal surgery. Pituitary function was assessed preoperatively, immediately postoperatively, and 3–6 months postoperatively. Adenohypophysis function was evaluated with hormonal tests (Cosyntropin stimulation test, TSH, fT3, fT4, prolactin, IGF-1, FSH, LH, and testosterone in men) and neurohypophysis function with fluid balance, plasma and urine osmolality, and serum and urinary sodium. (3) Results: Of the 34 patients (23 men, 11 women; average age 60.9 years), 5.9% in the ICG group developed diabetes insipidus postoperatively, compared to 23.5% in the control group. Adenohypophysis function worsened in 52.9% of the ICG group and in 35.3% of the control group. (4) Conclusions: Our study did not confirm the benefits of using ICG in these surgeries. Further research with a larger sample is needed.

Keywords: pituitary; adenohypophysis; neurohypophysis; non-functioning macroadenomas; ICG dye; endoscopic endonasal surgery; diabetes insipidus; pituitary–peripheral axis

1. Introduction

Pituitary adenomas are benign tumors of the anterior lobe of the pituitary gland. They account for approximately 18% of all intracranial neoplasms and are the most common tumors of the sellar region [1]. The prevalence of the disease in the general population is estimated at 16.7% [2]. They are the third most common intracranial neoplasm requiring surgery after gliomas and meningiomas [1]. Most pituitary adenomas are incidental findings and do not require intervention other than follow-up. Prolactinomas are most common (30–60%), followed by nonfunctioning adenomas (14–55%), growth-hormone-secreting adenomas (8–15%), and corticotropin-secreting adenomas (2–6%). Thyrotropin- and gonadotropin-secreting adenomas are extremely rare (<1%) [3]. Most of them occur sporadically (95%). A small minority are familial or part of a specific syndrome, such as multiple endocrine neoplasia types 1 and 4, McCune–Albright syndrome, Carney complex, and X-linked acrogigantism [4].

Pituitary adenomas are classified according to their size and hormonal overproduction. Those that are less than 1 cm in size are called microadenomas, those that are 1 cm or more in size are called macroadenomas, and those that are more than 4 cm in size are called giant [5].

Those pituitary adenomas that do not secrete hormones or whose hormone secretion does not cause clinical symptoms are called nonfunctioning adenomas. Hormonally active adenomas are referred to as functioning adenomas [6].

More sophisticated classifications have been developed to describe tumor invasion into the sella-adjacent structures. The Hardy classification describes the invasion of the sella floor [7]. A modified version by Willson, known as Hardy–Willson classification, describes the suprasellar invasion, but it lacks utility for the purposes of surgical cure and complication estimation [8]. Knosp's classification describes invasion of the parasellar space [9].

Patients with pituitary adenoma should be evaluated by a multidisciplinary team including endocrinologists, ophthalmologists, and neurosurgeons. Surgical therapy is indicated in cases where adenomas cause neurologic deficits due to the mass effect of the lesion, show growth on follow-up MRI, or cause hormonal dysfunction [10]. An exception is prolactionoma, where the first stage of treatment is conservative with dopamine agonists [11]. Historically, pituitary adenomas were removed through a transcranial approach followed by a microscopic transsphenoidal approach. In recent years, the endoscopic endonasal transsphenoidal approach has become the gold standard for pituitary adenoma surgery [12].

It is very important to distinguish normal pituitary tissue from adenoma. In this way, maximal resection of the tumor can be achieved safely and with little risk of postoperative complications due to pituitary damage. Histologic and imaging studies have shown that normal pituitary tissue and pituitary adenoma have different vascular densities [13]. Adenomas have significantly lower capillary density compared with normal pituitary tissue. Advances in intraoperative tumor imaging have demonstrated that the use of indocyanine green (ICG) is of great benefit in endoscopic endonasal transsphenoidal pituitary adenoma surgery [14]. After intravenous application, the dye binds to serum albumin and causes fluorescence of vascular structures. The maximum emission wavelength of ICG in plasma is 820 nm [15]. Due to the dense vasculature of the pituitary gland and the small vasculature of the adenoma, ICG is a promising pituitary marker [16].

In this study, we hypothesized that because of the easier intraoperative differentiation between pituitary adenoma and the normal gland through interoperative ICG, the incidence of postoperative hypopituitarism and fluid balance disorders should be lower. If this is true, ICG will prove to be a valuable adjunct to endoscopic endonasal pituitary adenoma surgery as it will provide better outcomes for patients.

2. Materials and Methods

Patients

This prospective randomized study was conducted at the Departments of Neurosurgery and of Endocrinology, Diabetes, and Metabolic Diseases, University Medical Centre (UMC) hospital in Ljubljana, Slovenia. It was approved by the Slovenian Medical Ethics committee (No. 0120-56/2019/6). In total, 34 patients were included in the study during the period between February 2019 and October 2023. Patients were randomly placed in two groups: a group that received ICG intraoperatively and a control group. All patients signed written informed consent forms for inclusion in this study. An endoscopic endonasal transsphenoidal approach for pituitary adenoma removal was performed on all patients.

Indocyanine green material

The ICG compound was acquired from Serb pharmaceuticals, Paris, France. First, 25 mg of the compound was dissolved in 10 mL of sterile water. After exposure of the intrasellar space, 5 mL of solution (12.5 mg of ICG) was injected intravenously as a bolus during surgery and after macroscopic removal of the macroadenoma.

Optics

At our institution, we use the Karl Storz rigid endoscope for endoscopic transsphenoidal surgeries. For the purpose of this study, an endoscope with ICG light detection was used. The light source can be switched between white and near-infrared light intraoperatively using a foot switch.

Hormonal testing

At the Department of Endocrinology, Diabetes and Metabolic Diseases of the UMC Ljubljana, pituitary function was examined before surgery, immediately after surgery, and 3–6 months after surgery. The function of the pituitary–peripheral axis was determined through routine hormone tests: Cosyntropin stimulation test with cortisol basal and after 30 min, thyrotropin (TSH), free triiodothyronine (fT3), free thyroxine (fT4), prolactin (PRL), insulin-like growth factor-1 (IGF-1), follicle-stimulating hormone (FSH), luteinizing hormone (LH), and, in men, testosterone. We measured the fluid balance, the osmolality of the first morning urine, plasma osmolality, and the serum sodium with the urinary sodium in order to check water metabolism and the function of the neurohypophysis.

Hypopituitarism was defined as a condition in which one or more aspects of the pituitary–peripheral axis was affected and the patient required hormone replacement therapy. The assessment of hypopituitarism immediately after surgery is approximate, as all patients receive prophylactic doses of hydrocortisone (10 mg at 8.00, 5 mg at 13.00, and 5 mg at 17.00). Improvement was defined as when the therapy was reduced 3–6 months after surgery compared with the preoperative or postoperative state. If the therapy 3–6 months postoperatively was equal to the preoperative or postoperative therapy, we defined the condition as being as stable as before surgery or after surgery. However, if the patient required higher doses of therapy 3–6 months postoperatively compared with the preoperative or postoperative state, we classified it as deterioration. Diabetes insipidus was defined as a condition where the patient required sublingual desmopressin therapy due to polyuria. In contrast, syndrome of inappropriate antidiuretic hormone secretion was defined as a condition in which the patient required fluid restriction due to low serum sodium levels in combination with other established diagnostic criteria.

Radiologic evaluation

Contrast-enhanced MRI imaging of the head was performed preoperatively and 3–6 months postoperatively in all patients according to the sella region pathology protocol. Tumor dimensions were measured in the transverse, sagittal, and coronal planes. Tumor volume was calculated as half of the product of all three dimensions. Knosp classification was determined using the coronal sequences, while the Hardy classification was determined using the sagittal sequences.

Statistical analysis of the data

We analyzed the data using the statistical software SPSS 25 (IBM Corp., Armonk, NY, USA). We considered *p*-values of less than 0.05 to be statistically significant.

Demographic and clinical characteristics of the patients, which were normally distributed, are presented with the mean and the standard deviation, while asymmetrically distributed variables are presented with the median and the first and third quartiles. The values of the descriptive variables are presented as relative and absolute frequencies.

To compare the proportions between the patient groups with and without ICG dye, we used the chi-square test or Fisher's exact test. The comparison of numerical variables between the study groups was performed using the *t*-test for independent samples or the non-parametric Mann–Whitney test. To compare the frequencies, we used the extended Fisher's exact test according to Freeman–Halton. To compare the total number of axes affected to the time of the control measurement, we used the dependent samples *t*-test and the Wilcoxon signed ranks test.

3. Results

In total, 34 patients were included in this study, 23 males (67.7%) and 11 females (23.3%), aged between 33 and 81 years, with an average of 60.9 years. Demographic and clinical data are presented in Table 1. There were no significant differences between the groups based on the patients' age, sex, or Knosp or Hardy classifications of the tumor. The sizes of tumors showed statistically significant differences.

Table 1. Demographic and clinical characteristics of patients with nonfunctioning pituitary adenoma, stratified by ICG application.

	All n = 34	ICG n = 17	No ICG n = 17	p-Value [1]
Age, years	60.9 ± 11.2	62.7 ± 9.9	59.1 ± 12.4	0.360
Gender, n (%)				0.714
Male	23 (67.7)	11 (64.7)	12 (70.6)	
Female	11 (32.4)	6 (35.3)	5 (29.4)	
Tumor size, mm^3	7802 (2577–11,261)	5130 (2344–6026)	10,473 (3753–16,273)	0.041
Knosp classification, n (%)				0.764
0	3 (8.8)	2 (11.8)	1 (5.9)	
1	18 (52.9)	8 (47.1)	10 (58.8)	
2	8 (23.5)	5 (29.4)	3 (17.6)	
3	5 (14.7)	2 (11.8)	3 (17.6)	
Hardy classification, n (%)				0.817
1	5 (14.7)	3 (17.6)	2 (11.8)	
2	9 (26.5)	4 (23.5)	5 (29.4)	
3	10 (29.4)	6 (35.3)	4 (23.5)	
4	10 (29.4)	4 (23.5)	6 (35.3)	

Numerical variables are presented as mean ± standard deviation or median (first–third quartile). ICG = indocyanine green dye. [1] p-value for comparison between patient groups with ICG and without ICG.

We assessed the function of the neurohypophysis by evaluating fluid balance, the osmolality of morning urine, the plasma osmolality, and the serum sodium with the urinary sodium. Table 2 shows a comparison of the two quantities measured between the two groups of patients and between the controls.

Table 2. Fluid balance before surgery, immediately after surgery, and 3–6 months after surgery.

	ICG Group			No ICG Group			p_1	p_2	p_3
	Pre-OP	Post-OP	3–6 Months Post-OP	Pre-OP	Post-OP	3–6 Months Post-OP	ICG vs. No ICG	Control Measurement	Interaction
Fluid balance, n (%)									
No complication	17/17 (100)	12/17 (70.6)	16/17 (94.1)	17/17 (100)	12/17 (70.6)	13/17 (76.5)	0.210	0.116	0.258
Complication	0/17 (0)	5/17 (29.4)	1/17 (5.9)	0/17 (0)	5/17 (29.4)	4/17 (23.5)			
Fluid balance complication, n (%)							-	-	
Diabetes insipidus	-	3/5	1/1	-	4/5	4/4	0.148	0.399	0.399
SIADH	-	2/5	0/1	-	1/5	0/4	-	-	

ICG = indocyanine green dye, OP = operation, SIADH = syndrome of inappropriate antidiuretic hormone secretion, $p_{1,2,3}$ = influence of ICG dye and control measurement time (only post-OP and 3–6 months post-OP) on fluid balance complication in a generalized linear model, p_1, p_2 = statistical significance of main effects, p_3 = statistical significance of interaction between main effects.

The presence of hypopituitarism was assessed at all three control measurements, i.e., before surgery, immediately after surgery and 3–6 months after surgery. The incidence of hypopituitarism, shown separately according to the patient group, is shown in Table 3. If hypopituitarism was compared between all three measurements, the output was categorised in five ways [2]. However, it is much less complicated if we only compare the preoperative state with the 3–6-month postoperative state. If we only compared those two states, the result was categorized in three ways [3].

Table 3. Incidence of hypopituitarism before adenoma surgery, immediately after surgery, and 3–6 months postoperatively after OP, separated according to ICG application.

	ICG n = 17	No ICG n = 17	*p*-Value [1]
HP before OP, n (%)			0.3
No	8 (47.1)	6 (35.3)	
Yes	9 (52.9)	11 (64.7)	
HP after OP, n (%)			-
No	0 (0)	0 (0)	
Yes	17 (100)	17 (100)	
HP 3–6 months after OP [2], n (%)			0.822
Not detectable	5/17 (33.3)	3/17 (18.8)	
Improvement	2/17 (13.3)	2/17 (12.5)	
As after OP (HP already before OP)	1/17(6.7)	3/17 (12.5)	
After OP (HP occurs after OP)	1/17 (6.7)	3/17 (18.8)	
Deterioration	8/17 (40.0)	6/17 (37.5)	
HP 3–6 months after OP [3], n (%)			1
Improvement	1/17 (5.9)	1/17 (5.9)	
Steady state	6/17 (35.3)	6/17 (35.3)	
Deterioration	10/17 (58.8)	10/17 (58.8)	

HP = hypopituitarism, ICG = indocyanine green dye, OP = operation. [1] *p*-values for comparison of proportions between patient groups with ICG and without ICG [2] comparison of the three control measurements. [3] Comparison of preoperative and 3–6-month postoperative status.

We compared the number of affected pituitary–peripheral axes before surgery and 3–6 months after surgery. A statistically significant difference in the number of affected axes between the two groups was confirmed in the control 3–6 months after surgery. No significant difference in the number of affected axes between the groups was confirmed in the preoperative examination (Table 4).

Table 4. Number of affected axes before operation (OP) and 3–6 months after OP in the groups with and without ICG dye.

Number of Axes Affected	Before OP			3–6 Months after OP		
	Total	ICG	No ICG	Total	ICG	No ICG
0	14 (41.2)	8 (47.1)	6 (35.3)	8 (23.5)	5 (29.4)	3 (17.6)
1	5 (14.7)	2 (11.8)	3 (17.6)	6 (17.6)	3 (17.6)	3 (17.6)
2	10 (29.4)	3 (17.6)	7 (41.2)	7 (20.6)	0 (0)	7 (41.2)
3	3 (8.8)	3 (17.6)	0 (0)	10 (29.4)	8 (47.1)	2 (11.8)
4	2 (5.9)	1 (5.9)	1 (5.9)	3 (8.8)	1 (5.9)	2 (11.8)
p-value		0.3			0.013	

ICG = indocyanine green dye, OP = operation. Values in the table are frequencies (%). *p*-value for comparison between groups with and without ICG using Fisher–Freeman–Halton exact test.

We also compared the mean number of affected axes between the two groups before surgery and 3–6 months after surgery. The number of affected axes was statistically significantly different between the two control groups: 3–6 months after surgery, the mean number of affected axes was statistically significantly higher (1.82) than before surgery (1.24). We did not confirm a difference in the mean number of axes affected between the two patient groups (Table 5).

We were also interested in how often each type of pituitary–peripheral axis is affected before surgery and 3–6 months after surgery. The results are presented in Table 6.

Table 5. Comparison of the mean value of the number of affected axes between the group with ICG and the group without ICG.

Number of Axes Affected	Before OP				3–6 Months after OP				p^2
	Total	ICG	No ICG	p^1	Total	ICG	No ICG	p^1	
Average ± SE	1.24 ± 0.22	1.24 ± 0.34	1.24 ± 0.28	1	1.82 ± 0.23	1.82 ± 0.36	1.82 ± 0.30	1	0.003
Median (first, third quartile)	1 (0, 2)	1 (0, 2.5)	1 (0, 2)	0.919	2 (0.75, 3)	3 (0, 3)	2 (1, 2.5)	0.892	0.003

[1]—p value for the comparison between the ICG group and the non-ICG group using t-test for independent samples and Mann–Whitney test. [2]—p value for the comparison between the total number of affected axes before and 3–6 months after OP with the t-test for the dependent sample and the Wilcoxon signed rank test. The interaction between the main factors 'control measurement' (before and 3–6 months after OP) and 'patient group' (with and without ICG) in the repeated measures analysis of variance model was statistically non-significant (p = 1). ICG = indocyanine green dye, OP = operation, SE = standard error.

Table 6. Type of affected axis before OP and 3–6 months after OP in groups with and without ICG dye.

Axis Type	Before OP			3–6 Months after OP		
	Total	ICG	No ICG	Total	ICG	No ICG
Tyroid axis	15	8	7	19	9	10
Adrenal axis	10	5	5	18	10	8
Gonadal axis	14	7	7	18	9	9
Somatotropic axis	2	1	1	7	3	4
Prolactin axis	0	0	0	0	0	0

The values in the table are absolute frequencies. ICG = indocyanine green dye, OP = operation.

Below are graphs comparing pituitary–peripheral axis involvement before and 3–6 months after surgery for all patients (Figure 1), the ICG group (Figure 2), and the control group (Figure 3) according to Table 6.

We were interested in the impact of demographic and clinical characteristics of patients on the outcome of pituitary adenoma surgery. The outcome was defined as the presence of the following conditions: hypopituitarism 3–6 months after surgery (yes vs. no) and diabetes insipidus 3–6 months after surgery (yes vs. no). The results are shown in Table 7.

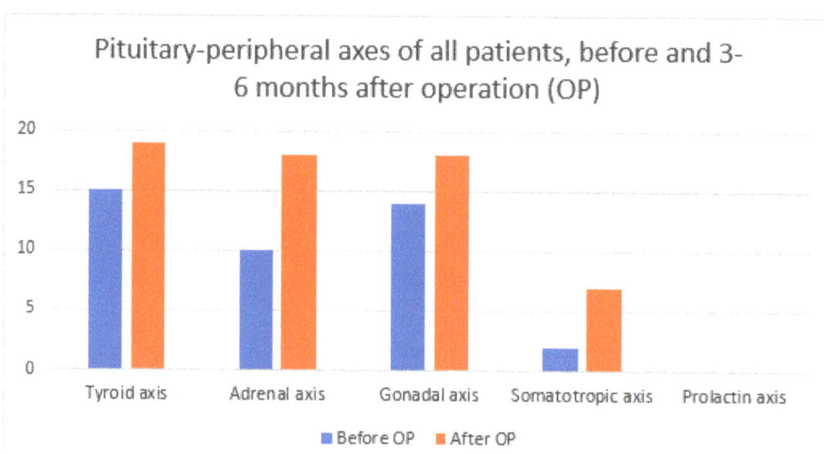

Figure 1. Pituitary–peripheral axis involvement before and 3–6 months after OP for all patients according to Table 6. OP = operation.

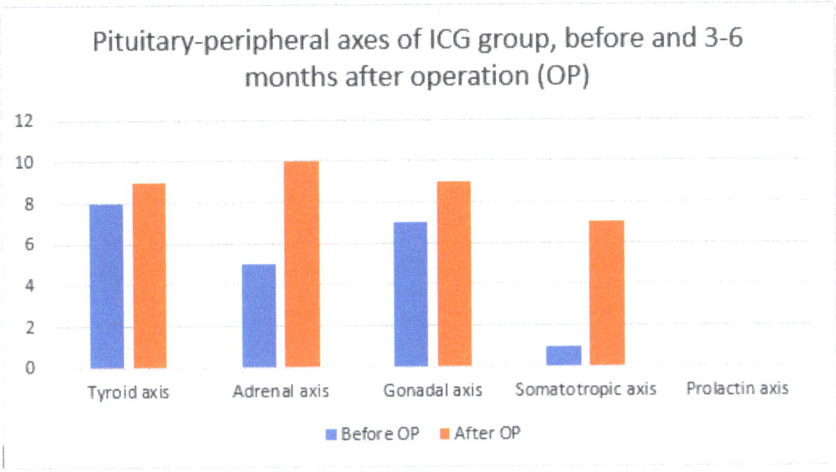

Figure 2. Pituitary–peripheral axis involvement before and 3–6 months after OP for ICG group according to Table 6. OP = operation.

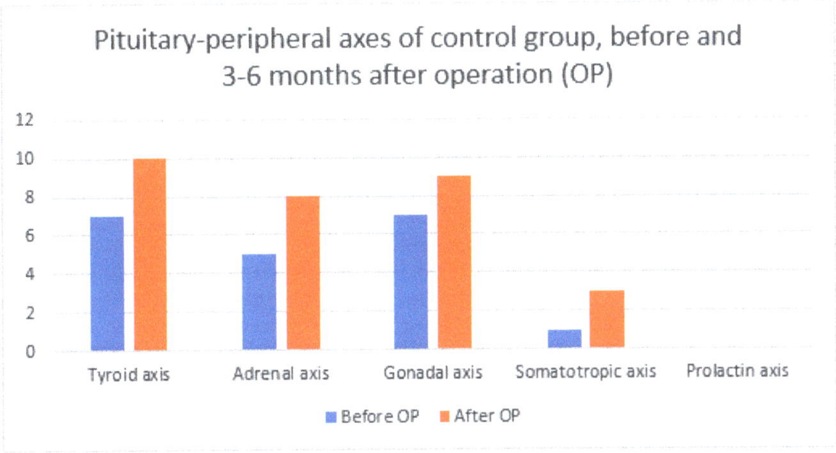

Figure 3. Pituitary–peripheral axis involvement before and 3–6 months after OP for control group according to Table 6. OP = operation.

Table 7. The impact of demographic and clinical characteristics on surgical outcome, assessed using a logistic regression model [1].

Factor	Hypopituitarism		Diabetes Insipidus	
	OR (95 % CI)	*p*	OR (95 % CI)	*p*
Age	1.04 (0.96–1.12)	0.337	1.03 (0.94–1.13)	0.518
Gender	2.86 (0.53–16.67)	0.223	2.18 (0.20–23.79)	0.522
Tumor size	1.00 (0.99–1.00)	0.101	1.00 (1.00–1.00)	0.169
Knosp	4.15 (0.96–17.86)	0.056	0.59 (0.16–2.13)	0.418
Hardy	2.48 (0.90–6.76)	0.078	0.53 (0.18–1.52)	0.235

ICG = indocyanine green dye, CI = confidence ratio, OR = odds ratio. [1] *p*-values for each factor are adjusted for the group of patients with and without ICG.

4. Discussion

The use of ICG dye in pituitary macroadenoma surgery is a relatively new technique. Some authors have already described the potential benefits of using this method [16–21]. We present the first prospective randomized trial comparing the outcomes of endoscopic endonasal transsphenoidal surgery with and without the use of ICG.

In our study, we did not find a better result of the operations with ICG dye compared to the conventional method. Litvac et al. have already shown in 2012 that ICG is a good potential marker for the pituitary gland [16]. This was confirmed in our study, as in all 17 patients who received ICG during surgery, the pituitary gland started to fluoresce after about half a minute, while the tumor tissue remained unstained. This is the so-called "early window". Jeon et al. described the concept of a late or second window [22]. If the patient receives the dye 16–30 h before surgery, it is thought that the dye is absorbed into the adenoma due to the increased permeability of the tumor microcirculation, but this was not tested in our study. Despite the fact that the pituitary gland stains better with ICG and is therefore easier to distinguish from the tumor, we did not find any statistically significant differences in postoperative outcomes between the two groups in our study. The differentiation between the adenoma and the pituitary gland is already reliable under white light. The adenoma tends to be pale grey, softer, and easier to aspirate [23,24]. Therefore, the surgical technique was not significantly different between the two groups. However, in the few cases in the control group, we encountered a piece of tissue when removing the adenoma where we were not sure whether it was healthy pituitary tissue or a tumor. In such cases, we are in a dilemma: either we remove the suspicious tissue and risk hypopituitarism or we leave it and risk a remnant or recurrence. These are the cases where the potential benefit of ICG could be demonstrated. However, as there are few such cases, the sample size would need to be much larger to collect a sufficient number of doubtful cases.

In our study, we did not find a lower incidence of diabetes insipidus with the use of ICG dye. Diabetes insipidus, which may be transient or permanent, is one of the more common complications of endoscopic transsphenoidal surgery for pituitary macroadenomas. Zhan et al. published a large study of a total of 313 patients in whom postoperative complications were observed after endoscopic surgery for nonfunctioning adenomas [25]. They observed that diabetes insipidus occurred in 15.6% in the early postoperative period, while persistent diabetes insipidus was observed in 3.8%. In our study, we observed a total of seven (20.6%) cases of early postoperative diabetes insipidus, of which three (17.6%) were in the ICG group and four (23.5%) were in the control group. Permanent diabetes insipidus was present in one (5.9%) patient in the ICG group and in four (23.5%) patients in the control group. The proportion of diabetes insipidus in the ICG group is comparable to the results of Zhan's study, but a higher proportion of patients with both transient and permanent insipidus was observed in the control group. Because Zhan et al. also included 53 (16.9%) patients with pituitary microadenomas, it is not unexpected that they obtained slightly better results. All of our patients had macroadenomas. The incidence of diabetes insipidus after endoscopic pituitary macroadenoma surgery was also studied by Kadir et al. [26]. They included 33 patients, which is almost identical to our sample size, so the results are more comparable. They described a 33.4% incidence of diabetes insipidus in the early postoperative period. Persistent diabetes insipidus was not described. In our study, as already stated above, 20.6% of patients had diabetes insipidus in the early postoperative period, of which 3/17 (17.6%) were from the ICG group and 4/17 (23.5%) were from the control group. Permanent diabetes insipidus was present in 1/17 (5.9%) patients from the ICG group and in 4/17 (23.5%) patients from the control group. Nevertheless, the statistical comparison of the samples showed no significant difference between the two groups, as shown in Table 2. We assume that a larger sample of patients could have shown a statistically significant difference. In their study of 271 patients with pituitary adenoma undergoing endoscopic surgery, Nayak et al. found that tumor size, suprasellar growth, and preoperative visual disturbances were positive predictors of the development of postoperative diabetes insipidus [27]. Our study partially confirmed this finding, as we found suprasellar tumor growth in four out of a total of five patients with persistent diabetes insipidus. Preoperative visual field loss was present in three of the five patients, but, in contrast, only one of our five patients with persistent diabetes insipidus had a tumor larger than the average of our sample.

In addition to diabetes insipidus, we also recorded the occurrence of SIADH. According to literature data, SIADH occurs in 4–23% of cases after endoscopic surgery of pituitary adenomas [28–30]. It is usually transient and resolves within a few weeks. In our study, we found three (8.8%) cases of SIADH, with two in the ICG group and one in the control group (Table 2). In all cases, it disappeared shortly after surgery. Our results regarding SIADH are therefore comparable with the literature. We could not find a statistically significant difference between the two groups, so we cannot claim that the intraoperative use of ICG leads to a better outcome regarding the occurrence of SIADH compared to the conventional method.

We also found no statistically significant difference between the two groups with regard to adenohypophysis function. In the literature, postoperative hypopituitarism has been reported in 1.4 to 19.8% [25]. In our study, the incidence of this complication was higher (Table 3). Preoperatively, the pituitary gland was functioning normally in only 14 of 34 patients (41.2%) and 3–6 months postoperatively in only 8/34 patients (23.5%). New-onset hypopituitarism was therefore noted in 6/14 patients (42.9%), 3 of whom were in the ICG group and 3 of whom were in the control group.

We were interested in the number of pituitary–peripheral axes affected (Table 4). Overall, 9/17 (52.9%) patients in the ICG group and 6/17 (35.3%) in the control group deteriorated after surgery. There is also a statistically significant difference in the number of affected axes between the two groups 3–6 months after surgery. However, upon closer analysis, we find that this statistically significant difference only means that the frequencies are differently distributed between the ICG and non-ICG groups, with the ICG group having a significantly higher proportion of cases of 0 and 3 pituitary–peripheral axis involvement, while the control group has a significantly higher proportion of 2 axis involvement. It cannot be argued that the final outcome of one group is better or worse compared to the other. When we compare the mean values of the affected axes, we see that there is no statistically significant difference between the groups (Table 6). A statistically significant difference occurs when comparing the mean number of affected axes of all patients before surgery with the mean number of affected axes after surgery. This means that our patients had a proven higher incidence of hypopituitarism 3–6 months after surgery regardless of the use of ICG. We also looked at the involvement of each pituitary–peripheral axis (Table 6). Mavromati et al. published a study in which they examined the surgical outcome of nonfunctioning pituitary macroadenomas according to the number of axes involved [31]. Patients were operated on using a combined microscopic–endoscopic approach. Of the 137 patients, 33% had no hypopituitarism preoperatively, 62.4% had hypogonadism, 41% had hypothyroidism, 30.8% had adrenal axis insufficiency, and 29.9% had growth hormone deficiency. Meanwhile, 3–6 months after surgery, 10% of patients had a new insufficiency of at least one of the pituitary–peripheral axes, 40.8% had hypogonadism, 29.3% had hypothyroidism, 27.4% had adrenal insufficiency, and 17% had growth hormone deficiency. In our study, we came to different results. The proportion of defects in the pituitary–peripheral axis before surgery is comparable, with 44.2% having hypogonadism, 44.1% with hypothyroidism, 29.4% with adrenal insufficiency, and 5.9% with growth hormone deficiency. However, 3–6 months after surgery, all of our axes showed deterioration in contrast to the study published by Mavromati et al. Postoperatively, 52.9% had hypogonadism, 55.9% had hypothyroidism, 52.9% had adrenal insufficiency, and 20.6% had growth hormone deficiency. There were no significant differences between our two groups. For each axis, approximately half of the patients were from the ICG group and the other half were from the control group.

We also investigated the influence of patient demographic and clinical characteristics on the outcomes of surgery for nonfunctioning pituitary macroadenomas, independent of the use of ICG. We were interested in hypopituitarism and diabetes insipidus as endpoints. The results are shown in Table 7. We were unable to demonstrate statistical significance in any of the parameters measured. However, borderline statistical significance ($p < 0.1$) was found in some cases. Regarding age, we cannot claim that it has an influence on the occurrence of hypopituitarism and diabetes insipidus. For gender and tumor size, we could not even detect borderline statistical significance. However, tumor size approached borderline statistical significance for postoperative hypopituitarism outcomes. For every one increase in the Knosp classification level, the probability of hypopituitarism 3–6 months after pituitary adenoma surgery increased 4.15-fold. Similarly, the probability of hypopituitarism 3–6 months after pituitary adenoma surgery increased 2.48-fold for every one increase in Hardy classification level. The Knosp and Hardy classifications showed no borderline significance for diabetes insipidus.

The main weakness of our study is the small number of patients included, which is partly due to the COVID-19 pandemic, when many patients with pituitary macroadenomas did not undergo surgery [32]. In addition, our results were affected by the initial inexperience of the surgical team in using the new equipment supporting ICG optics. We used a no-rinse endoscope, and it was often necessary to manually wipe the endoscopic camera during surgery, which disrupted the thread of the procedure. Also, when using ICG dye, the endoscope is slightly thicker than a conventional endoscope, so it provides less room for maneuvering, which can complicate the surgery. Another weakness of the study is the statistically significant higher volume of macroadenomas in the control group despite randomization in the group. We calculated the volume by measuring the largest dimensions of the tumor in the axial, sagittal, and coronal planes through magnetic resonance imaging according to the protocol for pituitary tumors, multiplied these measurements, and divided the result by half [33]. The mean volume in the ICG group was 5130 mm^3, and in the control group it was 10473 mm^3. When comparing the individual cases, we found that the largest case clearly stood out in terms of tumor size. The volume of the largest case was 34,965 mm^3, while the average volume was 7802 mm^3, which is more than four times smaller. When we excluded the largest case from the analysis, there was no longer a statistically significant difference in volume between the groups. Below are coronal images showing the largest case and a case that was closest in volume to the average value (Figure 4).

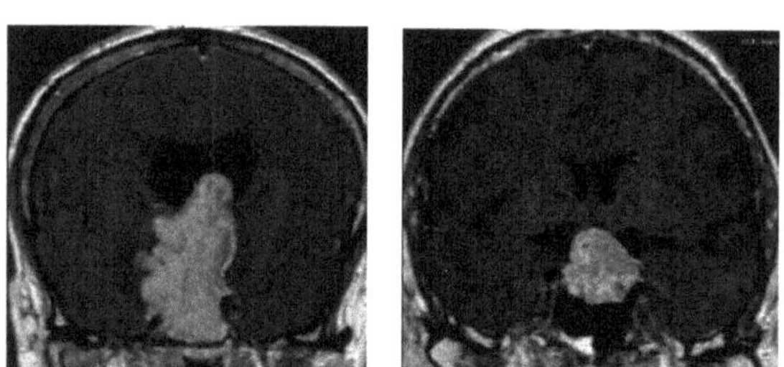

Largest case: 34,965 mm^3 Average case: 7439 mm^3

Figure 4. Coronal images showing the largest case (**left**) and average case (**right**).

The advantage of our study is that all patients were operated on by the same neurosurgeon, so there could not have been different results between the patients due to the different experience of the surgeons. Furthermore, the surgical approach and technique were always the same. All of the diagnostic laboratory and radiological measurements of the study are standard and performed in all related institutions, so the reproducibility and comparability of the study with other studies of this kind are very simple and practically perfect. It is also worth emphasizing once again that, to our knowledge, we present the first prospective, randomized study comparing conventional and fluorescence-guided endoscopic transsphenoidal surgery for pituitary macroadenomas. We hope that it will be a trigger for further research in this field.

5. Conclusions

The results of our study did not confirm that the use of ICG dye in endoscopic endonasal transsphenoidal surgery of nonfunctioning pituitary macroadenomas reduces the incidence of hypopituitarism, diabetes insipidus, or SIADH. Therefore, none of our hypotheses can be confirmed. We suggest that the benefit of ICG dye in this type of surgery could be better evaluated in prospective, randomized, and preferably multicenter trials with a larger number of patients.

Author Contributions: Conceptualization, T.F.; methodology, T.F. and T.K.; validation, T.V. and T.K.; formal analysis, T.F.; investigation, T.F.; resources, T.F. and T.K.; data curation, T.F.; writing—original draft preparation, T.F.; writing—review and editing, T.F., T.V. and T.K.; visualization, T.F.; supervision, T.V. and T.K.; project administration, T.F.; funding acquisition, T.V. All authors have read and agreed to the published version of the manuscript.

Funding: This research received no external funding.

Institutional Review Board Statement: This study was conducted in accordance with the Declaration of Helsinki and was approved by the Slovenian Medical Ethics committee (No. 0120-56/2019/6, 19 February 2019).

Informed Consent Statement: Informed consent was obtained from all subjects involved in the study.

Data Availability Statement: The raw data supporting the conclusions of this article will be made available by the authors upon request.

Acknowledgments: We are indebted to Roman Bošnjak who operated on the patients in the presented study. We also acknowledge the help of everybody else involved in the management of our patients with pituitary macroadenomas.

Conflicts of Interest: The authors declare no conflicts of interest.

References

1. Miller, K.D.; Ostrom, Q.T.; Kruchko, C.; Patil, N.; Tihan, T.; Cioffi, G.; Fuchs, H.E.; Waite, K.A.; Jemal, A.; Siegel, R.L.; et al. Brain and other central nervous system tumor statistics. *CA Cancer J. Clin.* **2021**, *71*, 381–406. [CrossRef] [PubMed]
2. Ezzat, S.; Asa, S.L.; Couldwell, W.T.; Barr, C.E.; Dodge, W.E.; Vance, M.L.; McCutcheon, I.E. The prevalence of pituitary adenomas: A systematic review. *Cancer* **2004**, *101*, 613–619. [CrossRef] [PubMed]
3. Melmed, S. Pituitary-Tumor Endocrinopathies. *N. Engl. J. Med.* **2020**, *382*, 937–950. [CrossRef] [PubMed]
4. Vandeva, S.; Vasilev, V.; Vroonen, L.; Naves, L.; Jaffrain-Rea, M.L.; Daly, A.F.; Zacharieva, S.; Beckers, A. Familial pituitary adenomas. *Ann. Endocrinol.* **2010**, *71*, 479–485. [CrossRef]
5. Tritos, N.A.; Miller, K.K. Diagnosis and Management of Pituitary Adenomas: A Review. *JAMA* **2023**, *329*, 1386–1398. [CrossRef]
6. Molitch, M.E. Diagnosis and Treatment of Pituitary Adenomas: A Review. *JAMA* **2017**, *317*, 516–524. [CrossRef]
7. Hardy, J. Transsphenoidal Neurosurgery of Intracranial Neoplasm—PubMed 1976. Available online: https://pubmed.ncbi.nlm.nih.gov/945663/ (accessed on 10 November 2023).
8. Araujo-Castro, M.; Acitores Cancela, A.; Vior, C.; Pascual-Corrales, E.; Rodríguez Berrocal, V. Radiological Knosp, Revised-Knosp, and Hardy–Wilson Classifications for the Prediction of Surgical Outcomes in the Endoscopic Endonasal Surgery of Pituitary Adenomas: Study of 228 Cases. *Front. Oncol.* **2021**, *11*, 807040. [CrossRef]
9. Knosp, E.; Steiner, E.; Kitz, K.; Matula, C. Pituitary adenomas with invasion of the cavernous sinus space: A magnetic resonance imaging classification compared with surgical findings. *Neurosurgery* **1993**, *33*, 610–618. [CrossRef] [PubMed]
10. Russ, S.; Anastasopoulou, C.; Shafiq, I. *Pituitary Adenoma. Preoperative Assessment: A Case-Based Approach*; Springer Nature: Berlin/Heidelberg, Germany, 2023; pp. 127–131.
11. Fukuhara, N.; Nishiyama, M.; Iwasaki, Y. Update in Pathogenesis, Diagnosis, and Therapy of Prolactinoma. *Cancers* **2022**, *14*, 3604. [CrossRef]
12. Messerer, M.; Cossu, G.; George, M.; Daniel, R.T. Endoscopic Endonasal Trans-sphenoidal Approach: Minimally Invasive Surgery for Pituitary Adenomas. *J. Vis. Exp.* **2018**, *2018*, 55896.
13. Jugenburg, M.; Kovacs, K.; Stefaneanu, L.; Scheithauer, B.W. Vasculature in Nontumorous Hypophyses, Pituitary Adenomas, and Carcinomas: A Quantitative Morphologic Study. *Endocr. Pathol.* **1995**, *6*, 115–124. [CrossRef] [PubMed]

14. Inoue, A.; Kohno, S.; Ohnishi, T.; Nishida, N.; Suehiro, S.; Nakamura, Y.; Matsumoto, S.; Nishikawa, M.; Ozaki, S.; Shigekawa, S.; et al. Tricks and traps of ICG endoscopy for effectively applying endoscopic transsphenoidal surgery to pituitary adenoma. *Neurosurg. Rev.* **2021**, *44*, 2133–2143. [CrossRef]
15. Reinhart, M.B.; Huntington, C.R.; Blair, L.J.; Heniford, B.T.; Augenstein, V.A. Indocyanine Green: Historical Context, Current Applications, and Future Considerations. *Surg. Innov.* **2016**, *23*, 166–175. [CrossRef] [PubMed]
16. Litvack, Z.N.; Zada, G.; Laws, E.R. Indocyanine green fluorescence endoscopy for visual differentiation of pituitary tumor from surrounding structures: Clinical article. *J. Neurosurg.* **2012**, *116*, 935–941. [CrossRef]
17. Amano, K.; Aihara, Y.; Tsuzuki, S.; Okada, Y.; Kawamata, T. Application of indocyanine green fluorescence endoscopic system in transsphenoidal surgery for pituitary tumors. *Acta Neurochir.* **2019**, *161*, 695–706. [CrossRef]
18. Vergeer, R.A.; Theunissen, R.E.; van Elk, T.; Schmidt, I.; Postma, M.R.; Tamasi, K.; van Dijk, J.M.C.; Kuijlen, J.M. Fluorescence-guided detection of pituitary neuroendocrine tumor (PitNET) tissue during endoscopic transsphenoidal surgery available agents, their potential, and technical aspects. *Rev. Endocr. Metab. Disord.* **2022**, *23*, 647–657. [CrossRef] [PubMed]
19. Catapano, G.; Sgulò, F.; Laleva, L.; Columbano, L.; Dallan, I.; de Notaris, M. Multimodal use of indocyanine green endoscopy in neurosurgery: A single-center experience and review of the literature. *Neurosurg. Rev.* **2018**, *41*, 985–998. [CrossRef]
20. Hide, T.; Yano, S.; Shinojima, N.; Kuratsu, J.I. Usefulness of the indocyanine green fluorescence endoscope in endonasal transsphenoidal surgery. *J. Neurosurg.* **2015**, *122*, 1185–1192. [CrossRef]
21. Lee, J.Y.; Cho, S.S.; Zeh, R.; Pierce, J.T.; Martinez-Lage, M.; Adappa, N.D.; Palmer, J.N.; Newman, J.G.; Learned, K.O. Folate receptor overexpression can be visualized in real time during pituitary adenoma endoscopic transsphenoidal surgery with near-infrared imaging. *J. Neurosurg.* **2018**, *129*, 390–403. [CrossRef]
22. Jeon, J.W.; Cho, S.S.; Nag, S.; Buch, L.; Pierce, J.; Su, Y.S.; Adappa, N.D.; Palmer, J.N.; Newman, J.G.; Singhal, S.; et al. Near-Infrared Optical Contrast of Skull Base Tumors During Endoscopic Endonasal Surgery. *Oper. Neurosurg.* **2019**, *17*, 32–42. [CrossRef]
23. Kamimura, K.; Nakajo, M.; Bohara, M.; Nagano, D.; Fukukura, Y.; Fujio, S.; Takajo, T.; Tabata, K.; Iwanaga, T.; Imai, H.; et al. Consistency of Pituitary Adenoma: Prediction by Pharmacokinetic Dynamic Contrast-Enhanced MRI and Comparison with Histologic Collagen Content. *Cancers* **2021**, *13*, 3914. [CrossRef]
24. Romano, A.; Coppola, V.; Lombardi, M.; Lavorato, L.; Di Stefano, D.; Caroli, E.; Rossi Espagnet, M.C.; Tavanti, F.; Minniti, G.; Trillò, G.; et al. Predictive role of dynamic contrast enhanced T1-weighted MR sequences in pre-surgical evaluation of macroadenomas consistency. *Pituitary* **2017**, *20*, 201–209. [CrossRef]
25. Zhan, R.; Ma, Z.; Wang, D.; Li, X. Pure Endoscopic Endonasal Transsphenoidal Approach for Nonfunctioning Pituitary Adenomas in the Elderly: Surgical Outcomes and Complications in 158 Patients. *World Neurosurg.* **2015**, *84*, 1572–1578. [CrossRef] [PubMed]
26. Incidence of Diabetes Insipidus in Postoperative Period among the Patients Undergoing Pituitary Tumour Surgery—PubMed. Available online: https://pubmed.ncbi.nlm.nih.gov/28919622/ (accessed on 13 May 2023).
27. Nayak, P.; Montaser, A.S.; Hu, J.; Prevedello, D.M.; Kirschner, L.S.; Ghalib, L. Predictors of Postoperative Diabetes Insipidus Following Endoscopic Resection of Pituitary Adenomas. *J. Endocr. Soc.* **2018**, *2*, 1010. [CrossRef] [PubMed]
28. Zoli, M.; Mazzatenta, D.; Faustini-Fustini, M. Transient Delayed Hyponatremia after Transsphenoidal Surgery: Attempting to Enlighten the Epidemiology and Management of a Still-Obscure Complication. *World Neurosurg.* **2016**, *90*, 654–656. [CrossRef]
29. Patel, K.S.; Chen, J.S.; Yuan, F.; Attiah, M.; Wilson, B.; Wang, M.B.; Bergsneider, M.; Kim, W. Prediction of post-operative delayed hyponatremia after endoscopic transsphenoidal surgery. *Clin. Neurol. Neurosurg.* **2019**, *182*, 87–91. [CrossRef] [PubMed]
30. Sorba, E.L.; Staartjes, V.E.; Voglis, S.; Tosic, L.; Brandi, G.; Tschopp, O.; Serra, C.; Regli, L. Diabetes insipidus and syndrome of inappropriate antidiuresis (SIADH) after pituitary surgery: Incidence and risk factors. *Neurosurg. Rev.* **2021**, *44*, 1503–1511. [CrossRef]
31. Mavromati, M.; Mavrakanas, T.; Jornayvaz, F.R.; Schaller, K.; Fitsiori, A.; Vargas, M.I.; Lobrinus, J.A.; Merkler, D.; Egervari, K.; Philippe, J.; et al. The impact of transsphenoidal surgery on pituitary function in patients with non-functioning macroadenomas. *Endocrine* **2023**, *81*, 340–348. [CrossRef]
32. Munda, M.; Velnar, T.; Bosnjak, R.; Zele, T.; Gradisnik, L.; Spazzapan, P.; Kos, N.; Kocivnik, N.; Benedicic, M.; Prestor, B. COVID-19 and Surgical Practice in Slovenia: Managing the Crisis in Neurosurgery during the COVID-19 Pandemic. *Life* **2023**, *13*, 2095. [CrossRef]
33. Lundin, P.; Pedersen, F. Volume of pituitary macroadenomas: Assessment by MRI. *J. Comput. Assist. Tomogr.* **1992**, *16*, 519–528. [CrossRef]

diagnostics

MDPI

Article

The Impact of Magnetic Resonance Imaging Findings in Predicting Neurological Status Pre- and Post-Treatment of Spinal Dural Arteriovenous Fistulas: A 22-Year Experience in a Neurovascular and Spine Center

Andreas Filis [1,†], Kay Engellandt [2,†], Sergio M. F. Romualdo [1], Ibrahim El-Battrawy [3], Dino Podlesek [1], Tareq A. Juratli [1], Ilker Y. Eyüpoglu [1] and Mido Max Hijazi [1,*]

1 Department of Neurosurgery, Technische Universität Dresden, Faculty of Medicine, and University Hospital Carl Gustav Carus, Fetscherstrasse 74, 01307 Dresden, Germany; afilis@neuromaster.gr (A.F.); sergiomiguelfernandes.romualdo@ukdd.de (S.M.F.R.); dino.podlesek@ukdd.de (D.P.); tareq.juratli@ukdd.de (T.A.J.); ilker.eyuepoglu@ukdd.de (I.Y.E.)

2 Institute of Diagnostic and Interventional Neuroradiology, Technische Universität Dresden, Faculty of Medicine, and University Hospital Carl Gustav Carus, Fetscherstrasse 74, 01307 Dresden, Germany; kay.engellandt@ukdd.de

3 Department of Cardiology, Bergmannsheil University Hospitals, Ruhr University Bochum, Bürkle de la Camp-Platz 1, 44789 Bochum, Germany; ibrahim.elbattrawy2006@gmail.com

* Correspondence: mido.hijazi@ukdd.de; Tel.: +49-1799847820

† These authors contributed equally to this work.

Abstract: Background: Successful treatment of spinal dural arteriovenous fistulas (SDAVF) requires prompt diagnosis with definitive fistula localization and non-delayed treatment. Magnetic resonance imaging (MRI) is used for the screening and follow-up of SDAVF, although the value of MRI signs such as myelopathy and flow voids is controversial. Therefore, we investigated the predictive value of MRI signs pre- and post-treatment and their correlation with the neurological status of SDAVF patients. Methods: We retrospectively analyzed the clinical records of 81 patients who underwent surgical or endovascular treatment for SDAVF at our hospital between 2002 and 2023. A total of 41 SDAVF patients with follow-up MRI of 4.6 [2.9–6.5] months (median [interquartile range]) post-treatment and clinical follow-up of 3, 6, and 12 months were included. Results: The extent of pretreatment myelopathy was seven [6–8] vertebral levels, with follow-up MRI showing no myelopathy in 70.7% of cases. The pretreatment flow voids extended over seven [4.5–10] vertebral levels and completely disappeared on follow-up MRI in 100% of cases. The modified Aminoff–Logue scale of disability (mALS) was four [2–7] pretreatment and two [0–4.5] at the third follow-up, with improvement in 65.9% of patients. The American Spinal Injury Association motor score (ASIA-MS) was 97 [88–100] pretreatment and 100 [95–100] at the third follow-up assessment, with 78% of patients improving. Pretreatment ASIA-MS correlated with the extent of myelopathy at admission (R^2: 0.179; 95% CI: −0.185, −0.033; $p = 0.006$) but not with flow voids at admission, while pretreatment mALS showed no correlation with either MRI signs. The improvement in ASIA-MS and mALS between admission and the last follow-up showed no correlation with the extent of pretreatment myelopathy and flow voids or with pos-treatment MRI changes. The diagnostic sensitivity of magnetic resonance angiography (MRA) for localization of the fistula was 68.3% (28/41). Conclusions: The severity of the clinical condition in SDAVF patients has a multifactorial cause, whereby the ASIA-MS correlates with the extent of myelopathy pretreatment. MRI changes after treatment showed no correlation with the clinical outcome and cannot be used as a prognostic factor.

Keywords: SDAVF; spinal arteriovenous fistula; myelopathy; endovascular treatment; surgical treatment; spinal cord edema; spinal angiography

1. Introduction

Spinal dural arteriovenous fistula (SDAVF) results from a spinal anomalous connection between radiculomeningeal arteries and radicular veins, leading to venous hypertension and myelopathy [1–7]. Diagnosis is often delayed and made after misdiagnosis has led to unnecessary invasive procedures or inadequate treatment [5,6,8]. Magnetic resonance imaging (MRI) is used for screening and follow-up of SDAVF, although digital subtraction angiography (DSA) remains the gold-standard diagnostic procedure and is needed to identify the spinal location of the fistula and confirm the diagnosis [9,10]. Treatment consists of surgical or endovascular closure of the fistula, with surgery being the treatment of choice [11–13].

A combination of gait disturbances, lower limb weakness, back pain, sensory disturbances (paresthesia, hypesthesia, anesthesia, or hyperesthesia), and bowel and bladder dysfunction characterizes the clinical manifestations of SDAVF [10]. The onset of these symptoms is progressive, with a gradual deterioration over a period of 6 months to 2 years, although rapid deterioration has also been reported [14]. The aim of treatment is to interrupt the fistulous arterial and venous points [15–19].

Prompt diagnosis with definitive localization of the fistula and timely treatment are required for clinical improvement in SDAVF patients [20–25]. The association between MRI signs such as myelopathy and flow voids on pre- and post-treatment MRIs on the one hand and the clinical condition and outcome of the SDAVF patient on the other remains unclear [26]. Some previous studies have reported that the extent of myelopathy and flow voids on pretreatment MRI reflects the severity of neurological dysfunction at admission [27,28]. Other studies claim the opposite [29,30]. Few studies have addressed the value of post-treatment MRI for the clinical outcome of SDAVF [26]. In the present study, we used a retrospective design to evaluate the predictive value of pre- and post-treatment MRI signs in patients with SDAVF after successful treatment.

2. Materials and Methods

2.1. Study Design and Patient Data

2.1.1. Study Design

We conducted a retrospective analysis of patients with SDAVF who underwent surgery or endovascular treatment at our endovascular and spine center between 2002 and 2023. Patients with suspected SDAVF on MRI (vascular myelopathy and flow voids), corresponding symptoms (gait dysfunction, sensory disturbances, motor deficits, bowel and bladder dysfunction, or back pain), and evidence of SDAVF on spinal DSA were included in the study. A total of 81 patients with SDAVF were identified, of whom 65 underwent follow-up MRI after surgical or endovascular occlusion of SDAVF. Follow-up MRI was only performed in 44 patients between three weeks and one year, with 3 patients presenting documented findings, but the images were no longer available in the picture archiving and communication system (PACS). A total of 41 patients with a successfully treated SDAVF and available follow-up MRI images between three weeks and one year were included (Figure 1). Patients without evidence of SDAVF or follow-up MRI within the first three weeks or after one year were excluded.

2.1.2. Patient Data and Institutional Review Board

The local ethics committee of the University Hospital Carl Gustav Carus in Dresden reviewed and approved our study (Ref: BO-EK-437102023). Patient data were collected via the ORBIS system (ORBIS, Dedalus, Bonn, Germany) and imaging examinations via the local PACS system (IMPAX, Impax Asset Management Group plc, London, UK). Spinal MRI, magnetic resonance angiography (MRA), and DSA were available in the IMPAX for review and assessment.

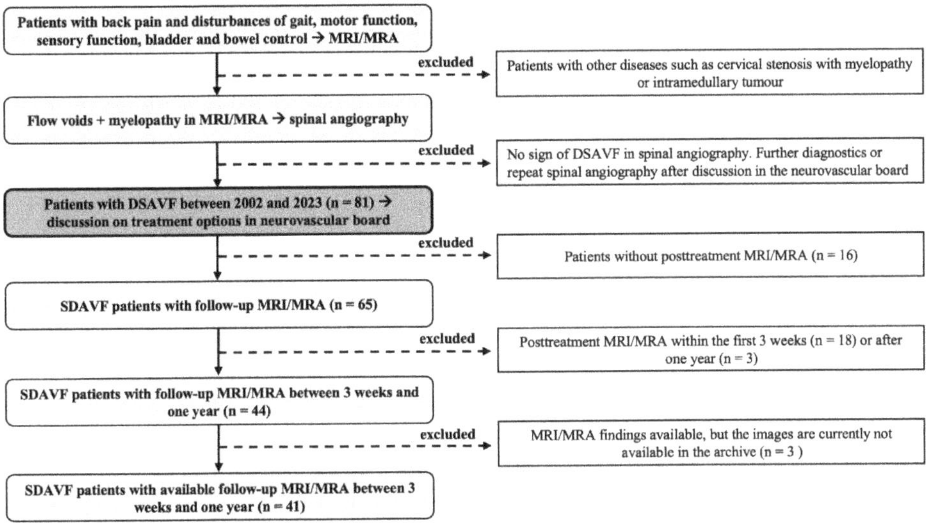

Figure 1. Study design: This figure shows our study design. MRI: magnetic resonance imaging; MRA: magnetic resonance angiography; DSA: digital subtraction angiography.

The following data were collected from the electronic medical records: age; gender; time from symptoms to MRI diagnosis; time from MRI diagnosis to surgery or embolization; history of comorbidities (vascular disease, coronary artery disease, stroke, hypertension, degenerative spine disease, bleeding medications, corticosteroid use and body mass index (BMI)); pre- or post-treatment MRI/MRA/DSA; number of incomplete or failed closures; number of secondary treatments performed (surgical or endovascular); complications related to treatment or hospitalization; side of fistula; location of fistula; first symptom; neurological status pretreatment, at the time of discharge, at first follow-up (3 months after treatment), at second follow-up (6 months after treatment), and at third follow-up (12 months after treatment); the American Spinal Injury Association motor score (ASIA-MS); and the modified Aminoff–Logue scale of disability (mALS).

2.2. Clinical Management

Clinical symptoms such as back pain and gait, sensory, motor, bowel, or bladder dysfunction, in conjunction with myelopathy and flow voids on MRI/MRA, are the basis for the diagnosis of SDAVF. Each case was discussed on a multidisciplinary board with neurointerventional radiologists and neurosurgeons, and the diagnosis was confirmed by spinal DSA. If two therapeutic options were considered, the patient was usually informed and educated about both treatment options, and the decision about the procedure was left to the patient. Endovascular treatment was preferred as a less invasive procedure in our hospital until around 2012. At that time, surgical treatment was suggested if endovascular treatment failed or was not feasible (vertebral artery or Adamkiewicz proximity with unintended risk of embolism). Since around 2012, surgical treatment has been the treatment of choice in our hospital, and endovascular therapy has been considered as an alternative.

In all cases, DSA and MRI/MRA were carefully reviewed by the neurosurgeon and a neurointerventional radiologist prior to treatment to determine the exact location and side of the fistula. Post-treatment spinal DSA and MRA/MRA were always performed after endovascular treatment. In most cases, a DSA and/or MRI/MRA were performed within the first three days after surgical treatment to assess fistula closure and any post-treatment complications. At 3, 6, and 12 months after surgical or endovascular treatment, an MRI/MRA was recommended to assess the disappearance of myelopathy and the regression of abnormal flow voids.

2.3. Illustrative Case

A 54-year-old woman presented with a one-month history of progressive gait disturbance, bowel and bladder dysfunction, and saddle anesthesia. The possible walking distance without a break was 200 m. There was also a slight paresis of the hip flexor and big toe extensor on the right side (ASIA-MS: 98, mALS: 6). The patient was admitted to the hospital by her general practitioner. On the day of admission, we performed a spinal MRI/MRA and DSA, which showed a DSAVF at the Th12/L1 level on the right. On the same day, the patient developed a rapidly progressing high-grade paraparesis with complete urinary and fecal incontinence (ASIA-MS: 70, mALS: 11). Emergency surgical treatment was performed via hemilaminectomy and closure of the right Th12 SDAVF without complications. Post-treatment DSA showed complete obliteration of the fistula, and MRI revealed no further flow voids and a reduction in myelopathy. The patient could be mobilized on the ward floor. After 2 months, the patient presented to the emergency room without motor deficits (ASIA-MS 100) but with a renewed deterioration of gait (gait score in mALS: 2) and persistent saddle anesthesia and leg paresthesia. The MRI showed further regression of the myelopathy and no signs of SDAVF recurrence. The gait disturbance improved spontaneously, and the patient was discharged home. At the second follow-up assessment (after 6 months), the MRI showed no myelopathy, but the patient still had a gait disturbance. A return to work was no longer possible. This case is the only one from our center with a rapid deterioration within one day, which we do not know in this form for this disease (Figures 2 and 3).

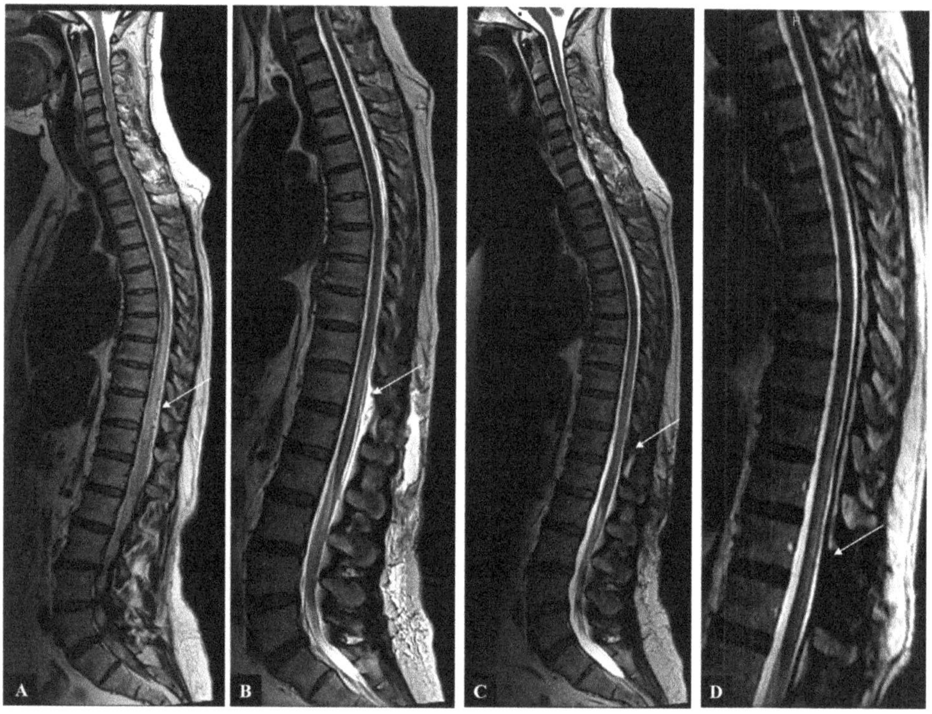

Figure 2. Case illustration: Sagittal T2-weighted MR image shows (**A**) preoperative spinal cord edema and flow voids (yellow arrow), (**B**) decrease in spinal cord edema and disappearance of flow voids immediately after operation (yellow arrow), (**C**) further decrease in spinal cord edema two months after operation (yellow arrow), (**D**) no myelopathy and no flow voids six months after operation (yellow arrow).

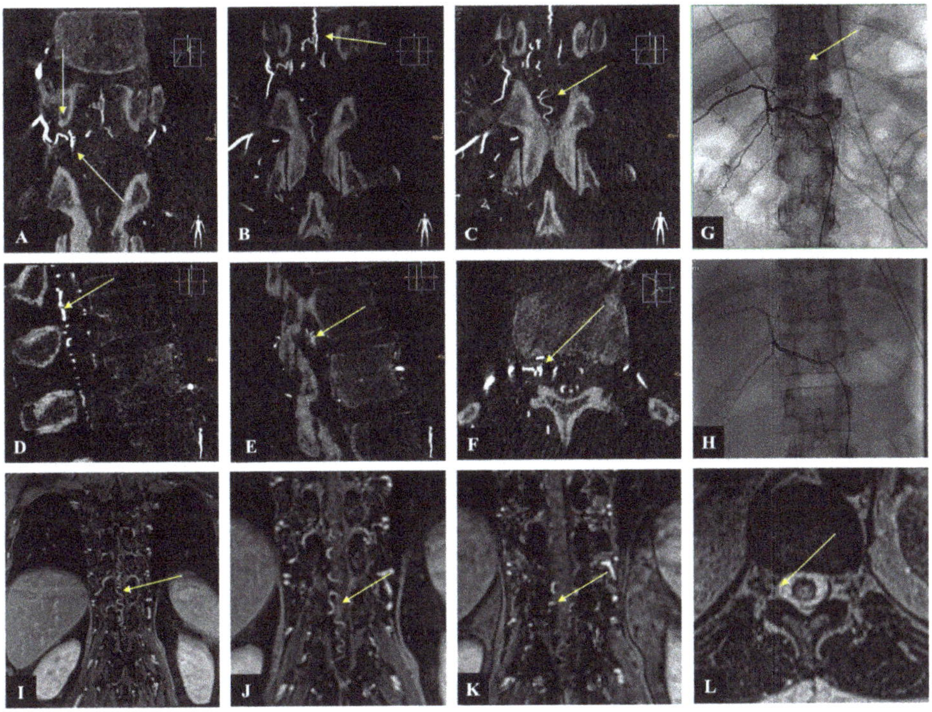

Figure 3. Case illustration: The images of three-dimensionally reconstructed digital subtraction angiography (DSA) of the spine ((**A–C**): coronary, (**D**,**E**): sagittal, and (**F**): axial) show the fistula location at the level of Th 12 on the right side as well as the flow voids (yellow arrows). Image (**G**) shows the preoperative SDAVF in conventional DSA with flow voids (yellow arrow), and image (**H**) demonstrates the postoperative absence of the SDAVF. The magnetic resonance angiography images ((**I–K**): coronary and (**L**): axial) show the fistulous point at the level of Th 12 on the right side as well as the flow voids (yellow arrow).

2.4. Statistical Analysis

Statistical analysis of the data was performed using the SPSS software package (SPSS Statistics 29, IBM, Armonk, New York, NY, USA). Descriptive statistics were used, and categorical variables were tested by Fisher exact tests or chi-square tests. Numerical variables were analyzed with Mann–Whitney U tests. All statistical tests were two-sided, and a p value < 0.05 was considered statistically significant.

A linear regression analysis was performed to evaluate the correlation between the extent of myelopathy and flow voids before treatment on the one hand and pretreatment mALS and ASIA-MS, post-treatment mALS and ASIA-MS, and improvement in mALS and ASIA-MS on the other hand. In addition, a binary logistic regression analysis was performed to determine the correlation between the improvement in myelopathy and flow voids at follow-up MRI and the improvement in mALS and ASIA-MS at the last follow-up.

3. Results

3.1. Patient Characteristics

Our study population consisted of 11 women (26.8%) and 30 men (73.2%) with an age of 65.9 [54.5–73.5] years (median [interquartile range]). The duration from symptoms to MRI diagnosis was 7 [2.5–24] months, and the time from suspected MRI diagnosis to surgical or endovascular treatment was 15 [9–34.5] days (Table 1).

Table 1. Baseline characteristics.

Variable	Value
Age, median [IQR]	65.9 [54.5–73.5] y
Female gender, *n* (%)	11 (26.8%)
Time from symptom to MRI diagnosis, median [IQR]	7 [2.5–24] m
Time from MRI diagnosis to treatment, median [IQR]	15 [9–34.5] d
Myelopathy extension at admission on MRI, median [IQR]	7 [6–8] v
Absence of myelopathy on FU MRI, *n* (%)	29 (70.7%)
Flow void extension at admission on MRI, median [IQR]	7 [4.5–10] v
Absence of flow voids on FU MRI, *n* (%)	41 (100%)
mALS at admission, median [IQR]	4 [2–7]
mALS at third FU, median [IQR]	2 [0–4.5]
ASIA-MS at admission, median [IQR]	97 [88–100]
ASIA-MS at third FU, median [IQR]	100 [95–100]
Interval between treatment and FU MRI, median [IQR]	4.6 [2.9–6.5] m
Fistulous point:	
Cervical, *n* (%)	3 (7.3%)
Upper thoracic, *n* (%)	7 (17.1%)
Lower thoracic, *n* (%)	17 (41.5%)
Lumbar, *n* (%)	12 (29.2%)
Sacral, *n* (%)	2 (4.9%)
Side of fistula, *n*	R: 22, L: 18, B: 1
Incomplete or failed occlusion, *n* (%)	2 (4.9%)
Treatment- or hospital-related complications, *n* (%)	6 (14.6%)
Improvement in mALS between admission and last FU, *n* (%)	27 (65.9%)
Improvement in ASIA-MS between admission and last FU, *n* (%)	32 (78%)
Diagnostic sensitivity of MRA to locate the fistula, *n* (%)	28 (68.3%)
Surgery vs. embolization, *n* (%)	36 (87.8%) vs. 5 (12.2%)
BMI	27.5 [24.9–30.3] kg/m^2

IQR: interquartile range; MRI: magnetic resonance imaging; MRA: magnetic resonance angiography; *n*: number; y: year; m: month; d: day; v: vertebral body; mALS: modified Aminoff–Logue scale of disability; ASIA-MS: American Spinal Injury Association motor score; FU: follow-up; BMI: body mass index; R: right; L: left; B: both.

The extent of myelopathy at admission was seven [6–8] vertebral levels, and in 70.7% of patients (*n*: 29), there was no evidence of myelopathy on follow-up MRI. The interval between treatment and follow-up MRI was 4.6 [2.9–6.5] months. The flow voids at admission were extended along seven [4.5–10] vertebral levels and were 100% completely absent on follow-up MRI (median 4.6 months).

The mALS score at admission was 4 [2–7] and 2 [0–4.5] at the third follow-up, with an improvement in mALS between admission and the last follow-up observed in 65.9% of patients (*n*: 27). The ASIA-MS at admission was 97 [88–100] and 100 [95–100] at the third follow-up, with an improvement in ASIA-MS between admission and the last follow-up seen in 32 patients (78%).

The majority of fistulas were located in the lower thoracic (17, 41.5%), followed by the lumbar (12, 29.2%), upper thoracic (7, 17.1%), cervical (3, 7.3%), and sacral (2, 4.9%). There were 18 left fistulas, 22 right fistulas, and 1 bilateral fistula. Two patients (4.9%) had an initial incomplete or failed occlusion, which was then occluded definitively with a second procedure.

Treatment- or hospital-related complications were reported in 14.6% of patients (*n*: 6). The diagnostic sensitivity of MRA to locate the fistula was 68.3% (*n*: 28). Surgery was performed in 36 patients (87.8%) and embolization in 5 patients (12.2%). The BMI was 27.5 [24.9–30.3] kg/m^2.

3.2. Myelopathy and Flow Voids

We used simple linear regression analysis to identify the correlation between the extent of myelopathy at admission on the one hand and clinical symptoms before treatment and one year after treatment using ASIA-MS and mALS on the other. A correlation was only observed between ASIA-MS and the extent of myelopathy (R2: 0.179; 95% CI: −0.185, −0.033; $p = 0.006$, Table 2). The improvement in ASIA-MS and mALS between admission and the last follow-up showed no correlation with the extent of myelopathy. The extent of flow voids showed no correlation to the clinical features or outcomes of SDAVF.

Table 2. Correlation between MRI signs and clinical features and outcomes of SDAVF patients.

Associated Variable	Simple Linear Regression					
	B	(95% CI)	SE	β	R^2	*p*
Extent of pre. myelopathy						
Pre. ASIA-MS	−0.109	−0.185, −0.033	0.037	−0.423	0.179	**0.006**
Third FU ASIA-MS	−0.058	−0.187, 0.071	0.062	−0.212	0.045	0.357
Improved ASIA-MS	0.410	−2.072, 2.892	1.227	0.053	0.003	0.740
Pre. mALS	0.319	−0.002, 0.641	0.159	0.306	0.094	0.052
Third FU mALS	0.331	−0.172, 0.834	0.240	0.302	0.091	0.184
Improved mALS	−0.503	−2.666, 1.661	1.070	−0.075	0.006	0.641
Extent of pre. Flow voids						
Pre. ASIA-MS	−0.075	−0.168, 0.018	0.046	−0.251	0.063	0.113
Third FU ASIA-MS	−0.003	−0.140, 0.134	0.065	−0.012	0.000	0.960
Improved ASIA-MS	−0.375	−3.229, 2.479	1.411	−0.430	0.002	0.792
Pre. mALS	0.195	−0.189, 0.578	0.189	0.162	0.026	0.311
Third FU mALS	0.117	−0.429, 0.662	0.261	0.102	0.010	0.660
Improved mALS	−0.011	−2.504, 2.483	1.233	−0.001	0.000	0.993

B: unstandardized coefficient, CI: confidence interval; SE: standard error; β: standardized coefficient; R^2: coefficient of determination; Pre.: pretreatment; mALS: modified Aminoff–Logue scale of disability; ASIA-MS: American Spinal Injury Association motor score; FU: follow-up. Bold values are significant results ($p < 0.05$) as indicated in the methods.

3.3. *Improvement in mALS and ASIA-MS*

Using binary logistic regression, no correlation was found between the absence of myelopathy in the follow-up MRI and the improvement in mALS or ASIA-MS in the last follow-up (Table 3). The analysis of a correlation between flow voids on follow-up MRI and the improvement in mALS or ASIA-MS in the last follow-up could not be performed as all patients had no flow voids in the follow-up MRI.

Table 3. Correlation between the absence of myelopathy on MRI and clinical improvement.

Associated Variable	Binary Logistic Regression	
	OR (95% CI)	*p* Value
Absence of myelopathy on FU MRI		
Improved mALS in the last FU	0.630 (0.157–2.533)	0.515
Improved ASIA-MS in the last FU	4.190 (0.463–37.938)	0.202

OR: odds ratio; CI: confidence interval; MRI: magnetic resonance imaging; mALS: modified Aminoff–Logue scale of disability; ASIA-MS: American Spinal Injury Association motor score; FU: follow-up.

4. Discussion

The main finding of our study and from our more than 20 years of monocentric experience with SDAVF showed that the extent of myelopathy on MRI at admission was related to patients' motor deficits but not to overall clinical conditions, such as gait, urination, and defecation function. In contrast, follow-up MRI changes showed no correlation with clinical outcome and cannot be used as a prognostic factor.

Our study population was predominantly men (three men to one woman) in the six decades of life, as reported in previous studies [10]. In our cohort, the diagnosis of SDAVF was delayed by a median of 7 months, and it took a median of 15 days before endovascular or surgical treatment was performed. The interval between treatment and follow-up MRI was 4.6 months. MRI was performed at the first follow-up (3 months) in some patients and at the second follow-up (6 months) in others, so there was no consistent performance of MRI for evaluation. Patients who received an MRI during their stay or after one year were excluded from the study due to standardization.

The extent of myelopathy on MRI at admission in our cohort was seven vertebral levels long. Shin et al. reported a 5.2 vertebral level average length of myelopathy in their cohort of 15 patients [9]. Luo et al. considered the length of myelopathy over five vertebral bodies as an indicator of severe neurological dysfunction and found a correlation with clinical outcome [26]. From our point of view, it is difficult to determine at what length of myelopathy severe neurological deficits are to be expected. Various factors are involved, such as the localization of the myelopathy in the spinal cord (cervical and conus) and the degree of spinal stenosis due to the flow voids. The absence of myelopathy on follow-up MRI was found in 70% of our patients, as in an earlier study (73%, 4/15 patients) [9]. The extent of flow voids in our study was similar to myelopathy and was seven vertebral levels long, supporting the pathophysiology of myelopathy based on venous hypertension. No flow voids were seen on follow-up MRIs in all patients. If these persist, incomplete or failed fistula closure is conceivable.

Our cohort has shown that almost half of SDAVFs are localized in the lower thoracic spine, and there is no side preference, although some studies claim that the pathology occurs predominantly on the left side [31,32]. The diagnostic sensitivity of MRA for the fistula location has not yet been investigated. We compared the results of the MRA examination before DSA with the DSA result for the fistula location and found a diagnostic sensitivity of 68.3% (28/41) for the fistula location and side. This is an unsatisfactory result overall but offers good sensitivity for a non-invasive and radiation-free examination and should be used to reduce the radiation exposure of angiography beforehand.

In our cohort, the mALS was 4 at admission and improved to 2 at the third follow-up. Overall, 65.9% of patients had an improvement in mALS between admission and the last follow-up. The mALS values are consistent with previous studies and showed the main improvement between admission and hospital discharge [6,9,26]. In course, even after one year, there was only a slight improvement in the mALS values. The median ASIA-MS was 97 at admission and 100 at the third follow-up, with overall improvement between admission and the last follow-up in 78% of patients. To our knowledge, the use of ASIA-MS in SDAVF has not yet been performed. The reason we have used this detailed score is because mALS does not provide conclusive information about the motor deficits that we have observed more frequently in severe myelopathy. The regression analysis in our study showed a significant correlation between ASIA-MS and the extent of myelopathy on MRI at admission, confirming our clinical hypothesis.

In our study, we could not confirm the discussed correlation of MRI signs (myelopathy and flow voids) with mALS at admission and the correlation of their change on follow-up MRI with the clinical outcome. Therefore, we agree with the prevailing opinion that the change in the follow-up MRI does not allow any conclusions to be drawn about the clinical condition of the patients.

A post-treatment DSA is the method of choice to confirm the closure of the fistula. An MRI examination remains optional as long as the patient shows clinical improvement. The flow voids usually disappear after approximately one week. A reduction in myelopathy can be observed after one week, and a complete disappearance can be seen after three months, which shows no clinical correlation. We recommend postoperative DSA and MRI examinations in 3 months. If the clinical symptoms worsen or persist, we recommend prompt MRI control.

Limitations and Strengths of This Study

The monocentric, retrospective nature of our analysis, the long inclusion interval, and the limited number of SDAVF patients (41 patients) might reduce the external validity of our study. Furthermore, our analysis could be affected by a possible selection bias due to our treatment flow charts, as our experience has been to favor surgery over embolization.

Nevertheless, our cohort analysis is based on a 20-year treatment period of SDAVF in a large university neurosurgery center, suggesting a high internal validity of our study. The clinical follow-up and the follow-up MRI examination were not performed at the same time. Therefore, our observations may be useful to understand the clinical and radiologic characteristics of SDAVF.

5. Conclusions

SDAVF is a rare but well-treatable disease in which mALS and ASIA-MS improve over the disease course. Although MRI forms the basis for the diagnosis of SDAVF, it does not provide sufficient diagnostic sensitivity for the localization of the fistula. It offers a good non-invasive and radiation-free option for narrowing down the potential localization in advance and should be used to reduce the radiation exposure of angiography.

The severity of the clinical condition of SDAVF patients has a multifactorial reason, whereby the motor deficits correlate with the extent of the myelopathy. MRI changes at follow-up showed no correlation with the clinical outcome and cannot be used as a prognostic factor.

Author Contributions: K.E., A.F. and M.M.H.: conceptualization, methodology, validation, formal analysis, writing—original draft preparation, visualization, and supervision. I.Y.E., T.A.J., D.P., I.E.-B. and S.M.F.R.: writing—review and editing. All authors have read and agreed to the published version of the manuscript.

Funding: The Article Processing Charges (APC) were funded by the Open Access Publication Fund of the SLUB/TU Dresden. The SLUB/TU Dresden was neither involved in the drafting of this study nor in the decision to publish it.

Institutional Review Board Statement: This study was conducted in accordance with the Declaration of Helsinki and approved by the Institutional Review Board of the local ethics committee at the University Hospital Dresden (protocol code: BO-EK-437102023, January 2023).

Informed Consent Statement: Patient consent was waived due to the retrospective, anonymous nature of this study.

Data Availability Statement: The original contributions presented in this study are included in the article. Further inquiries can be directed to the corresponding author.

Acknowledgments: We would like to thank Silke Hennig for her support.

Conflicts of Interest: The authors declare no conflicts of interest.

References

1. Aminoff, M.J.; Logue, V. Clinical features of spinal vascular malformations. *Brain* **1974**, *97*, 197–210. [CrossRef]
2. Aminoff, M.J.; Barnard, R.O.; Logue, V. The pathophysiology of spinal vascular malformations. *J. Neurol. Sci.* **1974**, *23*, 255–263. [CrossRef]
3. Hurst, R.W.; Kenyon, L.C.; Lavi, E.; Raps, E.C.; Marcotte, P. Spinal dural arteriovenous fistula: The pathology of venous hypertensive myelopathy. *Neurology* **1995**, *45*, 1309–1313. [CrossRef]
4. Narvid, J.; Hetts, S.W.; Larsen, D.; Neuhaus, J.; Singh, T.P.; McSwain, H.; Lawton, M.T.; Dowd, C.F.; Higashida, R.T.; Halbach, V.V. Spinal dural arteriovenous fistulae: Clinical features and long-term results. *Neurosurgery* **2008**, *62*, 159–166; discussion 166–167. [CrossRef]
5. Muralidharan, R.; Saladino, A.; Lanzino, G.; Atkinson, J.L.; Rabinstein, A.A. The clinical and radiological presentation of spinal dural arteriovenous fistula. *Spine* **2011**, *36*, E1641–E1647. [CrossRef]
6. Muralidharan, R.; Mandrekar, J.; Lanzino, G.; Atkinson, J.L.; Rabinstein, A.A. Prognostic value of clinical and radiological signs in the postoperative outcome of spinal dural arteriovenous fistula. *Spine* **2013**, *38*, 1188–1193. [CrossRef]
7. Klopper, H.B.; Surdell, D.L.; Thorell, W.E. Type I spinal dural arteriovenous fistulas: Historical review and illustrative case. *Neurosurg. Focus* **2009**, *26*, E3. [CrossRef] [PubMed]
8. Jellema, K.; Tijssen, C.C.; van Gijn, J. Spinal dural arteriovenous fistulas: A congestive myelopathy that initially mimics a peripheral nerve disorder. *Brain* **2006**, *129*, 3150–3164. [CrossRef]
9. Shin, D.A.; Park, K.Y.; Ji, G.Y.; Yi, S.; Ha, Y.; Park, S.W.; Yoon, D.H.; Kim, K.N. The use of magnetic resonance imaging in predicting the clinical outcome of spinal arteriovenous fistula. *Yonsei Med. J.* **2015**, *56*, 397–402. [CrossRef]

10. Marcus, J.; Schwarz, J.; Singh, I.P.; Sigounas, D.; Knopman, J.; Gobin, Y.P.; Patsalides, A. Spinal dural arteriovenous fistulas: A review. *Curr. Atheroscler. Rep.* **2013**, *15*, 335. [CrossRef]
11. Bretonnier, M.; Henaux, P.L.; Gaberel, T.; Roualdes, V.; Kerdiles, G.; Le Reste, P.J.; Morandi, X. Spinal Dural Arteriovenous Fistulas: Clinical Outcome After Surgery Versus Embolization: A Retrospective Study. *World Neurosurg.* **2019**, *127*, e943–e949. [CrossRef]
12. Cesak, T.; Adamkov, J.; Poczos, P.; Kanta, M.; Krajina, A.; Krajickova, D.; Herzig, R.; Valis, M. Multidisciplinary approach in the treatment of spinal dural arteriovenous fistula-results of endovascular and surgical treatment. *Acta Neurochir.* **2018**, *160*, 2439–2448. [CrossRef]
13. Bakker, N.A.; Uyttenboogaart, M.; Luijckx, G.J.; Eshghi, O.S.; Mazuri, A.; Metzemaekers, J.D.; Groen, R.J.; Van Dijk, J.M. Recurrence Rates After Surgical or Endovascular Treatment of Spinal Dural Arteriovenous Fistulas: A Meta-analysis. *Neurosurgery* **2015**, *77*, 137–144; discussion 144. [CrossRef]
14. Willinsky, R.; TerBrugge, K.; Lasjaunias, P.; Montanera, W. The variable presentations of craniocervical and cervical dural arteriovenous malformations. *Surg. Neurol.* **1990**, *34*, 118–123. [CrossRef]
15. Brinjikji, W.; Colombo, E.; Cloft, H.J.; Lanzino, G. Clinical and Imaging Characteristics of Spinal Dural Arteriovenous Fistulas and Spinal Epidural Arteriovenous Fistulas. *Neurosurgery* **2021**, *88*, 666–673. [CrossRef]
16. Oh, Y.; Heo, Y.; Jeon, S.R.; Roh, S.W.; Park, J.H. Microsurgery Versus Endovascular Treatment—Which Is Adequate for Initial Treatment of Spinal Dural Arteriovenous Fistula: A Case Series. *Neurospine* **2021**, *18*, 344–354. [CrossRef]
17. Acerbi, F.; Ferroli, P. Surgery versus embolization in spinal dural arteriovenous fistulas: The ideal competition to improve the care of patients. *World Neurosurg.* **2013**, *80*, e191–e193. [CrossRef]
18. Kirsch, M.; Berg-Dammer, E.; Musahl, C.; Bazner, H.; Kuhne, D.; Henkes, H. Endovascular management of spinal dural arteriovenous fistulas in 78 patients. *Neuroradiology* **2013**, *55*, 337–343. [CrossRef]
19. Krings, T.; Geibprasert, S. Spinal dural arteriovenous fistulas. *AJNR Am. J. Neuroradiol.* **2009**, *30*, 639–648. [CrossRef]
20. Tacconi, L.; Lopez Izquierdo, B.C.; Symon, L. Outcome and prognostic factors in the surgical treatment of spinal dural arteriovenous fistulas. A long-term study. *Br. J. Neurosurg.* **1997**, *11*, 298–305. [CrossRef]
21. Ushikoshi, S.; Hida, K.; Kikuchi, Y.; Miyasaka, K.; Iwasaki, T.; Abe, H. Functional prognosis after treatment of spinal dural arteriovenous fistulas. *Neurol. Med. Chir.* **1999**, *39*, 206–212; discussion 212–213. [CrossRef]
22. Shinoyama, M.; Endo, T.; Takahash, T.; Shimizu, H.; Takahashi, A.; Suzuki, M.; Tominaga, T. Long-term outcome of cervical and thoracolumbar dural arteriovenous fistulas with emphasis on sensory disturbance and neuropathic pain. *World Neurosurg.* **2010**, *73*, 401–408. [CrossRef]
23. Safaee, M.M.; Clark, A.J.; Burkhardt, J.K.; Winkler, E.A.; Lawton, M.T. Timing, severity of deficits, and clinical improvement after surgery for spinal dural arteriovenous fistulas. *J. Neurosurg. Spine* **2018**, *29*, 85–91. [CrossRef]
24. Ronald, A.A.; Yao, B.; Winkelman, R.D.; Piraino, D.; Masaryk, T.J.; Krishnaney, A.A. Spinal Dural Arteriovenous Fistula: Diagnosis, Outcomes, and Prognostic Factors. *World Neurosurg.* **2020**, *144*, e306–e315. [CrossRef]
25. Niimi, Y.; Berenstein, A.; Setton, A.; Neophytides, A. Embolization of spinal dural arteriovenous fistulae: Results and follow-up. *Neurosurgery* **1997**, *40*, 675–682; discussion 682–683. [CrossRef]
26. Luo, M.; Li, J.; Wu, C.; He, M. Prognostic value of magnetic resonance imaging in spinal dural arteriovenous fistulas. *Acta Neurochir.* **2022**, *164*, 49–54. [CrossRef]
27. Hetts, S.W.; Moftakhar, P.; English, J.D.; Dowd, C.F.; Higashida, R.T.; Lawton, M.T.; Douglas, V.C.; Halbach, V.V. Spinal dural arteriovenous fistulas and intrathecal venous drainage: Correlation between digital subtraction angiography, magnetic resonance imaging, and clinical findings. *J. Neurosurg. Spine* **2012**, *16*, 433–440. [CrossRef]
28. Lee, J.; Lim, Y.M.; Suh, D.C.; Rhim, S.C.; Kim, S.J.; Kim, K.K. Clinical presentation, imaging findings, and prognosis of spinal dural arteriovenous fistula. *J. Clin. Neurosci.* **2016**, *26*, 105–109. [CrossRef]
29. Fugate, J.E.; Lanzino, G.; Rabinstein, A.A. Clinical presentation and prognostic factors of spinal dural arteriovenous fistulas: An overview. *Neurosurg. Focus* **2012**, *32*, E17. [CrossRef]
30. Kaufmann, T.J.; Morris, J.M.; Saladino, A.; Mandrekar, J.N.; Lanzino, G. Magnetic resonance imaging findings in treated spinal dural arteriovenous fistulas: Lack of correlation with clinical outcomes. *J. Neurosurg. Spine* **2011**, *14*, 548–554. [CrossRef]
31. Van Dijk, J.M.; TerBrugge, K.G.; Willinsky, R.A.; Farb, R.I.; Wallace, M.C. Multidisciplinary management of spinal dural arteriovenous fistulas: Clinical presentation and long-term follow-up in 49 patients. *Stroke* **2002**, *33*, 1578–1583. [CrossRef] [PubMed]
32. Patsalides, A.; Knopman, J.; Santillan, A.; Tsiouris, A.J.; Riina, H.; Gobin, Y.P. Endovascular treatment of spinal arteriovenous lesions: Beyond the dural fistula. *AJNR Am. J. Neuroradiol.* **2011**, *32*, 798–808. [CrossRef] [PubMed]

diagnostics

MDPI

Article

Minimally Invasive Surgery Versus Conventional Neurosurgical Treatments for Patients with Subcortical Supratentorial Intracerebral Hemorrhage: A Nationwide Study of Real-World Data from 2016 to 2022

Huanwen Chen [1,2,†], Matthew K. McIntyre [3,†], Mihir Khunte [4], Ajay Malhotra [5], Mohamed Labib [2], Marco Colasurdo [6] and Dheeraj Gandhi [2,*]

1 Department of Neurology, MedStar Georgetown University Hospital, Washington, DC 20007, USA
2 Neurosurgery, University of Maryland Medical Center, Baltimore, MD 21201, USA
3 Department of Neurological Surgery, Oregon Health & Science University, Portland, OR 97239, USA
4 Warren Alpert Medical School, Brown University, Providence, RI 02903, USA
5 Radiology, Yale New Haven Hospital, New Haven, CT 06510, USA
6 Interventional Radiology, Oregon Health & Science University, Portland, OR 97239, USA
* Correspondence: dheeraj.gandhi@som.umaryland.edu
† These authors contributed equally to this work.

Abstract: Background: Neurosurgical interventions are often indicated for patients with subcortical, supratentorial intracerebral hemorrhage (ICH); however, the optimal treatment modality is controversial. Whether minimally invasive surgery (MIS) may be superior to conventional craniotomy (CC) or decompressive craniectomy (DC) in real-world clinical practice is unknown. **Methods**: This was a retrospective cohort study of hospitalization data from the 2016–22 Nationwide Readmissions Database. International Classification of Diseases—10th edition (ICD-10) codes were used to identify patients with primary supratentorial subcortical ICH who underwent neurosurgical treatment. Patients with ICH in other brain compartments (other than intraventricular hemorrhage) were excluded. Coprimary outcomes were routine discharge to home without rehabilitation needs (excellent outcome) and in-hospital mortality. Outcomes were compared between MIS versus CC and MIS versus DC, with multivariable adjustments for patient demographics and comorbidities. **Results**: A total of 3829 patients were identified; 418 underwent MIS (10.9%), 2167 (56.6%) underwent CC, and 1244 (32.5%) underwent DC. Compared to CC patients, MIS patients were less likely female (p = 0.004) but otherwise had similar patient characteristics; compared to DC patients, MIS patients were older, less likely female, more likely to have mental status abnormalities, more likely to have underlying dementia, less likely to undergo external ventricular drainage, more likely to have vascular risk factors (hypertension, hyperlipidemia, diabetes), and less likely to have underlying coagulopathy (all $p < 0.05$). After multivariable adjustments, MIS patients had higher odds of excellent outcomes compared to CC (OR 1.99 [95%CI 1.06–3.30], p = 0.039), and similar odds compared to DC (OR 1.10 [95%CI 0.66–1.86], p = 0.73). In terms of in-hospital mortality, MIS had lower odds compared to DC (OR 0.63 [95%CI 0.41–0.96], p = 0.032) and similar odds compared to CC (OR 0.81 [95%CI 0.56–1.18], p = 0.26). **Conclusions**: For patients with subcortical, supratentorial ICH requiring surgical evacuation, MIS was associated with higherhigher rates of excellent outcomes compared to CC and lower rates of in-hospital mortality compared to DC. However, since key variables such as hematoma size and symptom severity were not available, residual confounding could not be excluded, and results should be interpreted cautiously. Dedicated prospective or randomized studies are needed to confirm these findings.

Diagnostics **2025**, *15*, 1308 https://doi.org/10.3390/diagnostics15111308

Keywords: intracerebral hemorrhage; intracranial hemorrhage; minimally invasive; neurosurgery; evacuation; real-world; nationwide readmissions database

1. Introduction

Spontaneous intracranial hemorrhage (ICH) affects over 3 million patients annually and represents nearly 30% of incident strokes and 50% of stroke-related deaths worldwide [1]. Despite high rates of neurological disability and death, treatment options are limited. More specifically, for patients with supratentorial, subcortical ICH, the role of surgical management is controversial. In 2005, the STICH trial reported negative results for early surgery with conventional craniotomy (CC) versus conservative management for patients with ICH, and subgroup analyses revealed that there may be significant treatment heterogeneity depending on ICH location where surgery may be less effective for subcortical hemorrhages compared to lobar locations [2]. More recently, the SWITCH trial investigated the effectiveness of decompressive hemicraniectomy (DC) in this population [3]; while results were marginally positive, the efficacy of DC was primarily driven by the prevention of extremely poor neurological outcomes (bedridden state or death), and it did not appear to be effective in meaningfully improving the odds of good neurological recovery.

To limit procedural harms associated with surgical ICH treatments, minimally invasive surgery (MIS), which can involve various devices and techniques, has been proposed as a safer alternative to CC or DC [4–6]. In 2018, Scaggiante et al. reported in a meta-analysis of randomized trials that MIS techniques may be favorable to conventional treatment including medical management and conventional craniotomy [6]. More recently, in 2024, the randomized controlled MSICH trial results demonstrated that ICH evacuation with MIS techniques (either with endoscopic or stereotactic aspiration) was associated with more favorable clinical outcomes compared with conventional craniotomy, particularly for subcortical hemorrhages [7]. Finally, in 2024, Huan et al. reported in an updated network meta-analysis that MIS, either using endoscopic or minimally invasive puncture approaches, may be superior to conservative management, CC, or DC for patients with ICH [8]. While these data are promising, they largely originate from large academic teaching centers and outcome measurements may be biased from the investigators. Thus, the generalizability of these findings to real-world practice is unknown.

In this retrospective study of nationwide hospitalization records in the United States, we sought to investigate the real-world effectiveness of MIS versus CC and DC for patients with subcortical supratentorial ICH. We hypothesized that MIS would yield superior clinical outcomes compared to CC and DC.

2. Methods

2.1. Database Characteristics

This was a retrospective analysis of the 2016 to 2022 Nationwide Readmissions Database (NRD), which is part of the Healthcare Cost and Utilization Project (HCUP). The NRD provides information on all hospitalization records of admitted and readmitted patients across 30 geographically dispersed states, representing real-world data across all hospital types and practice settings. In total, NRD captures over 16 million records per year, representing roughly 50% of all hospitalizations in the United States. Patient identifiers are not included in the NRD. As such, this study was exempt from institutional review board approval under the Health Insurance Portability and Accountability Act or informed consent.

2.2. Patient Population

All patient diagnoses and procedures were identified using the International Classification of Disease, 10th revision (ICD-10) codes for diagnoses and procedures. Adult patients with a primary diagnosis code for subcortical intracerebral hemorrhage (ICH) who underwent neurosurgical treatment were included; patients with intracranial tumor, subdural hematoma, subarachnoid hemorrhage, ischemic stroke, multi-compartment ICH (except intraventricular hemorrhage) or missing discharge destination data were excluded. Patients were divided into three cohorts: minimally invasive surgery (MIS), conventional craniotomy (CC), and decompressive craniectomy (DC). MIS patients were identified by the presence of ICD-10 codes specifying endoscopic or percutaneous hematoma evacuation, whereas CC was identified by codes specifying open evacuation. DC patients were identified by the presence of codes specifying craniectomy, regardless of the presence of other codes pertaining to hematoma evacuation. Patient demographics (age, sex) were recorded. The presence of intraventricular hemorrhage and the placement of external ventricular drain were identified. Prior anticoagulant use, prior antiplatelet use, and other medical comorbidities (atrial fibrillation, hypertension, hyperlipidemia, diabetes, chronic liver disease, chronic kidney disease, coagulopathy, dementia) were also recorded. Elixhauser comorbidity index was calculated for each patient to estimate the overall medical comorbidity burden [9].

2.2.1. Study Outcomes

The primary outcome is routine discharge to home with self-care, which is a surrogate marker for excellent neurological outcomes [10–12]. Other outcomes include discharge to home (with or without in-home care services, a surrogate marker for good outcomes for patients with pre-existing disability [13–15]), discharge to a facility (acute rehabilitation, skilled nursing facility, long-term care or any other non-home setting), and in-hospital death (regardless of goals-of-care or hospice services). Other outcomes included hospital length of stay and cost of hospitalization, adjusted for inflation. All ICD-10 codes used for this study were included in Table S1.

2.2.2. Statistical Methods

The number of patients was calculated using discharge-level weights. Patients with missing data were excluded from the analysis. Continuous data were expressed as median and quartiles and compared using Wilcoxon rank-sum tests. Categorical data were represented as percentages and compared using chi-squared tests. Patients treated with MIS were compared to those treated with CC and DC. Multivariable logistic and linear regression models accounting for patient age, sex, intraventricular hemorrhage, external ventricular drain, antithrombotic medication use, captured comorbidities, Elixhauser comorbidity index, and treatment year were used to provide adjusted estimates of differences between MIS and other treatment modalities in terms of discharge outcomes, hospital length of stay, and hospitalization costs. Overall, two-sided p-values less than 0.05 were deemed statistically significant. All statistical analyses were performed using R, Version 3.6.2.

3. Results

3.1. Patient Characteristics

A total of 6352 patients with subcortical supratentorial ICH who underwent neurosurgical treatment were identified. After excluding 193 patients with intracranial tumors, 64 with endocarditis, 60 with cerebral amyloid angiopathy, 275 with concurrent subdural hematoma, 625 with concurrent subarachnoid hemorrhage, 515 with multi-compartment

ICH, 761 with concurrent ischemic stroke, and 30 patients with missing data, 3829 patients were included for analysis. Overall, 418 underwent MIS (10.9%), 2167 (56.6%) underwent CC, and 1244 (32.5%) underwent DC. The study flowchart is presented in Figure 1.

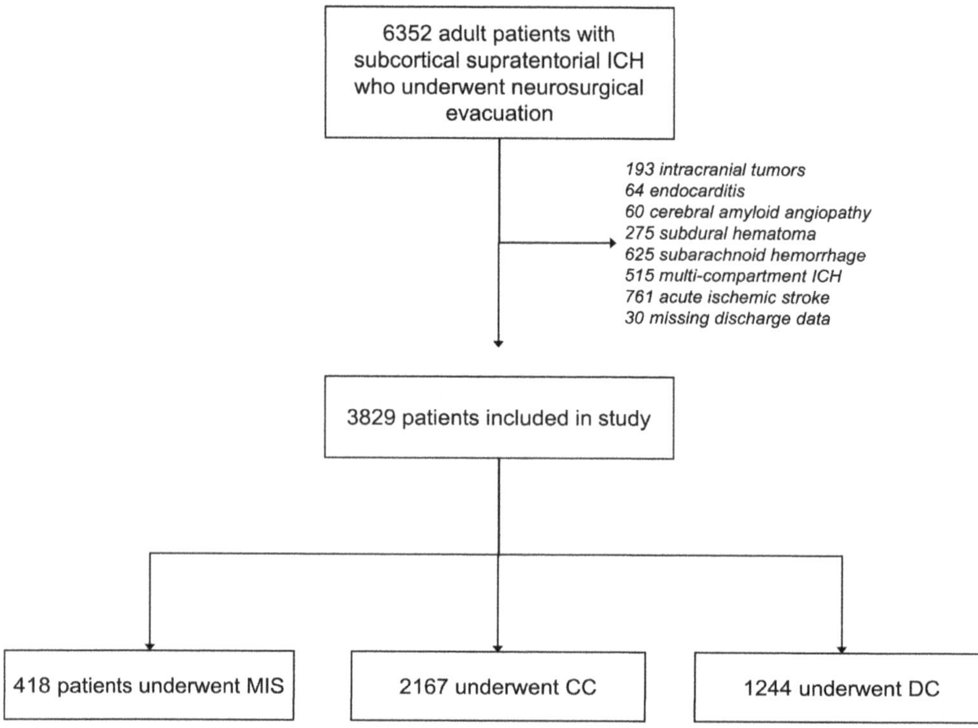

Figure 1. Study flow chart. Abbreviations: ICH—intracerebral hemorrhage; MIS—minimally invasive surgery; CC—conventional craniotomy; DC—decompressive hemicraniectomy.

In terms of patient characteristics, MIS patients were less likely female compared to CC patients (27.2% vs. 36.1%, $p < 0.001$) but otherwise had similar patient characteristics (all $p > 0.05$). Compared to DC patients, MIS patients were older (median 58 vs. 52 years, $p < 0.001$), less likely female (27.2% vs. 36.9%, $p = 0.008$), more likely to have underlying dementia (2.9% vs. 0.3%, $p < 0.001$), less likely to undergo external ventricular drainage (25.1% vs. 35.7%, $p = 0.009$), more likely to have vascular risk factors (hypertension, hyperlipidemia, diabetes, all $p < 0.05$), and less likely to have underlying coagulopathy (11.9% vs. 17.1%, $p = 0.039$). All patient characteristics and comparisons are detailed in Table 1.

Table 1. Patient characteristics.

	Total	**MIS**	**CC**	**DC**	***p*-Values**	
Characteristic—Median (Q1–Q3) or % (n)	**N = 3829**	**N = 418**	**N = 2167**	**N = 1244**	**MIS vs. CC**	**MIS vs. DC**
Age (years)	55 (45–64)	58 (49–65)	56 (47–65)	52 (42–62)	0.34	**<0.001** *
Female sex	35.4% (1356)	27.2% (114)	36.1% (783)	36.9% (459)	**0.004** *	**0.008** *
Intraventricular extension	31.8% (1217)	32.2% (135)	31.2% (676)	32.6% (406)	0.79	0.92
External ventricular drain	28.5% (1093)	25.1% (105)	25.1% (543)	35.7% (445)	1.00	**0.009** *

Table 1. *Cont.*

	Total	MIS	CC	DC	p-Values	
Characteristic—Median (Q1–Q3) or % (n)	**N = 3829**	**N = 418**	**N = 2167**	**N = 1244**	**MIS vs. CC**	**MIS vs. DC**
Antithrombotic medications						
Anticoagulant use	6.1% (233)	4.0% (17)	6.1% (133)	6.7% (83)	0.20	0.15
Antiplatelet use	2.0% (78)	0.7% (3)	2.4% (51)	1.9% (24)	0.087	0.15
Comorbidities						
Atrial fibrillation	8.6% (328)	7.1% (30)	9.8% (211)	7.0% (87)	0.18	0.93
Hypertension	80.1% (3068)	83.8% (350)	83.8% (1817)	72.4% (901)	0.99	**<0.001** *
Hyperlipidemia	26.4% (1010)	29.7% (124)	28.6% (620)	21.4% (266)	0.74	**0.015** *
Diabetes	23.2% (890)	24.9% (104)	25.8% (559)	18.2% (227)	0.78	**0.013** *
Chronic liver disease	5.3% (203)	5.6% (23)	4.8% (105)	6.1% (75)	0.61	0.75
Chronic kidney disease	17.0% (653)	16.3% (68)	17.7% (384)	16.1% (200)	0.60	0.94
Coagulopathy	15.0% (574)	11.9% (50)	14.4% (312)	17.1% (212)	0.31	**0.039** *
Dementia	1.7% (63)	2.9% (12)	2.2% (47)	0.3% (4)	0.57	**<0.001** *
Elixhauser comorbidity index	16 (11–21)	15 (11–21)	16 (10–21)	17 (10–23)	0.71	0.41
Treatment year					0.40	**0.004** *
2016	9.1% (349)	11.3% (47)	11.3% (245)	4.6% (57)		
2017	11.5% (440)	13.5% (56)	11.7% (254)	10.5% (130)		
2018	13.1% (501)	9.2% (38)	14.7% (319)	11.5% (143)		
2019	16.6% (636)	17.4% (73)	16.6% (360)	16.3% (203)		
2020	17.1% (653)	19.1% (80)	14.7% (318)	20.5% (255)		
2021	17.4% (667)	12.4% (52)	16.8% (364)	20.2% (252)		
2022	15.2% (583)	17.2% (72)	14.1% (306)	16.4% (205)		

Bold and * denotes statistical significance ($p < 0.05$) for emphasis.

3.2. MIS vs. CC Outcomes

In unadjusted analyses, MIS was significantly associated with higher rates of routine discharge compared to CC (12.0% vs. 7.2%, $p = 0.026$; Table 2), and this association remained statistically significant after multivariable adjustments (OR 1.99 [95%CI 1.06–3.30], $p = 0.039$; Table 2). MIS was also associated with higher hospitalization costs than CC (median 89,866 vs. 80,418 USD, $p = 0.003$; Table 2), which also remained statistically significant after multivariable adjustments (+ 10,767 USD [95%CI +702 to +20,831], $p = 0.03$; Table 2). Finally, MIS was associated with longer hospital stays (median 21 vs. 19 days, $p = 0.042$; Table 2); however, this association was no longer statistically significant after multivariable adjustments ($p = 0.80$, Table 2). There were no statistically significant differences between MIS and CC for home discharge or in-hospital death, both before and after multivariable adjustments (all $p > 0.05$, Table 2). Aisual representation of discharge outcomes is presented in Figure 2.

Table 2. MIS vs. CC outcomes.

	Unadjusted Comparisons			With Multivariable Adjustments	
Outcome	**MIS (n = 418)**	**CC (n = 2167)**	***p*-value**	**OR or B [95%CI]**	***p*-Value**
Routine discharge	12.0% (50)	7.2% (157)	**0.026** *	1.99 [1.06 to 3.30]	**0.039** *
Home discharge	19.3% (81)	15.5% (336)	0.16	1.35 [0.94 to 2.00]	0.097
In-hospital mortality	18.5% (77)	21.4% (464)	0.30	0.81 [0.56 to 1.18]	0.26
Length of hospital stay (days)	21 (13–37)	19 (11–34)	**0.042** *	0.43 [−2.91 to 3.77]	0.80
Cost of hospitalization (USD)	89,866 (60,656–139,896)	80,418 (52,437–123,765)	**0.003** *	10,767 [702 to 20,831]	**0.036** *

Bold and * denotes statistical significance ($p < 0.05$) for emphasis.

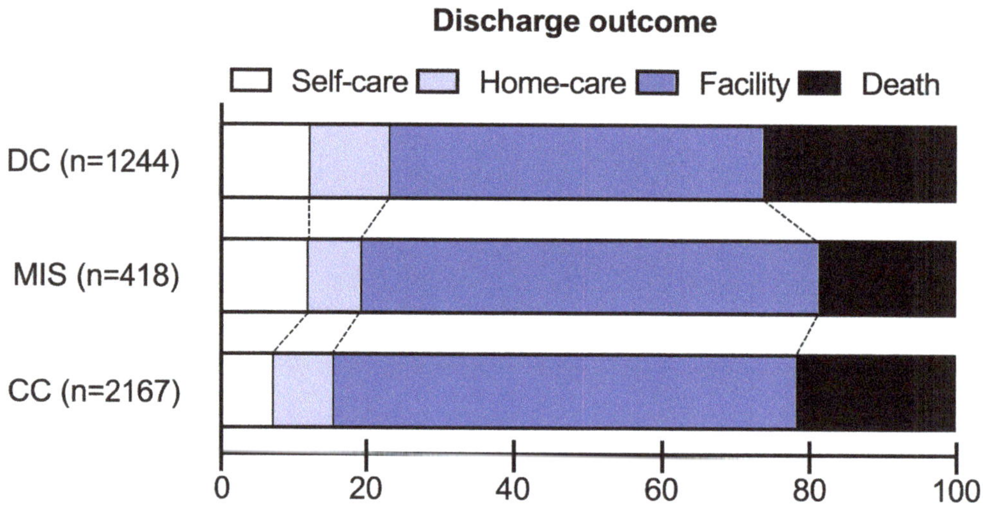

Figure 2. Discharge outcomes of surgical supratentorial subcortical ICHs stratified by treatment modality. Self-care indicates discharge to home with no in-home rehabilitation needs; home-care indicates discharge to home with no in-home rehabilitation services.

3.3. MIS vs. DC Outcomes

In unadjusted analyses, MIS was significantly associated with lower rates of in-hospital death compared to DC (18.5% vs. 26.0%, $p = 0.026$; Table 3), which remained statistically significant after multivariable adjustments (OR 0.63 [95%CI 0.41–0.96], $p = 0.032$; Table 3). There were no statistically significant differences between MIS and DC for routine discharge, home discharge, hospital length of stay, or hospitalization cost, both before and after multivariable adjustments (all $p > 0.05$; Table 3). Visual representation of discharge outcomes are presented in Figure 2.

Table 3. MIS vs. DC outcomes.

	Unadjusted Comparisons			With Multivariable Adjustments	
Outcome	**MIS (n = 418)**	**DC (n = 1244)**	***p*-Value**	**OR or B [95%CI]**	***p*-Value**
Routine discharge	12.0% (50)	12.2% (152)	0.94	1.10 [0.66 to 1.86]	0.73
Home discharge	19.3% (81)	23.2% (289)	0.23	0.82 [0.54 to 1.25]	0.35
In-hospital mortality	18.5% (77)	26.0% (323)	**0.026 ***	0.63 [0.41 to 0.96]	**0.032 ***
Length of hospital stay (days)	21 (13–37)	19 (9–36)	0.077	2.10 [−1.59 to 5.80]	0.26
Cost of hospitalization (USD)	89,866 (60,656–139,896)	88,000 (56,766–144,319)	0.9	2984 [−10,045 to 16,014]	0.65

Bold and * denotes statistical significance ($p < 0.05$) for emphasis.

4. Discussion

In this nationwide retrospective study of supratentorial subcortical ICH patients who underwent neurosurgical treatment, we found that MIS evacuation waswas associated with higher rates of favorable neurological outcomes compared to CC, and lower rates of in-hospital death compared to DC. This study provides real-world data suggesting that MIS evacuation may be preferred over conventional neurosurgical treatments for patients undergoing surgery for supratentorial subcortical ICHs.

Our overall finding that MIS was associated with superior outcomes in real-world clinical practice in the United States is consistent with the current literature [6–8]. Specifically, when compared to conventional craniotomy, MIS was associated with higher rates of excellent short-term neurological outcomes; this effect may be driven by less iatrogenic injury to healthy brain tissue during surgical exploration. In contrast, MIS was associated with lower rates of in-hospital mortality compared to DC. This may have been driven by an overall less invasive nature of MIS; however, the possible effect of residual confounding where DC patients may have larger and clinically more severe ICHs cannot be excluded.

Of note, while MIS may be preferable to other surgical modalities, whether MIS evacuation is superior to medical management alone is unclear. Due to the lack of information on ICH size and neurological exam within the NRD, it was not feasible to compare medically managed patients to surgical patients as the former would inevitably be associated with milder cases which would confound associations with discharge outcomes. Recently, two trials have explored MIS evacuation of ICH patients compared to conservative management. ENRICH, which compared MIS evacuation (with an endoscopic, trans-sulcal, parafascicular approach) within 24 h to medical management, found a significant treatment benefit associated with MIS evacuation of lobar hemorrhages [16]; however, due to the triggering of a pre-determined adaptation rule, recruitment of anterior basal ganglia hemorrhages was halted early due to lack of observed clinical benefit in this subgroup early in the trial. As such, while the overall results of ENRICH were positive in favor of MIS, the study was underpowered to detect treatment benefits for patients with subcortical ICH. In parallel with ENRICH, the MIND study also sought to investigate the MIS versus medical management for ICH patients, and the study population consisted mostly of subcortical hemorrhages [17]. However, due to the publication of ENRICH, the MIND study was halted early due to concerns regarding equipoise, which also compromised its statistical power. Thus, overall, there is currently a lack of high-level clinical trial data on MIS for the treatment of subcortical supra-tentorial ICHs. Future dedicated trials of MIS for subcortical ICHs compared to medical management are needed to further demonstrate its effectiveness.

Another interesting finding in our study was that MIS was associated with significantly increased cost of hospitalization compared to conventional craniotomy. The more specialized procedure and associated equipment may likely be driving this difference between MIS and CC. Future studies are needed to investigate the cost-effectiveness of MIS for ICH. More importantly, the higher costs of MIS may limit the accessibility of this treatment in rural or socio-economically challenged locales. Future studies are also needed to identify potential discrepancies in access to MIS treatment across the United States and worldwide, especially considering recent positive results from ENRICH and MIND trial results for lobar hemorrhages [16,17]. One possible bottleneck for access to MIS treatments may be the limited neurosurgery workforce in the United States [18]. Given recent increases in the neuro-interventional workforce as a result of the advent of stroke thrombectomy and chronic subdural hematoma treatments [19–23], it has been suggested that, with appropriate procedural training, MIS evacuation could be performed by neurointerventionalists [24]. Future efforts are needed to assess whether MIS evacuation of ICHs can be safely performed by neurointerventionalists.

Limitations

Our study has several limitations. First, as a retrospective analysis of a large administrative database, we were unable to obtain disease-specific measures such as hemorrhage volume, radiographic features, ICH score, clinical exam, and other hidden/unmeasured confounders [25–27]. As such, our analysis was limited to only surgical patients, and comparison with medically managed patients was not feasible. Importantly, lack of information on hematoma size is a major limitation, as this factor may have introduced significant confounding by indication (larger hematomas may be associated with CC/DC and therefore worse outcomes). Future prospective or randomized studies are needed to confirm our study findings. Second, while discharge destinations can be used as a surrogate measure of neurological outcomes following cerebrovascular events, more dedicated long-term outcomes such as modified Rankin scale [28] and patient quality of life [29,30] are not available. Furthermore, a majority of patients were discharged to a facility; however, information on the type of facility (e.g., acute rehabilitation, nursing home, hospice care, etc.) is not reported in the NRD. Third, the study period is limited to 2016 to 2022 due to data availability, which predates the publication of ENRICH and the presentation of MIND, which may have impacted current clinical practice. Future studies are needed to further confirm our study findings in more contemporary settings.

5. Conclusions

In this retrospective study of nationwide real-world hospitalization data in the United States, MIS was associated with higher rates of excellent outcomes compared to CC and lower rates of in-hospital mortality compared to DC for patients with subcortical, supratentorial ICH requiring surgical evacuation. However, since key variables such as hematoma size and symptom severity were not available, residual confounding could not be excluded, and results should be interpreted cautiously, Dedicated prospective or randomized studies are needed to confirm these findings.

Supplementary Materials: The following supporting information can be downloaded at https://www.mdpi.com/article/10.3390/diagnostics15111308/s1, Table S1: ICD-10 codes.

Author Contributions: H.C., M.C. and D.G. conceived the study idea. H.C. and M.K. analyzed and visualized the data. H.C. and M.K.M. wrote the manuscript. A.M., M.L., M.C. and D.G. revised the manuscript. H.C. and M.K.M. contributed equally to the manuscript and are co-first authors. All authors approve the final submission. All authors have read and agreed to the published version of the manuscript.

Funding: This research received no external funding.

Institutional Review Board Statement: Patient identifiers are not included in the NRD. As such, this study was exempt from institutional review board approval under the Health Insurance Portability and Accountability Act.

Informed Consent Statement: Patient identifiers are not included in the NRD. As such, this study was exempt from informed consent.

Data Availability Statement: Data used in this study are publicly availbe for purchase at https://hcup-us.ahrq.gov/.

Conflicts of Interest: DG receives research grants from the Focused Ultrasound Foundation, NIH, University of Maryland Medical Center, and Microvention, and is a consultant for Navigantis. Other authors have no relevant disclosures to report.

References

1. Parry-Jones, A.R.; Krishnamurthi, R.; Ziai, W.C.; Shoamanesh, A.; Wu, S.; Martins, S.O.; Anderson, C.S. World Stroke Organization (WSO): Global intracerebral hemorrhage factsheet 2025. *Int. J. Stroke* **2025**, *20*, 145–150. [CrossRef] [PubMed]
2. Mendelow, A.D.; Gregson, B.A.; Fernandes, H.M.; Murray, G.D.; Teasdale, G.M.; Hope, D.T.; Karimi, A.; Shaw, N.D.M.; Barer, D.H. Early surgery versus initial conservative treatment in patients with spontaneous supratentorial intracerebral haematomas in the International Surgical Trial in Intracerebral Haemorrhage (STICH): A randomised trial. *Lancet* **2005**, *365*, 387–397. [CrossRef] [PubMed]
3. Beck, J.; Fung, C.; Strbian, D.; Bütikofer, L.; Z'Graggen, W.J.; Lang, M.F.; Beyeler, S.; Gralla, J.; Ringel, F.; Schaller, K.; et al. Decompressive craniectomy plus best medical treatment versus best medical treatment alone for spontaneous severe deep supratentorial intracerebral haemorrhage: A randomised controlled clinical trial. *Lancet* **2024**, *403*, 2395–2404. [CrossRef]

4. Hannah, T.C.; Kellner, R.; Kellner, C.P. Minimally Invasive Intracerebral Hemorrhage Evacuation Techniques: A Review. *Diagnostics* **2021**, *11*, 576. [CrossRef]
5. Hou, D.; Lu, Y.; Wu, D.; Tang, Y.; Dong, Q. Minimally Invasive Surgery in Patients With Intracerebral Hemorrhage: A Meta-Analysis of Randomized Controlled Trials. *Front. Neurol.* **2022**, *12*, 789757. [CrossRef]
6. Scaggiante, J.; Zhang, X.; Mocco, J.; Kellner, C.P. Minimally Invasive Surgery for Intracerebral Hemorrhage. *Stroke* **2018**, *49*, 2612–2620. [CrossRef]
7. Xu, X.; Zhang, H.; Zhang, J.; Luo, M.; Wang, Q.; Zhao, Y.; Gan, Z.; Xu, B.; Chen, X. Minimally invasive surgeries for spontaneous hypertensive intracerebral hemorrhage (MISICH): A multicenter randomized controlled trial. *BMC Med.* **2024**, *22*, 244. [CrossRef]
8. Huan, J.; Yao, M.; Ma, Y.; Mei, F.; Liu, Y.; Ma, L.; Luo, X.; Liu, J.; Xu, J.; You, C.; et al. Surgical interventions for spontaneous supratentorial intracerebral haemorrhage: A systematic review and network meta-analysis. *eClinicalMedicine* **2025**, *79*, 102999. [CrossRef]
9. Quan, H.; Sundararajan, V.; Halfon, P.; Fong, A.; Burnand, B.; Luthi, J.-C.; Saunders, L.D.; Beck, C.A.; Feasby, T.E.; Ghali, W.A. Coding Algorithms for Defining Comorbidities in ICD-9-CM and ICD-10 Administrative Data. *Med. Care* **2005**, *43*, 1130–1139. [CrossRef]
10. Chen, H.; Khunte, M.; Colasurdo, M.; Malhotra, A.; Gandhi, D. Thrombectomy vs Medical Management for Posterior Cerebral Artery Stroke: Systematic Review, Meta-Analysis, and Real-World Data. *Neurology* **2024**, *102*, e209315. [CrossRef]
11. Chen, H.; Khunte, M.; Malhotra, A.; Gandhi, D.; Colasurdo, M. Endovascular thrombectomy versus medical management for moderate-to-severe anterior cerebral artery occlusion stroke. *J. Neurol.* **2024**, *271*, 6247–6254. [CrossRef]
12. Chen, H.; Colasurdo, M.; Khunte, M.; Malhotra, A.; Gandhi, D. Post-Thrombectomy Subarachnoid Hemorrhage: Incidence, Predictors, Clinical Relevance, and Effect Modulators. *Diagnostics* **2024**, *14*, 1856. [CrossRef]
13. Chen, H.; Khunte, M.; Colasurdo, M.; Jindal, G.; Malhotra, A.; Gandhi, D.; Chaturvedi, S. Associations of Osteoarthritis With Thrombectomy Utilization and Outcomes for Large Vessel Acute Ischemic Stroke. *Stroke* **2023**, *54*, 518–526. [CrossRef]
14. Chen, H.; Colasurdo, M.; Khunte, M.; Malhotra, A.; Gandhi, D. Endovascular thrombectomy versus medical management for acute basilar artery occlusion stroke in the elderly. *Am. J. Neuroradiol.* **2025**, *46*, 278–284. [CrossRef]
15. Chen, H.; Khunte, M.; Colasurdo, M.; Malhotra, A.; Gandhi, D. Intravenous thrombolysis prior to endovascular thrombectomy in elderly stroke patients: An analysis of the National Inpatient Sample database. *J. Neurol. Sci.* **2023**, *454*, 120842. [CrossRef]
16. Pradilla, G.; Ratcliff, J.J.; Hall, A.J.; Saville, B.R.; Allen, J.W.; Paulon, G.; McGlothlin, A.; Lewis, R.J.; Fitzgerald, M.; Caveney, A.F.; et al. Trial of Early Minimally Invasive Removal of Intracerebral Hemorrhage. *N. Engl. J. Med.* **2024**, *390*, 1277–1289. [CrossRef]
17. Arthur, A.S.; Fiorella, D. Procedural, safety, and functional outcomes following minimally invasive surgery for deep and lobar intracranial hemorrhages: MIND study results. In Proceedings of the International Stroke Conference 2025, Los Angeles, CA, USA, 5–7 February 2025.
18. Singh, R.; Parikh, P.P.; De La Peña, N.M.; Bhandarkar, A.R.; Doan, M.K.; Patel, N.P.; Meyer, F.B. Trends in the Neurosurgical Workforce and Implications in Providing for an Aging Population. *World Neurosurg.* **2022**, *160*, e261–e266. [CrossRef]
19. Chen, H.; Marino, J.; Stemer, A.B.; Singh, I.P.; Froehler, M.T. Emerging Subspecialties in Neurology: Interventional Neurology. *Neurology* **2023**, *101*, e1939–e1942. [CrossRef]
20. Kan, P.; Fiorella, D.; Dabus, G.; Samaniego, E.A.; Lanzino, G.; Siddiqui, A.H.; Chen, H.; Khalessi, A.A.; Pereira, V.M.; Fifi, J.T.; et al. ARISE I Consensus Statement on the Management of Chronic Subdural Hematoma. *Stroke* **2024**, *55*, 1438–1448. [CrossRef]
21. Chen, H.; Colasurdo, M.; Kan, P. Middle Meningeal Artery Embolization for Subdural Hematoma. *Neurosurg. Clin. N. Am.* **2025**, *36*, 73–82. [CrossRef]
22. Nguyen, T.N.; Abdalkader, M.; Fischer, U.; Qiu, Z.; Nagel, S.; Chen, H.-S.; Miao, Z.; Khatri, P. Endovascular management of acute stroke. *Lancet* **2024**, *404*, 1265–1278. [CrossRef] [PubMed]
23. Steiger, K.; Singh, R.; Fox, W.C.; Koester, S.; Brown, N.; Shahrestani, S.; Miller, D.A.; Patel, N.P.; Catapano, J.S.; Srinivasan, V.M.; et al. Procedural, workforce, and reimbursement trends in neuroendovascular procedures. *J. Neurointerv. Surg.* **2023**, *15*, 909–913. [CrossRef]
24. Tekle, W.; Benites, G.; Miller, S.; Betancourt, A.; Hassan, A.E. Minimally invasive surgery for evacuation of intracerebral hematoma by neurointerventionalists: Initial experience. *J. Neurointerv. Surg.* **2025**. *online ahead of print*. [CrossRef]
25. Teasdale, G.; Jennett, B. Assessment of Coma and Impaired Consciousness. *Lancet* **1974**, *304*, 81–84. [CrossRef]
26. Hemphill, J.C.; Bonovich, D.C.; Besmertis, L.; Manley, G.T.; Johnston, S.C. The ICH Score. *Stroke* **2001**, *32*, 891–897. [CrossRef]
27. Wada, R.; Aviv, R.I.; Fox, A.J.; Sahlas, D.J.; Gladstone, D.J.; Tomlinson, G.; Symons, S.P. CT Angiography "Spot Sign" Predicts Hematoma Expansion in Acute Intracerebral Hemorrhage. *Stroke* **2007**, *38*, 1257–1262. [CrossRef]
28. van Swieten, J.C.; Koudstaal, P.J.; Visser, M.C.; Schouten, H.J.; van Gijn, J. Interobserver agreement for the assessment of handicap in stroke patients. *Stroke* **1988**, *19*, 604–607. [CrossRef]

29. Lins, L.; Carvalho, F.M. SF-36 total score as a single measure of health-related quality of life: Scoping review. *SAGE Open Med.* **2016**, *4*. [CrossRef]
30. Balestroni, G.; Bertolotti, G. EuroQol-5D (EQ-5D): An instrument for measuring quality of life. *Monaldi Arch. Chest Dis.* **2015**, *78*, 155–159. [CrossRef]

diagnostics

MDPI

Systematic Review

The Value of Cerebral Blood Volume Derived from Dynamic Susceptibility Contrast Perfusion MRI in Predicting IDH Mutation Status of Brain Gliomas—A Systematic Review and Meta-Analysis

José Pablo Martínez Barbero [1,2], Francisco Javier Pérez García [1,2], Paula María Jiménez Gutiérrez [1,3], Marta García Cerezo [1,4], David López Cornejo [1,5], Gonzalo Olivares Granados [6,7], José Manuel Benítez [1,5,†] and Antonio Jesús Láinez Ramos-Bossini [1,2,7,*,†]

1 Advanced Medical Imaging Group (TeCe22), Instituto de Investigación Biosanitaria de Granada (ibs.GRANADA), 18012 Granada, Spain; josep.martinez.sspa@juntadeandalucia.es (J.P.M.B.); wajaviray@gmail.com (F.J.P.G.); paulajg@correo.ugr.es (P.M.J.G.); martagarcia_99@outlook.com (M.G.C.); davidlc@correo.ugr.es (D.L.C.); j.m.benitez@decsai.ugr.es (J.M.B.)

2 Department of Radiology, Hospital Universitario Virgen de las Nieves, 18014 Granada, Spain

3 Department of Anesthesiology, Hospital Universitario Virgen de las Nieves, 18014 Granada, Spain

4 Centro de Genómica e Investigación Oncológica (GENYO), 18016 Granada, Spain

5 Department of Computer Science and Artificial Intelligence, University of Granada, 18071 Granada, Spain

6 Department of Neurosurgery, Hospital Universitario Virgen de las Nieves, 18014 Granada, Spain; gonzalo.olivares@ugr.es

7 Department of Human Anatomy and Embryology, School of Medicine, University of Granada, 18016 Granada, Spain

* Correspondence: ajbossini@ugr.es

† These authors contributed equally to this work.

Abstract: Background: Dynamic susceptibility contrast perfusion MRI (DSC-MRI) is a promising non-invasive examination to predict histological and molecular characteristics of brain gliomas. However, the diagnostic accuracy of relative cerebral blood volume (rCBV) is heterogeneously reported in the literature. This systematic review and meta-analysis aims to assess the diagnostic accuracy of mean rCBV derived from DSC-MRI in differentiating Isocitrate Dehydrogenase (IDH)-mutant from IDH-wildtype gliomas. **Methods:** A comprehensive literature search was conducted in PubMed, Web of Science, and EMBASE up to January 2025, following PRISMA guidelines. Eligible studies reported mean CBV values in treatment-naïve gliomas with histologically confirmed IDH status. Pooled estimates of standardized mean differences (SMDs), diagnostic odds ratios (DOR), and area under the receiver-operating characteristic curve (AUC) were computed using a random-effects model. Heterogeneity was assessed via I^2 statistic. Meta-regression analyses were also performed. **Results:** An analysis of 18 studies ($n = 1733$) showed that mean rCBV is significantly lower in IDH-mutant gliomas (SMD = −0.86; $p < 0.0001$). The pooled AUC was 0.80 (95% CI, 0.75–0.90), with moderate sensitivity and specificity. Meta-regression revealed no significant influence of DSC-MRI acquisition parameters, although a flip angle showed a trend toward significance ($p = 0.055$). **Conclusions:** Mean rCBV is a reliable imaging biomarker for IDH mutation status in gliomas, demonstrating good diagnostic performance. However, heterogeneity in acquisition parameters and post-processing methods limits generalizability of results. Future research should focus on standardizing DSC-MRI protocols.

https://doi.org/10.3390/diagnostics15070896

Keywords: glioma; brain; magnetic resonance imaging; dynamic susceptibility contrast; cerebral blood volume; neuroimaging

1. Introduction

Gliomas are the most common primary malignant brain tumors [1,2], prompting extensive research to improve their characterization. Traditionally, the most relevant factors considered in glioma classification, established by the World Health Organization, were based on histological characteristics. However, a fundamental paradigm shift occurred in the 2016 WHO classification, which emphasized molecular such as Isocitrate Dehydrogenase (IDH) mutation status and 1p/19q codeletion to improve diagnostic accuracy and prognostic stratification of gliomas [3]. This change was consolidated and further extended in the most recent WHO classification (2021) [4]. Therefore, differentiating IDH-mutant from IDH-wild type gliomas is of paramount importance, since these subtypes have distinct prognostic and therapeutic implications

Considering the need for assessing tumor biomarkers in order to establish the WHO grade of a glioma, invasive methods to obtain a histological specimen of the tumor are necessary, with stereotactic biopsy being the most frequent procedure [5]. However, this technique entails patient risks, including intracranial hemorrhage, infection, or neurological deficits [6]. Additionally, small biopsied tissue samples may not fully capture the heterogeneity of gliomas, potentially leading to misclassification or underestimation of aggressive components within the tumor [7]. These limitations have warranted the search for non-invasive imaging techniques capable of providing reliable molecular characterization of brain glioma without the need for tissue sampling.

Magnetic Resonance Imaging (MRI) is an essential examination in glioma assessment, offering insights into tumor morphology, vascularization, and metabolic activity [8]. Conventional MRI sequences, including T1-weighted, T2-weighted, and FLAIR imaging, are widely used for glioma detection and anatomical delineation. However, these sequences provide limited information regarding tumor biology as they only offer structural information [9,10]. Advanced MRI techniques, such as Diffusion-Weighted Imaging (DWI), Magnetic Resonance Spectroscopy (MRS), and Perfusion-Weighted Imaging (PWI), have gained increasing attention for their ability to assess tumor microstructure, metabolism, and hemodynamics, respectively [10]. Among these, Dynamic Susceptibility Contrast perfusion MRI (DSC-MRI) has demonstrated particular promise in evaluating glioma vascular properties, distinguishing tumor subtypes [11,12], and differentiating progression from pseudoprogression [13].

Cerebral Blood Volume (CBV), derived from DSC-MRI, has been extensively studied as a biomarker of tumor vascularity, particularly as a normalized measure (rCBV) [14]. This perfusion metric is calculated by measuring the area under the curve (AUC) of the signal-intensity–time curve during the first pass of a bolus of gadolinium-based contrast agent, which is usually normalized to the mean value of normal-appearing white matter (NAWM) in the contralateral hemisphere to account for inter-patient variability [15]. In biological terms, rCBV measures the volume of blood within a given amount of brain tissue, reflecting tumor vascularity. Thus, high rCBV values indicate increased tumor angiogenesis, which is a hallmark of high-grade tumors [16].

Accordingly, brain gliomas with higher vascular proliferation, such as IDH-wildtype glioblastomas, exhibit elevated rCBV values, whereas IDH-mutant gliomas, known for their lower angiogenic activity, tend to have lower rCBV values [17]. This biological distinction supports that rCBV may serve as a reliable non-invasive imaging biomarker for predicting

IDH mutation status, offering a potential alternative to invasive biopsy. In fact, several studies have reported promising results regarding the utility of rCBV in glioma molecular stratification [18].

However, significant variability exists in reported diagnostic performance, likely due to differences in imaging acquisition parameters, post-processing techniques, or tumor segmentation strategies [19]. Similarly, there is significant variability in the reported specific rCBV values that offer the best diagnostic performance in terms of probabilistic distribution. Mean rCBV, max rCBV, and different specific percentiles of rCBV have been studied, with variable outcomes across studies [20,21]. Overall, this heterogeneity limits the generalizability and consistency of rCBV as a surrogate biomarker for IDH mutation status.

Understanding the impact of technical and methodological variations on rCBV measurements is crucial for standardizing its use in clinical practice [22]. Currently, the most widely used rCBV metric in clinical practice is mean rCBV, which is commonly calculated in an automatic or semi-automatic fashion by most commercial software packages. Although previous works have analyzed the role of different rCBV parameters in differentiating IDH-mutant- vs. IDH-wild-type gliomas, to our knowledge, no previous meta-analyses have been performed specifically aimed at assessing mean rCBV in this diagnostic challenge.

In this study, we performed a comprehensive systematic review and meta-analysis to determine the between-group differences in CBV and the diagnostic accuracy of mean rCBV in distinguishing IDH-mutant from IDH-wildtype gliomas. Additionally, we explored the influence of DSC-MRI acquisition parameters on mean rCBV diagnostic performance. This synthesis will be helpful not only in terms of increasing supporting evidence but also in emphasizing the need for standardization of DSC-MRI performance.

2. Materials and Methods

2.1. Eligibility Criteria

The design of the meta-analysis and the selection criteria were based on the PICO search strategy. The population was formed by patients with histologically confirmed brain glioma; the intervention was DSC-MRI with derived CBV values; the comparator was the IDH mutation status (mutant vs. wild-type); the primary outcomes were the difference in mean CBV values and the predictive value of mean rCBV. The Preferred Reporting Items for Systematic Reviews and Meta-Analyses (PRISMA) [23] guidelines were followed in the design and writing of the study (the PRISMA checklist can be consulted in Supplementary File S1). The protocol of the study was registered in the Open Science Framework registry [24].

Accordingly, the inclusion criteria were the following: published observational or experimental studies evaluating DSC-MRI-derived CBV values in treatment-naive gliomas with known IDH status. The exclusion criteria were studies not providing mean (r)CBV values or other CBV values permitting a reliable estimation of mean (r)CBV, studies not reporting IDH mutation status, studies solely reporting outcomes of MRI perfusion modalities other than T2*-DSC, and studies focused on machine learning methods that did not provide diagnostic yield metrics of CBV following conventional statistical approaches. In addition, case reports, editorials, and other article formats different from original studies were excluded.

2.2. Information Sources and Search Strategy

Two authors (FJPG and DLC) searched the PubMed, Web of Science, and EMBASE databases. Different search equations were carried out, and a final consistent equation was constructed, including combinations derived from a main equation as follows: "(perfusion OR dynamic) AND (magnetic resonance imaging OR MRI) AND (brain OR cerebr* OR "central nervous system") AND (glioma) AND (gene* OR IDH OR 1p/19q deletion OR MGMT) (the full search strategies in PubMed, Web of Science, and EMBASE can be consulted in Supplementary Files S2, S3 and S4, respectively)". To increase the sensitivity of the search, a cluster search was performed examining the references of all fully read articles. No language restrictions were established. The search was updated to 1 January 2025.

All titles and abstracts of interest were screened, and those which did not meet the eligibility criteria were excluded. Next, the screened studies were read in full to assess whether they met all eligibility criteria. Discrepancies during the article selection process were solved by a third author (JPMB).

2.3. Measured Variables

For each study, the main characteristics were collected, including first author, year, country, study design, sample size (total and in each IDH group), and number of MRI machines involved in the study. In addition, we gathered available information on MRI acquisition parameters (TE, TR, Flip Angle, Slice Thickness, Slice Gap, Matrix, Field of View, contrast agent dose) and post-processing information (commercial software used, arterial input function modality, tumor segmentation modality). The primary outcomes were the mean CBV values for mutated and wild-type IDH and the diagnostic test performance (AUC) of mean rCBV to differentiate between them.

2.4. Data Extraction

Two authors (PMJG and FJPG) independently extracted the data from the selected articles, and a third author (AJLRB) reviewed the data and solved any discrepancies. If a study reported data for a subgroup of patients from the main cohort, only data related to patients with known IDH mutation status were collected. All data were annotated in a spreadsheet for ulterior analysis.

2.5. Meta-Regression Analyses

To explore the potential moderating influence of DSC-MRI acquisition parameters as a source of heterogeneity in the main primary outcomes, we performed meta-regression analyses, including echo time (TE), repetition time (TR), flip angle (FA), slice thickness (ST) and gap (ST), acquisition time, and number of images per DSC sequence (dynamic images).

2.6. Quality and Publication Bias Assessment

The QUADAS-2 tool [25] was used to systematically assess the existence of potential risks of bias and applicability concerns. For each study, two authors (PMJG and FJPG) classified the risk of bias as low, unclear, or high in each of the four risk of bias items and in the three applicability concern items. An overall risk of bias estimation was provided by a consensus. In case of discrepancy, a third author (AJLRB) was consulted. On the other hand, the publication bias was analyzed using funnel plots and Egger's tests.

2.7. Statistical Analysis

To ensure a robust estimation of the overall effect size, we applied a random-effects model using the restricted maximum likelihood (REML) method to estimate standard mean differences (SMD) of mean (r)CBV between IDH-mutant- and IDH-wild-type gliomas. To assess the diagnostic accuracy of rCBV, we performed a hierarchical-summary receiver-operating characteristic (HSROC) analysis complemented with calculation of the pooled Youden J Index (Sensitivity + Specificity − 1), as well as bivariate random-effects meta-analysis for sensitivity and specificity. Additionally, we computed the pooled AUC, diagnostic odds ratio (DOR), and Youden index for each study when available. Importantly, the analyses were performed separately for studies reporting AUC values for continue (r)CBV values or for specific cutoffs.

When a study reported data for a given glioma WHO grade, it was sub-divided into different subsets as if they were individual studies for data analysis. When data were not explicitly provided, but were presented in graphs, extraction of visual data using the free version of PlotDigitizer tool [26] was performed. Moreover, to avoid excluding relevant studies from analysis, when mean (r)CBV values or other essential metrics, such as AUC, were not explicitly reported, they were estimated to obtain reliable data in accordance with the recommendations of the Cochrane Handbook for Systematic Reviews of Interventions [27,28], as follows:

- Estimation of mean and standard deviation

If a study did not provide the mean and standard deviation of (r)CBV, we estimated these values based on the median and IQR using the method proposed by Wan et al. (2014) for asymmetric distributions [29], as follows:

$$\mu = Q2 + 0.2\cdot(Q3 - Q1)$$

where μ is the mean; Q1, Q2, and Q3 are the first, second (i.e., median), and third quartile values of the distribution. Similarly, for the SD (σ), the following formula was applied:

$$\sigma = \frac{Q3 - Q1}{1.35}$$

Finally, in some studies, mean/SD (r)CBV values were provided for subgroup comparisons involving a third group (e.g., IDH-mutated with and without 1p19q codeletion). In these cases, combined values were also estimated for the IDH-mutated group (merging both subgroups), weighting the means and standard deviations according to their respective sample sizes.

- Estimation of missing AUC values from different sources

In some studies, AUC values were not directly reported but were instead provided for different percentiles or could be inferred from other performance metrics. Since excluding these studies could have entailed an underestimation of the pooled AUC, we applied well-established statistical methods (e.g., Monte Carlo simulations) to estimate AUC values in those studies where they were not explicitly reported. Such estimations allowed us to retain valuable data and minimize the risk of selection bias, improving the robustness of the analyses. Specifically, based on the available information in each study, we applied the following approaches to estimate AUC values:

If a study reported AUC values for different (r)CBV percentiles rather than a single metric of AUC value for mean (r)CBV, we calculated an overall AUC estimate by computing a weighted average of the reported percentiles. The initial weight was assigned assuming that the percentiles represented equal strata of the (r)CBV distribution. This was further refined using a weighting proportional to the total sample size. The standard error of the estimated AUC was derived following the approach of Hanley & McNeil (1982) [30], according to the following formula:

$$SE_{AUC} = \sqrt{\frac{AUC\cdot(1 - AUC) + (N_1 - 1)\cdot\left(Q_1 - AUC^2\right) + (N_2 - 1)\cdot\left(Q_2 - AUC^2\right)}{N_1\cdot N_2}}$$

Similarly, a study reported mean (r)CBV values for different percentiles in each IDH subgroup but did not provide the AUC corresponding to the mean, limiting itself to indicating that this metric did not differentiate ($p > 0.05$) between the mutated- and wild-type IDH groups. To estimate the AUC of the mean rCBV, a simulation method based on Monte Carlo was used, which is widely used in diagnostic accuracy studies when individual data are not available and only summary statistics are available [31,32].

First, normal distributions were modeled for each group using the reported mean and SD values, under the assumption that rCBV follows an approximately normal distribution within each group. Based on these distributions, simulated values of rCBV were generated for each group according to their respective sample sizes, ensuring that the variability within each group was consistent with the reported SD. Subsequently, this simulated sample was used to calculate the receiver-operating characteristics (ROCs) curve and obtain the estimated AUC. To evaluate the uncertainty associated with this estimate, a bootstrap resampling analysis was performed (1000 iterations), obtaining a 95% confidence interval (95% CI). In addition, the optimum cut-off point for the mean rCBV was determined using the Youden index.

Finally, when only the odds ratio or β coefficient values were reported, an estimation of the AUC was made based on the coefficient β obtained in the univariate logistic regression. To do this, the relationship between the coefficient β and the OR was used, following the method described by Zhou et al. (2002) [33], where the AUC can be calculated from the OR using the formula:

$$AUC = \frac{OR^{0.5}}{1 + OR^{0.5}}$$

When AUC 95% CIs were not explicitly provided in a given study, they were estimated based on the standard error (SE) according to the Hanley & McNeil formulae [30], as follows:

$$SE = \frac{\sqrt{AUC \cdot (1 - AUC)}}{\sqrt{N}} \qquad 95\%CI = AUC \pm 1.96 \cdot SE$$

- Estimation of other diagnostic performance metrics

Other relevant values assessed in this meta-analysis that were not directly reported in the original study were estimated. For OR, the weighted overall OR was calculated using an adjusted mean of the values provided at each percentile, applying a logarithmic adjustment for the 95% confidence interval. Similarly, when the sensitivity and specificity values were not directly reported, they were calculated from the predictive values collected in the study.

Finally, we applied the I^2 and tau^2 statistics to assess heterogeneity among studies with non-relevant, moderate, and considerable cut-off values set at $I^2 < 40\%$, $40\% < I^2 < 75\%$, and $I^2 > 75\%$, respectively [34–37]. Sensitivity analyses were performed to evaluate the robustness of the results. First, a sensitivity analysis was carried out based on the exclusion of studies with imputed data, comparing the SMD and AUC estimates with and without these studies, evaluating changes in effect size and heterogeneity. In addition, an overall sensitivity analysis was performed using the leave-one-out technique, in which each study was sequentially excluded to determine its individual impact on the pooled estimates. Changes in point estimates and heterogeneity were analyzed to identify potentially influential studies and to assess the stability of the results. To visually display the results, forest plots were generated, showing the effect sizes and 95% CIs for individual studies as well as the overall pooled estimates.

3. Results

3.1. Search Results and Main Characteristics of the Included Studies

The initial search in the three databases identified a total of 3184 articles. After duplicate removal (879 articles) and title/abstract screening, 113 articles were fully read. Following the inclusion and exclusion criteria, a total of 18 studies were finally included in the quantitative synthesis. The PRISMA flow chart of the study can be consulted in Figure 1.

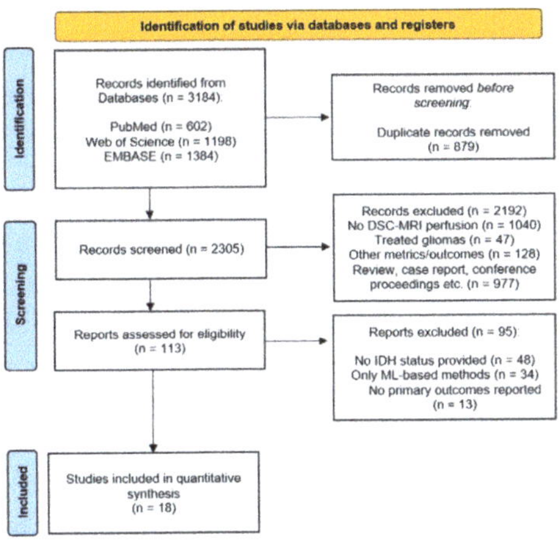

Figure 1. PRISMA flow diagram of the systematic review and meta-analysis.

The main characteristics of each study are described in Table 1. Further information regarding DSC-MRI post-processing data and MRI acquisition parameters in each study can be consulted in Supplementary Tables S1 and S2, respectively.

Table 1. Main characteristics of the included studies. * No data provided for each subgroup, but all gliomas were "high-grade gliomas". ^ Number of women with respect to the total sample of the study, which was larger than the analyzed patients (i.e., those with known IDH status).

Study (Year) [Reference]	Country	N	Age	Women	WHO-II	WHO-III	WHO-IV	IDH-M	IHD-wt
Ahn et al. (2023) [38]	Republic of Korea	132	46 ± 13	66	54	78	0	87	45
Brendle et al. (2020) [39]	Germany	56	48 ± 16	23	29	20	7	32	24
Choi et al. (2019) [40]	Republic of Korea	463	52.2 ± 14.8	191	32	142	289	125	338
Cindil et al. (2022) [41]	Turkey	58	49 ± 17 (IDHm); 58 ± 14 (IDHwt)	27	0	29 *	29 *	23	35
Guo et al. (2022) [42]	China	102	43.5 (18–74)	46	37	22	43	54	48
Hempel et al. (2018) [43]	Germany	100	51.4 ± 15.2	45	40	30	30	54	46
Hong et al. (2021) [44]	Republic of Korea	76	47.69 (19–68)	29	0	76	0	47	29
Kickingereder et al. (2015) [45]	Germany	73	43 ± 14	31	34	49	0	60	13
Lee et al. (2015) [46]	Republic of Korea	52	49.8 ± 14.5	20	0	36	16	16	36
Lee et al. (2019) [47]	Republic of Korea	110	47.44 ± 13.40	54	45	65	0	19	45
Lee_MH et al. (2019) [48]	Republic of Korea	88	52 (20–80)	41	0	0	88	12	76
Lu et al. (2021) [49]	China	71	53 (18.0–74.0)	36	0	0	71	45	26
Ozturk et al. (2021) [50]	USA	47	54 (20–90)	24	0	0	47	7	40

Table 1. *Cont.*

Study (Year) [Reference]	Country	N	Age	Women	WHO-II	WHO-III	WHO-IV	IDH-M	IHD-wt
Pruis et al. (2022) [51]	The Netherlands	99	53.4 ± 15.3	36	78	17	4	81	18
Prysiazhniuk et al. (2024) [52]	Norway	66	47.07 ± 14.84	36 ^	19	13	34	33	33
Song et al. (2020) [53]	China	52	51.23 ± 15.59	21	16	6	30	22	30
Tan et al. (2016) (WHO II) [54]	China	31	38.94 ± 10.31 (IDHm); 51.57 ± 17.71 (IDHwt)	14	31	0	0	17	14
Tan et al. (2016) (WHO III) [54]	China	24	44.56 ± 43.33 (IDHm); 43.33 ± 13.85 (IDHwt)	10	0	24	0	9	15
Tan et al. (2016) (WHO IV) [54]	China	36	39.50 ± 10.10 (IDHm); 51.77 ± 13.57 (IDHwt)	12	0	0	36	6	30
Zhang et al. (2020) [55]	China	43	47 ± 13	23	14	14	15	20	23

3.2. *Quality Assessment*

The 18 studies included in the meta-analysis showed a low overall risk of bias, except for three [49,53,55] that were categorized as having an unclear risk due to some concerns in patient selection (Figure 2). Further details on the assessment of risk of bias and applicability concerns domains can be found in Supplementary Table S3.

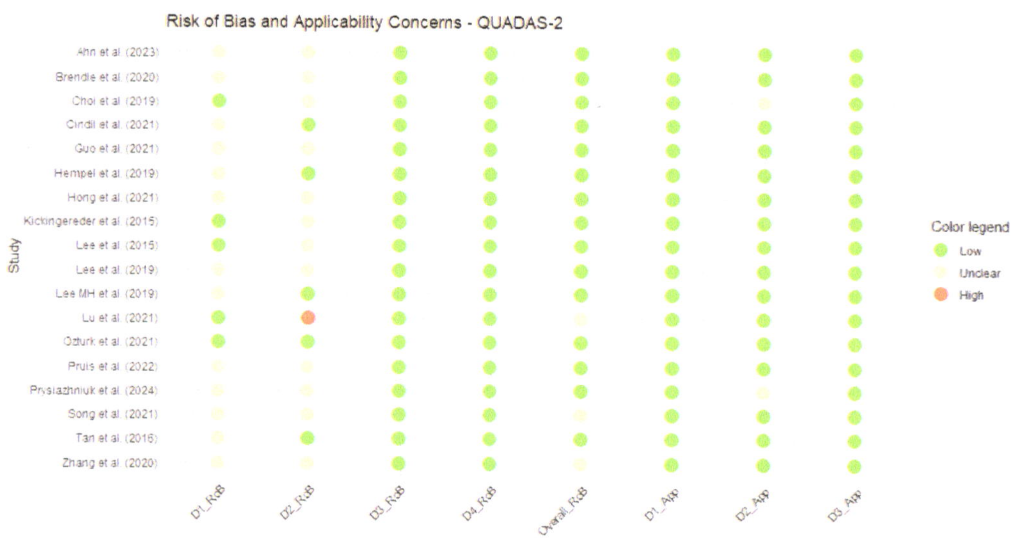

Figure 2. Traffic light plot of the QUADAS-2 assessment for the studies included in the meta-analysis. Ahn et al. (2023) [38], Brendle et al. (2020) [39], Choi et al. (2019) [40], Cindil et al. (2022) [41], Guo et al. (2022) [42], Hempel et al. (2018) [43], Hong et al. (2021) [44], Kickingereder et al. (2015) [45], Lee et al. (2015) [46], Lee et al. (2019) [47], Lee MH et al. (2019) [48], Lu et al. (2021) [49], Ozturk et al. (2021) [50], Pruis et al. (2022) [51], Prysiazhniuk et al. (2024) [52], Song et al. (2020) [53], Tan et al. (2016) [54], Zhang et al. (2020) [55].

3.3. *Differences in Mean Cerebral Blood Volume Based on the IDH Status*

Statistically significant differences were found in the SMD, being lower in the IDH-mutant group, both overall (SMD = −0.86; $p < 0.0001$) and in each individual study. The greatest between-group difference was found in Kickingereder et al. [45]: (SMD = −1.90), whereas the smallest difference was observed in Lee et al. (2015) [46]: (SMD = −0.30). In five studies [44,46–48,50], the 95%CI for SMD included positive SMD values. The overall heterogeneity was moderate (I^2 = 62.8%; tau^2 = 0.11), indicating that there are methodological or population differences between the included studies. Figure 3 shows the forest plot of the studies included in the analysis.

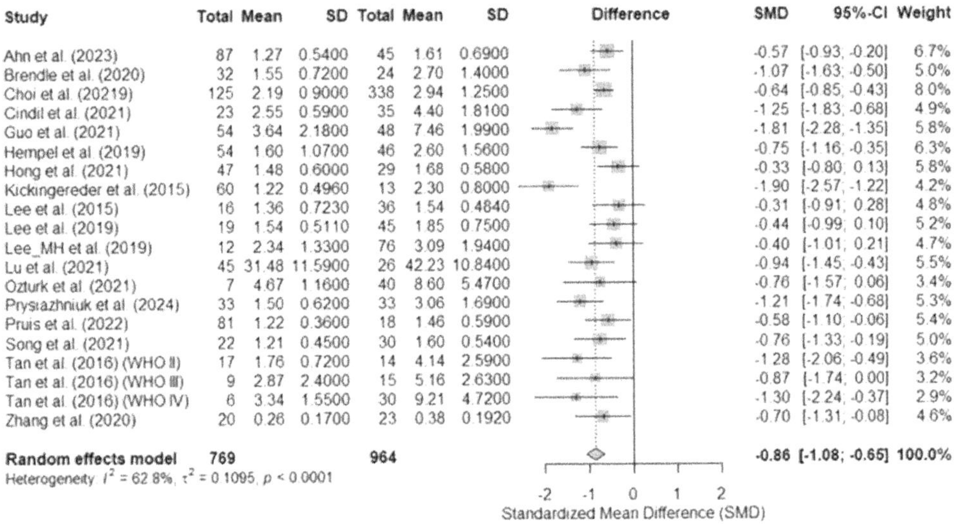

Figure 3. Forest plot for the standard mean difference (SMD) in mean relative cerebral blood volume between IDH-mutated- (left columns) vs. IDH-wild-type brain gliomas (right columns). The horizontal lines indicate the 95% confidence intervals (95% CI). The pooled SMD was −0.86, indicating significantly lower rCBV in IDH-mutant gliomas. WHO II–IV, 2007 World Health Organization central nervous system tumor grades II–IV. Ahn et al. (2023) [38], Brendle et al. (2020) [39], Choi et al. (2019) [40], Cindil et al. (2022) [41], Guo et al. (2022) [42], Hempel et al. (2018) [43], Hong et al. (2021) [44], Kickingereder et al. (2015) [45], Lee et al. (2015) [46], Lee et al. (2019) [47], Lee_MH et al. (2019) [48], Lu et al. (2021) [49], Ozturk et al. (2021) [50], Prysiazhniuk et al. (2024) [52], Pruis et al. (2022) [51], Song et al. (2020) [53], Tan et al. (2016) (WHO II) [54], Tan et al. (2016) (WHO III) [54], Tan et al. (2016) (WHO IV) [54], Zhang et al. (2020) [55].

3.4. *Diagnostic Performance of Mean rCBV*

3.4.1. Pooled AUC Based on Reported Mean rCBV Cutoff Values

The analysis of the studies that reported an AUC for a specific cut-off value showed a pooled AUC estimate of 0.83 (95% CI: 0.75–0.90), indicating that the mean rCBV value has a good discriminatory capacity for differentiating gliomas with mutated vs. wild-type IDH. However, the heterogeneity between studies was moderate (I^2 = 68.0%, p = 0.0009), suggesting that there are methodological or population differences between the included studies.

The individual studies reported AUCs ranging from 0.50 to 0.94, reflecting variability in the selected rCBV thresholds and in the populations studied. Figure 4 shows the forest plot of this analysis.

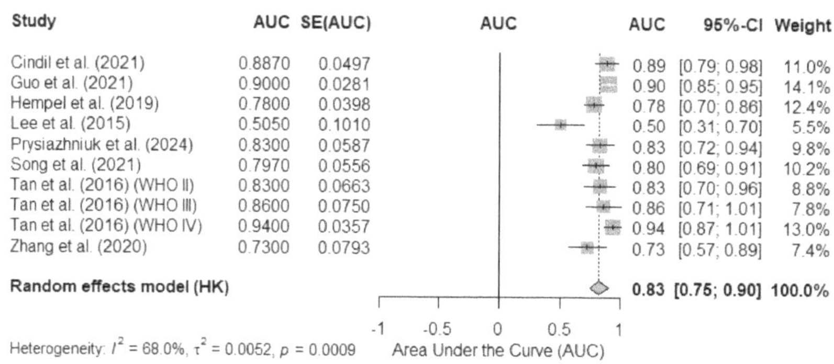

Figure 4. Forest plot of the area under the curve (AUC) in studies reporting a cut-off value for the mean rCBV in the differentiation of gliomas with mutated- vs. wild-type IDH. Each study is represented by a square, the size of which is proportional to the weight of the study in the meta-analysis. The horizontal lines indicate the 95% confidence intervals (95% CIs). The pooled AUC estimate under a random-effects model is represented by the diamond at the bottom of the figure. SE, standard error. Cindil et al. (2022) [41], Guo et al. (2022) [42], Hempel et al. (2018) [43], Lee et al. (2015) [46], Prysiazhniuk et al. (2024) [52], Song et al. (2020) [53], Tan et al. (2016) (WHO II) [54], Tan et al. (2016) (WHO III) [54], Tan et al. (2016) (WHO IV) [54], Zhang et al. (2020) [55].

3.4.2. Pooled AUC in Studies Reporting rCBV as Continuous Values

The meta-analysis of the studies that reported an AUC for rCBV as a continuous variable showed a pooled AUC estimate of 0.78 (95% CI: 0.39–1.16). However, the heterogeneity between studies was considerable ($I^2 = 91.8\%$, $p < 0.0001$). Individual studies reported AUCs ranging from 0.60 to 0.89, indicating significant dispersion in the discriminatory capacity of rCBV when analyzed as a continuous variable. Figure 5 shows the forest plot of this analysis.

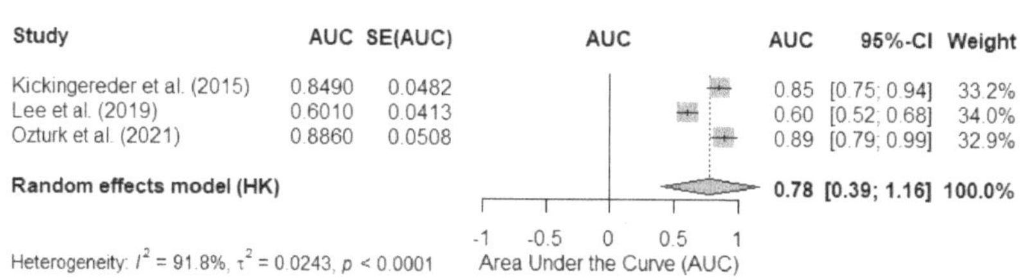

Figure 5. Forest plot of the area under the curve (AUC) in studies reporting the mean rCBV value as a continuous variable to differentiate gliomas with IDH-mutant- vs. IDH-wild-type. Each study is represented by a square, the size of which is proportional to the weight of the study in the meta-analysis. The horizontal lines indicate the 95% confidence intervals (95% CIs). The pooled AUC estimate under a random-effects model is represented by the diamond at the bottom of the figure. SE, standard error. Kickingereder et al. (2015) [45], Lee et al. (2019) [47], Ozturk et al. (2021) [50].

3.4.3. Bivariate Meta-Analysis of Sensitivity and Specificity: HSROC Analysis

The forest plots in Figure 6 illustrate the pooled sensitivity and specificity of mean rCBV for distinguishing IDH-mutant- from IDH-wild-type gliomas across multiple studies. Individual sensitivity values were variable, with a pooled sensitivity estimate of 0.80 (95% CI: 0.56–0.96). Similarly, the pooled specificity was 0.80 (95% CI: 0.53–0.99). For individual studies, the ones reporting highest sensitivity and specificity values were those by Guo et al. (2021) [42] and Tan et al. (2016, WHO IV) [54] (0.98 and 1, respectively). Conversely, the studies reporting lowest sensitivity and specificity values were Hempel et al. (2019) [43] and Lee et al. (2015) [46] (0.52 and 0.50, respectively).

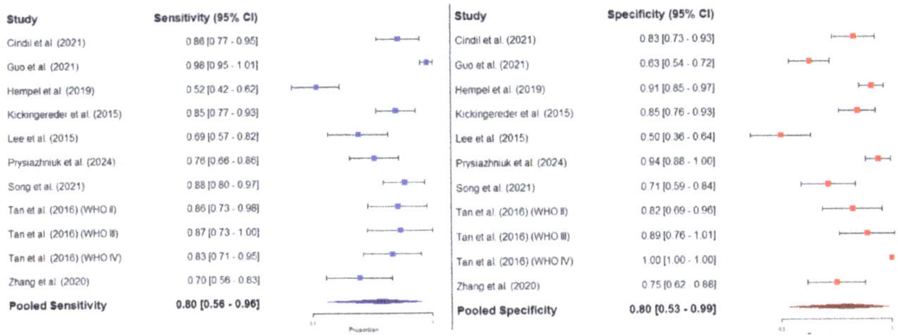

Figure 6. Pooled estimates of sensitivity and specificity for rCBV in predicting IDH mutation status. **Left panel**: Forest plot of sensitivity estimates from individual studies, together with the pooled sensitivity derived from the meta-analysis using a random-effects model. **Right panel:** Forest plot of specificity estimates from individual studies, together with the pooled specificity derived from the meta-analysis using a random-effects model. Each square represents the point estimate of a single study, with horizontal lines indicating the 95% confidence intervals (CI). The combined estimates are shown as diamonds at the bottom of each panel, and their width represents the 95% CI. Cindil et al. (2022) [41], Guo et al. (2022) [42], Hempel et al. (2018) [43], Kickingereder et al. (2015) [45], Lee et al. (2015) [46], Prysiazhniuk et al. (2024) [52], Song et al. (2020) [53], Tan et al. (2016) (WHO II) [54], Tan et al. (2016) (WHO III) [54], Tan et al. (2016) (WHO IV) [54], Zhang et al. (2020) [55].

The results of the HSROC analysis were similar to those of the bivariate meta-analysis, with pooled sensitivity and specificity values of 0.784 (95%CI, 0.674–0.865) and 0.787 (95%CI, 0.678–0.867), respectively, and a pooled AUC of 0.789 (95%CI, 0.779–0.794). Figure 7 shows the HSROC curve of diagnostic performance.

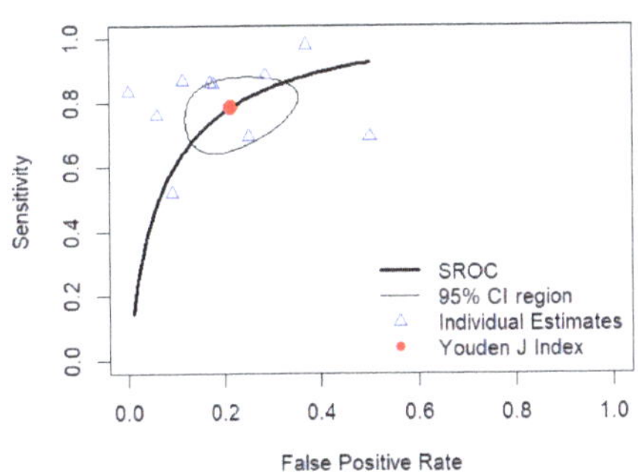

Figure 7. Hierarchical-summary receiver-operating characteristics (HSROC) curve of the diagnostic performance of mean rCBV to classify brain gliomas into IDH-mutant- vs. IDH-wild-type for the studies reporting mean rCBV cutoff values that were included in the meta-analysis.

3.4.4. Diagnostic Odds Ratio of Mean rCBV

The individual results of the studies show considerable variability, with DOR values ranging from 2.00 [0.62–6.43] to 93.00 [7.23–1196.69]. The combined DOR estimate using a random-effects model was 14.21 [7.67–26.35]. The pooled Youden J Index was 0.58, with considerable variability ranging from 0.54 to 0.62. Figure 8 shows the forest plot of the DOR analysis, and Figure 9 shows the forest plot of the Youden J Index of individual and pooled data.

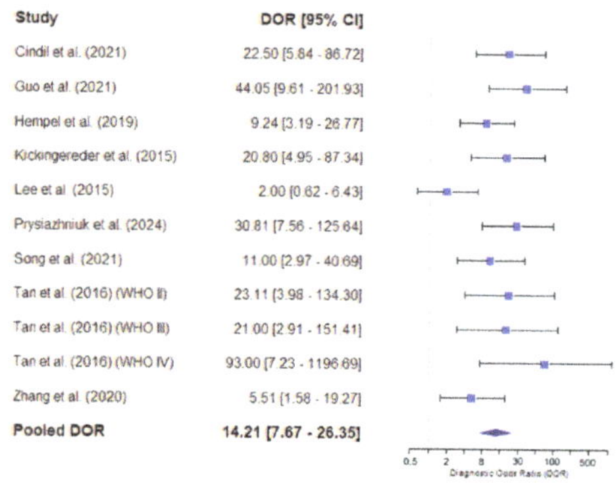

Figure 8. Forest plot showing the diagnostic odds ratio (DOR) and its 95% confidence interval (95% CI) for each individual study included in the meta-analysis. The squares represent the point estimates of the DOR for each study, and the horizontal lines indicate the 95% CIs. The size of the squares is proportional to the weight of each study in the analysis. The blue diamond represents the combined estimate of the pooled DOR using a random-effects model, with its corresponding confidence interval. Cindil et al. (2022) [41], Guo et al. (2022) [42], Hempel et al. (2018) [43], Kickingereder et al. (2015) [45], Lee et al. (2015) [46], Prysiazhniuk et al. (2024) [52], Song et al. (2020) [53], Tan et al. (2016) (WHO II) [54], Tan et al. (2016) (WHO III) [54], Tan et al. (2016) (WHO IV) [54], Zhang et al. (2020) [55].

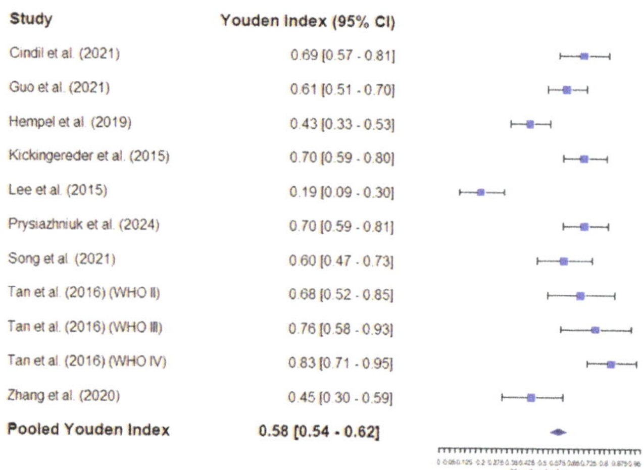

Figure 9. Forest plot of the Youden J index and its 95% confidence interval (95% CI) for each individual study included in the meta-analysis. The squares represent the point estimates of the DOR for each study, and the horizontal lines indicate the 95% CIs. The size of the squares is proportional to the weight of each study in the analysis. The blue diamond represents the combined estimate of the pooled DOR using a random-effects model, with its corresponding confidence interval. Cindil et al. (2022) [41], Guo et al. (2022) [42], Hempel et al. (2018) [43], Lee et al. (2015) [46], Kickingereder et al. (2015) [45], Prysiazhniuk et al. (2024) [52], Song et al. (2020) [53], Tan et al. (2016) (WHO II) [54], Tan et al. (2016) (WHO III) [54], Tan et al. (2016) (WHO IV) [54], Zhang et al. (2020) [55].

3.5. Meta-Regression Analyses

None of the DSC-MRI acquisition parameters showed significant influence in the primary outcomes, but the flip angle showed a trend toward significance ($p = 0.055$) in the SMD meta-regression, with decreasing units being associated with reduced SMD values (β) = −0.009). Heterogeneity was moderate in all cases, ranging from 66.7% to 78.27%

in SMD, and from 44.4% to 84.2% in AUC. Tables 2 and 3 show the results of the meta-regression analyses for SMD and AUC estimates, respectively.

Table 2. Meta-regression analysis results for standard mean difference. TRH, test for residual heterogeneity.

Variable	β Coefficient (95%CI)	p-Value	I²	Tau²	p-Value (TRH)
TE	−0.0011 (−0.0311, 0.0289)	0.9441	68.61%	0.1440	<0.0001
TR	−0.0004 (−0.0012, 0.0004)	0.345	67.71%	0.1349	<0.0001
FA (°)	−0.0091 (−0.0183, 0.0002)	0.0551	66.68%	0.1355	0.0002
Slice thickness	0.0301 (−0.3125, 0.3727)	0.8634	71.12%	0.1533	<0.0001
Slice gap	0.4497 (−0.1306, 1.0301)	0.1288	68.48%	0.1358	0.0007
N. images	−0.0352 (−0.1188, 0.0484)	0.4089	76.30%	0.2355	<0.0001
Scan time	0.0031 (−0.0124, 0.0187)	0.6922	78.27%	0.1880	<0.0001

Table 3. Meta-regression analysis results for area under the curve. TRH, test for residual heterogeneity.

Variable	β Coefficient (95%CI)	p-Value	I²	Tau²	p-Value (TRH)
TE	0.0009 (−0.0075, 0.0092)	0.8424	72.60%	0.0069	0.0007
TR	0.0001 (0.0002, 0.0004)	0.6953	72.37%	0.0069	0.0009
FA (°)	0 (−0.0048, 0.0047)	0.9856	44.42%	0.0021	0.1047
Slice thickness	0.0102 (−0.0796, 0.0999)	0.8241	70.49%	0.0071	0.0008
Slice gap	−0.0152 (−0.1863, 0.1559)	0.8620	74.03%	0.0092	0.0025
N. images	−0.0032 (−0.0307, 0.0244)	0.8213	84.19%	0.0164	0.0016
Scan time	0.0021 (−0.0059, 0.0101)	0.6099	50.46%	0.0036	0.1329

3.6. Publication Bias and Sensitivity Analyses

Regarding publication bias, the shape of the funnel plot for the 20 studies included in the SMD analysis indicated no significant biases, which was supported by the results of the Egger's test (t = −1.45; $p = 0.166$). The variance of residual heterogeneity ($tau^2 = 2.541$) indicated high variability between studies, in agreement with the dispersion observed in the funnel plot. Similar results were observed in the funnel plot of the 10 studies reporting mean rCBV cutoff values that were used to estimate pooled AUC (Egger's test, t = −2.81; $p = 0.0227$; $tau^2 = 1.765$). Figure 10 shows the corresponding funnel plots.

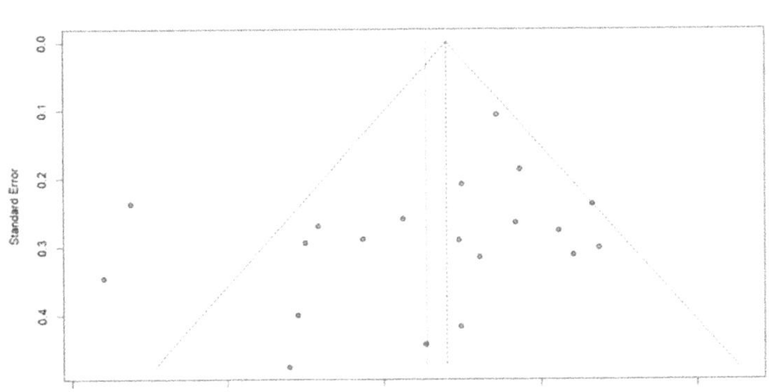

Figure 10. *Cont.*

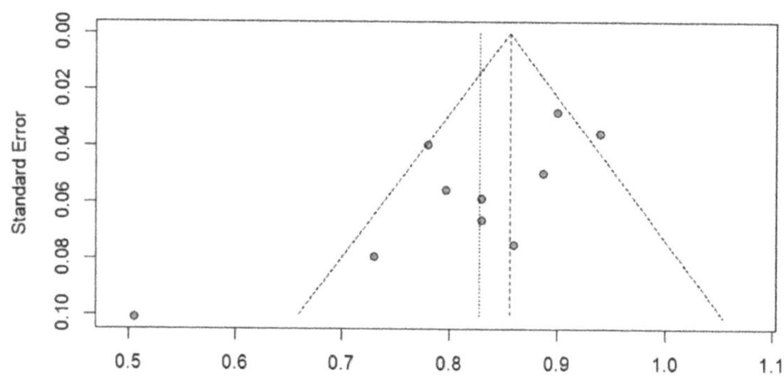

Figure 10. Funnel plots for studies included in the standardize mean difference (**top**) and area under the curve (**bottom**) analyses. The line centered at the vertex of the triangle indicates the estimation according to the random-effects model, and the parallel vertical line on the left refers to the estimation according to a common-effects model.

Finally, leave-one-out sensitivity analyses showed that the exclusion of individual studies did not substantially alter the global estimates for SMD (range: −0.897 to −0.789) or for AUC (range: 0.812 to 0.851), indicating stability in the results. However, heterogeneity (I^2) decreased slightly when certain studies were excluded, particularly Guo et al. (2021) [42] for SMD and Lee et al. (2015) [46] for AUC, suggesting that they contributed more to the observed variability. In addition, the exclusion of studies with imputed data did not significantly alter the association between rCBV and IDH mutational status (SMD = −0.874 vs. −0.865; pooled AUC for studies with reported rCBV cutoff = 0.857 vs. 0.828) and led to a very slight decrease in heterogeneity in SMD (I^2 = 59.2% vs. 62.8%) and a mild decrease in pooled AUC (I^2 = 68.0% vs. 50.6%), suggesting that these studies did not significantly contribute to the observed variability. Figure 11 shows the results of the leave-one-out sensitivity analyses for SMD and AUC.

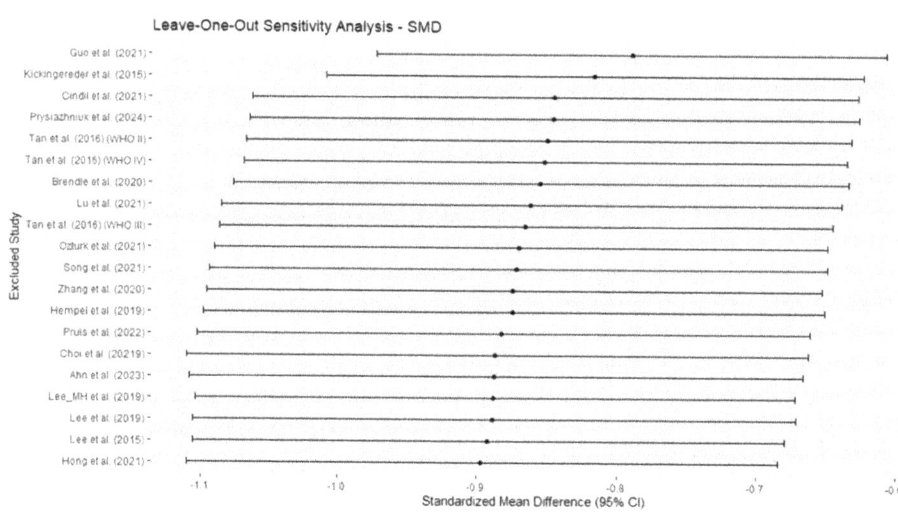

Figure 11. *Cont.*

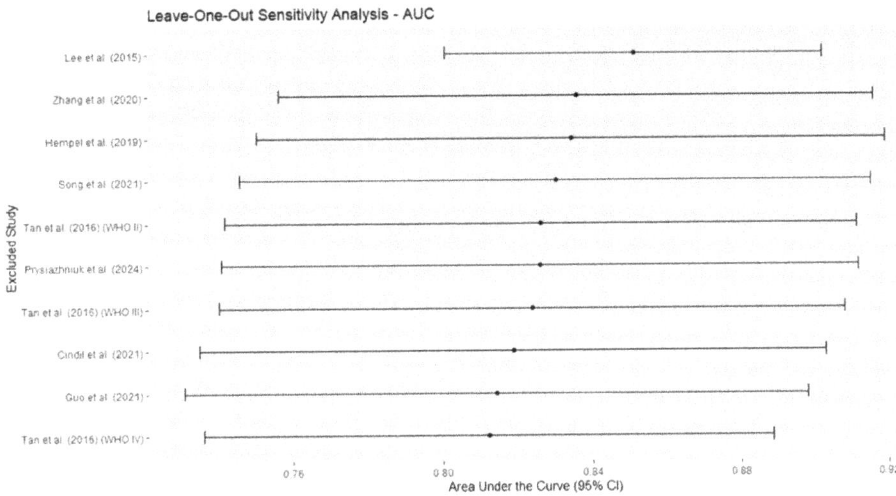

Figure 11. This figure illustrates the results of the leave-one-out sensitivity analysis for the standardized mean difference (SMD) (**top**) and the area under the curve (AUC) (**bottom**). Each point represents the pooled-effect estimate after excluding a single study, with horizontal lines indicating the corresponding 95% confidence intervals (95% CIs). Ahn et al. (2023) [38], Brendle et al. (2020) [39], Choi et al. (2019) [40], Cindil et al. (2022) [41], Guo et al. (2022) [42], Hempel et al. (2018) [43], Hong et al. (2021) [44], Kickingereder et al. (2015) [45], Lee et al. (2015) [46], Lee et al. (2019) [47], Lee_MH et al. (2019) [48], Lu et al. (2021) [49], Ozturk et al. (2021) [50], Prysiazhniuk et al. (2024) [52], Pruis et al. (2022) [51], Song et al. (2020) [53], Tan et al. (2016) (WHO II) [54], Tan et al. (2016) (WHO III) [54], Tan et al. (2016) (WHO IV) [54], Zhang et al. (2020) [55].

4. Discussion

This study focused on evaluating the diagnostic performance of mean rCBV obtained in DSC-MRI to differentiating between IDH-mutant- and IDH-wild-type brain gliomas. We included a total of 18 studies encompassing 1733 patients. We found that, despite moderate heterogeneity, the overall diagnostic accuracy of mean rCBV is high, with pooled sensitivity, specificity and AUC values of approximately 0.80. These results were consistent between different statistical approaches (pooled AUC, sensitivity and specificity, HSROC, and bivariate random-effects meta-analysis). Moreover, our analysis was further supported by a pooled DOR of 14.2, indicating a moderate-to-high discriminative power. In addition, meta-regression analyses did not reveal any significant influence of DSC-MRI acquisition parameters, although a trend toward significance was found for the flip angle. However, the relatively low number of included studies limit the reliability of meta-regression analyses. In sum, this meta-analysis not only supports the utility of mean rCBV to differentiate between IDH-mutant- vs. -wild-type gliomas but also quantifies its diagnostic performance through consistent and complimentary analyses.

Two previous meta-analyses explored the role of DSC-MRI perfusion metrics in predicting IDH mutation status. Van Santwijk et al. [56] conducted a meta-analysis including studies exploring T1-DCE and DSC MRI perfusion parameters in the differentiation of low- and high-grade glioma, as well as IDH mutation status. They included 12 studies with 1384 patients and found that CBV, ktrans, Ve, and Vp values were, in general, significantly higher in IDH-wild-type compared to IDH. The reported AUC for CBV values was 0.85 (95%-CI 0.75–0.93), but only three studies with DSC-MRI were included in their analysis. In addition, they included studies that reported CBV-related values not conventionally used in radiological practice, such as leakage (i.e., CBV-uncorrected—CBV corrected) [57], which represents a notable limitation.

Siakallis et al. [58] reviewed 16 studies including 1819 patients and analyzed a number of CBV-related metrics (e.g., mean rCBV, max rCBV, 75th percentile rCBV) and reported that the highest pooled specificity to differentiate between IDHm and IDHwt was observed for mean rCBV (82%), whereas rCBV 10th percentile showed maximum pooled-sensitivity, AUC, and DOR values (92%, 0.91, and 0 20.96, respectively). However, only two studies reported the latter measure, limiting its generalizability. In clinical practice, most software packages for image post-processing offer mean rCBV values, which seem more intuitive and stable compared to low and high percentiles, which may be affected by errors (e.g., inadequate tumor segmentation).

Our results align with those of the above-mentioned meta-analyses but focused on mean rCBV. Of note, all but one [49] of the included studies in our meta-analysis permitted a reliable estimation of mean rCBV. The study that only reported mean CBV values was only included in the SMD meta-analysis, since the statistical assumptions of this specific analysis allow for using mean CBV—not rCBV—to pool between-group differences. The pooled-sensitivity, specificity, and AUC values for the mean rCBV (80%) reinforce the validity of using mean rCBV as a biomarker for decision-making in clinical and radiological practice.

Nevertheless, the substantial variability found between the included studies calls for caution, since the range of reported AUCs for mean rCBV ranged from almost null (0.50 in Lee et al. (2015) [46]) to almost perfect (0.94 for Tan et al. (2016) [54] in WHO IV patients), and significant heterogeneity (I^2 ranging from 62.8% to 91.8%) was observed. Such variability led us to explore possible modulating factors, particularly DSC-MRI acquisition parameters, which have been previously reported to influence mean rCBV measures. In fact, it is known that different MRI acquisition parameters may influence signal intensity of DSC-MRI perfusion, with subsequent variations in rCBV. For instance, Leu et al. (2017) showed that varying these parameters can impact the estimation of relative cerebral blood volume (rCBV) in gliomas, with different acquisition strategies yielding varying degrees of fidelity in CBV estimation [59]. Siakallis et al. [58] found that shorter TEs and smaller slice gaps were associated with higher sensitivities of mean rCBV.

Meta-regression analyses did not identify a dominant factor explaining this heterogeneity, precluding us from supporting Siakallis et al.'s findings in the specific context of mean rCBV, probably due to the low number of studies. However, we found statistical cues (p = 0.055) that lower flip-angle values are associated with smaller SMDs, suggesting that technical variability may contribute to differences in reported diagnostic performance. In fact, previous studies have found that a lower flip angle can reduce T1-weighting effects from contrast agent leakage, potentially yielding more accurate rCBV estimations in tumors with significant blood–brain barrier disruption [60,61]. Conversely, a higher flip angle may enhance signal-to-noise ratio (SNR), which, based on our results, seems to improve the discriminatory ability of mean rCBV—despite potential bias due to residual T1 effects. Notably, a balance between leakage contamination and SNR can be reached with different acquisition parameter configurations [62]. In sum, the observed trend toward significance in our meta-regression suggests that flip angle is a relevant parameter when standardizing DSC-MRI acquisition protocols for glioma assessment and, future studies should further investigate the impact of flip angle variations on rCBV reproducibility and diagnostic accuracy.

Be that as it may, the lack of standardization in parameter acquisition is evident in the included studies, and this underlying problem is further complicated considering the variability depending upon magnetic field [19], contrast agent doses [63], or imaging post-processing software [64]. In fact, another potential source of bias lies in the post-processing method used in each study, a problem that widely affects a number of neuroimaging-related clinical challenges, both in CT [65] and MRI. Up to seven different software packages were used in the included studies, the most frequent of which was NordicIce. Each of these packages include a specific pipeline and internal algorithms for parameter estimation. Moreover, each software tool may include a variety of post-processing algorithms. For instance, the NeuroPerfusion module of IntelliSpace Portal v. 11.0 (Phillips®) includes four different reconstruction algorithms, namely gamma-variate, model-free, manual AIF, and leakage correction [66]. Each of these reconstruction methods include mathematical nuances that result in different rCBV quantifications. The variability in rCBV based on different post-processing algorithms has also been demonstrated in the literature. For instance, Kudo et al. found that rCBV values of tumor and cutoff values for discriminating low- and high-grade gliomas differed between software packages, suggesting that optimal software-specific cutoff values should be used for diagnosis of high-grade gliomas [67].

Although limited by the relatively low number of included studies, the significant heterogeneity observed, along with existing knowledge on the influence of acquisition parameters (TE, TR, FA, etc.) and post-processing strategies, calls for the need of standardizing DSC-MRI parameter acquisition and harmonization of post-processing methodologies across different software platforms to improve the generalizability of rCBV as a biomarker for IDH mutation status. Multi-center prospective studies using uniform imaging and analysis pipelines will be essential to validate rCBV as a reproducible and clinically actionable biomarker. In sum, there is an emerging need for standardization not only in acquisition parameters but also in post-processing methods.

In the context of brain gliomas, significant efforts have been made to further extend the interpretability of rCBV in biological terms. An outstanding example is represented by studies exploring the so-called tumor vascular habitats, which are linked to different biological tumor features, as demonstrated by transcriptomic correlations [68–70]. For instance, Álvarez-Torres et al. applied complex clustering algorithms to delineate four vascular habitats within brain gliomas and peritumoral edema based on a mixture of rCBV and rCBF data. These vascular habitats are heuristically dichotomized into high and low angiogenic tumor habitats and have been found to significantly differentiate between IDH-wild-type glioblastoma and IDH-mutant astrocytoma [71].

In the current AI paradigm, a number of studies are increasingly exploiting the advantages of machine learning methods to extract information of perfusion MRI metrics that escapes conventional approaches [72]. We excluded these studies, as they are currently circumscribed to the research field, and the variability in methodological approaches precludes withdrawing generalizable conclusions. Notably, the studies by Kickingereder et al. (2015) [45] and Lee et al. (2019) [48] included in our meta-analysis applied machine learning algorithms to improve the diagnostic yield of perfusion MRI in diagnosing IDH mutation status as well as the 1-year overall survival in patients with brain glioma. They found that their developed ML model significantly outperformed the diagnostic yield of rCBV applied as per conventionally performed in clinical practice.

Similarly, radiomics has emerged as a novel methodology to extract meaningful quantitative features from imaging studies [73]. The application of radiomics to predict genomic data (i.e., radiogenomics) has shown promising results in the clinical problem approached in this study [74–76]. For instance, Bhandari et al. [77] found pooled-sensitivity and specificity values close to 90% in predicting IDH and 1p19q codeletion status of brain gliomas. In this context, interesting insights can be drawn from the combination between radiomics and perfusion MRI, since the latter provides temporal information that is absent in conventional MRI sequences [78–80]. Therefore, future meta-analysis should also explore the role of these recently developed approaches.

This study has several limitations: First of all, this meta-analysis aimed to focus on mean rCBV obtained in T2*-DSC perfusion MRI. This specific nature precludes us from withdrawing any conclusion regarding other MRI sequences (e.g., dynamic contrast enhancement, arterial spin labeling) or other rCBV metrics. Second, some studies did not report direct mean rCBV values, which implied the need to estimate them indirectly. Although the formulae applied for such conversion are widely accepted and used in the literature, estimation errors cannot be excluded. Third, although we did not detect significant publication bias, the presence of unpublished studies or studies reporting negative results could still influence the overall conclusions. Finally, some potentially relevant variables, such as the WHO glioma grade, were not considered in our analyses due to the heterogeneity in the edition of the WHO classification among the included studies, which varied from the 2007 edition [54] to the current 2021 edition [52]. These limitations should be overcome in future studies.

5. Conclusions

Mean rCBV is a reliable DSC-MRI parameter for differentiating between IDH-mutated- and IDH-wild-type brain gliomas, with significantly lower values in the former. Pooled sensitivity, specificity and AUC values of 80%, and DOR of 14.21 were observed. However, considerable heterogeneity in acquisition parameters, post-processing methods, and tumor segmentation limit optimal comparability between studies. Our results highlight the need for standardizing DSC-MRI perfusion to establish generalizable cutoff values of mean rCBV.

Supplementary Materials: The supporting information can be downloaded at: https://www.mdpi.com/article/10.3390/diagnostics15070896/s1. Supplementary File S1 (Prisma Checklist); Supplementary Files S2–S4 (Search equations in PubMed, Web of Science and EMBASE, respectively); Supplementary Table S1 (Number of MRI scanners and post-processing information of the included studies); Supplementary Table S2 (Acquisition parameters according to the MRI scanners in each study); Supplementary Table S3 (QUADAS-2 Assessment by items).

Author Contributions: Conceptualization, A.J.L.R.-B. and F.J.P.G.; methodology, A.J.L.R.-B. and J.P.M.B.; software, A.J.L.R.-B. and J.M.B.; validation, J.P.M.B., P.M.J.G. and D.L.C.; formal analysis, A.J.L.R.-B.; investigation, F.J.P.G., A.J.L.R.-B. and D.L.C.; resources, J.M.B.; data curation, P.M.J.G. and M.G.C.; writing—original draft preparation, F.J.P.G.; writing—review and editing, A.J.L.R.-B., J.P.M.B. and G.O.G.; visualization, P.M.J.G. and G.O.G.; supervision, J.P.M.B. and J.M.B.; project administration, A.J.L.R.-B.; funding acquisition, J.M.B. All authors have read and agreed to the published version of the manuscript.

Funding: This research was funded by grant number PID2020-118224RB-I00 and grant number PID2023-151336OB-I00, both funded by MICIU/AIE/10.13039/501100011033 and by FEDER, EU.

Institutional Review Board Statement: Not applicable.

Informed Consent Statement: Not applicable.

Data Availability Statement: All data are available as Supplementary Materials. For specific extracted information of the review process, data are available upon reasonable request to the corresponding author.

Acknowledgments: The authors wish to thank Ángela Rivera Izquierdo for revising the English writing of the manuscript.

Conflicts of Interest: The authors declare no conflicts of interest.

References

1. Price, M.; Ballard, C.; Benedetti, J.; Neff, C.; Cioffi, G.; Waite, K.A.; Kruchko, C.; Barnholtz-Sloan, J.S.; Ostrom, Q.T. CBTRUS Statistical Report: Primary Brain and Other Central Nervous System Tumors Diagnosed in the United States in 2017–2021. *Neuro Oncol.* **2024**, *26*, vi1–vi85. [CrossRef] [PubMed]
2. Ostrom, Q.T.; Bauchet, L.; Davis, F.G.; Deltour, I.; Fisher, J.L.; Langer, C.E.; Pekmezci, M.; Schwartzbaum, J.A.; Turner, M.C.; Walsh, K.M.; et al. The Epidemiology of Glioma in Adults: A "State of the Science" Review. *Neuro Oncol.* **2014**, *16*, 896–913. [CrossRef] [PubMed]
3. Louis, D.N.; Perry, A.; Reifenberger, G.; von Deimling, A.; Figarella-Branger, D.; Cavenee, W.K.; Ohgaki, H.; Wiestler, O.D.; Kleihues, P.; Ellison, D.W. The 2016 World Health Organization Classification of Tumors of the Central Nervous System: A Summary. *Acta Neuropathol.* **2016**, *131*, 803–820. [CrossRef]
4. Gritsch, S.; Batchelor, T.T.; Gonzalez Castro, L.N. Diagnostic, Therapeutic, and Prognostic Implications of the 2021 World Health Organization Classification of Tumors of the Central Nervous System. *Cancer* **2022**, *128*, 47–58. [CrossRef]
5. Nabors, L.B.; Portnow, J.; Ahluwalia, M.; Baehring, J.; Brem, H.; Brem, S.; Butowski, N.; Campian, J.L.; Clark, S.W.; Fabiano, A.J.; et al. Central Nervous System Cancers, Version 3.2020, NCCN Clinical Practice Guidelines in Oncology. *J. Natl. Compr. Cancer Netw.* **2020**, *18*, 1537–1570. [CrossRef]
6. Riche, M.; Marijon, P.; Amelot, A.; Bielle, F.; Mokhtari, K.; Chambrun, M.P.d.; Le Joncour, A.; Idbaih, A.; Touat, M.; Do, C.-H.; et al. Severity, Timeline, and Management of Complications after Stereotactic Brain Biopsy. *J. Neurosurg.* **2022**, *136*, 867–876. [CrossRef]
7. Mikkelsen, V.E.; Solheim, O.; Salvesen, Ø.; Torp, S.H. The Histological Representativeness of Glioblastoma Tissue Samples. *Acta Neurochir.* **2021**, *163*, 1911–1920. [CrossRef]
8. Kang, K.M.; Song, J.; Choi, Y.; Park, C.; Park, J.E.; Kim, H.S.; Park, S.-H.; Park, C.-K.; Choi, S.H. MRI Scoring Systems for Predicting Isocitrate Dehydrogenase Mutation and Chromosome 1p/19q Codeletion in Adult-Type Diffuse Glioma Lacking Contrast Enhancement. *Radiology* **2024**, *311*, e233120. [CrossRef]
9. Bonm, A.V.; Ritterbusch, R.; Throckmorton, P.; Graber, J.J. Clinical Imaging for Diagnostic Challenges in the Management of Gliomas: A Review. *J. Neuroimaging* **2020**, *30*, 139–145. [CrossRef]
10. Hirschler, L.; Sollmann, N.; Schmitz-Abecassis, B.; Pinto, J.; Arzanforoosh, F.; Barkhof, F.; Booth, T.; Calvo-Imirizaldu, M.; Cassia, G.; Chmelik, M.; et al. Advanced MR Techniques for Preoperative Glioma Characterization: Part 1. *J. Magn. Reson. Imaging* **2023**, *57*, 1655–1675. [CrossRef]
11. Wu, H.; Tong, H.; Du, X.; Guo, H.; Ma, Q.; Zhang, Y.; Zhou, X.; Liu, H.; Wang, S.; Fang, J.; et al. Vascular Habitat Analysis Based on Dynamic Susceptibility Contrast Perfusion MRI Predicts IDH Mutation Status and Prognosis in High-Grade Gliomas. *Eur. Radiol.* **2020**, *30*, 3254–3265. [CrossRef] [PubMed]
12. Venugopal, K.; Arzanforoosh, F.; van Dorth, D.; Smits, M.; van Osch, M.J.P.; Hernandez-Tamames, J.A.A.; Warnert, E.A.H.; Poot, D.H.J. MR Vascular Fingerprinting with Hybrid Gradient-Spin Echo Dynamic Susceptibility Contrast MRI for Characterization of Microvasculature in Gliomas. *Cancers* **2023**, *15*, 2180. [CrossRef] [PubMed]
13. Fu, R.; Szidonya, L.; Barajas, R.F.J.; Ambady, P.; Varallyay, C.; Neuwelt, E.A. Diagnostic Performance of DSC Perfusion MRI to Distinguish Tumor Progression and Treatment-Related Changes: A Systematic Review and Meta-Analysis. *Neurooncol. Adv.* **2022**, *4*, vdac027. [CrossRef] [PubMed]
14. Arzanforoosh, F.; Croal, P.L.; van Garderen, K.A.; Smits, M.; Chappell, M.A.; Warnert, E.A.H. Effect of Applying Leakage Correction on RCBV Measurement Derived From DSC-MRI in Enhancing and Nonenhancing Glioma. *Front. Oncol.* **2021**, *11*, 648528. [CrossRef]
15. Cha, S.; Lu, S.; Johnson, G.; Knopp, E.A. Dynamic Susceptibility Contrast MR Imaging: Correlation of Signal Intensity Changes with Cerebral Blood Volume Measurements. *J. Magn. Reson. Imaging* **2000**, *11*, 114–119. [CrossRef]
16. Price, S.J.; Green, H.A.L.; Dean, A.F.; Joseph, J.; Hutchinson, P.J.; Gillard, J.H. Correlation of MR Relative Cerebral Blood Volume Measurements with Cellular Density and Proliferation in High-Grade Gliomas: An Image-Guided Biopsy Study. *Am. J. Neuroradiol.* **2011**, *32*, 501–506. [CrossRef]
17. Shiroishi, M.S.; Erickson, B.J.; Hu, L.S.; Barboriak, D.P.; Becerra, L.; Bell, L.C.; Boss, M.A.; Boxerman, J.L.; Cen, S.; Cimino, L.; et al. The QIBA Profile for Dynamic Susceptibility Contrast MRI Quantitative Imaging Biomarkers for Assessing Gliomas. *Radiology* **2024**, *313*, e232555. [CrossRef]
18. Tyurina, A.N.; Vikhrova, N.B.; Batalov, A.I.; Kalaeva, D.B.; Shults, E.I.; Postnov, A.A.; Pronin, I.N. Radiological Biomarkers of Brain Gliomas. *Zh. Vopr. Neirokhir. Im. N. N. Burdenko* **2022**, *86*, 121–126. [CrossRef]
19. Shiroishi, M.S.; Weinert, D.; Cen, S.Y.; Varghese, B.; Dondlinger, T.; Prah, M.; Mendoza, J.; Nazemi, S.; Ameli, N.; Amini, N.; et al. A Cross-Sectional Study to Test Equivalence of Low- versus Intermediate-Flip Angle Dynamic Susceptibility Contrast MRI Measures of Relative Cerebral Blood Volume in Patients with High-Grade Gliomas at 1.5 Tesla Field Strength. *Front. Oncol.* **2023**, *13*, 1156843. [CrossRef]

20. Jain, R.; Poisson, L.; Narang, J.; Gutman, D.; Scarpace, L.; Hwang, S.N.; Holder, C.; Wintermark, M.; Colen, R.R.; Kirby, J.; et al. Genomic Mapping and Survival Prediction in Glioblastoma: Molecular Subclassification Strengthened by Hemodynamic Imaging Biomarkers. *Radiology* **2013**, *267*, 212–220. [CrossRef]
21. Pons-Escoda, A.; Garcia-Ruiz, A.; Naval-Baudin, P.; Martinez-Zalacain, I.; Castell, J.; Camins, A.; Vidal, N.; Bruna, J.; Cos, M.; Perez-Lopez, R.; et al. Differentiating IDH-Mutant Astrocytomas and 1p19q-Codeleted Oligodendrogliomas Using DSC-PWI: High Performance through Cerebral Blood Volume and Percentage of Signal Recovery Percentiles. *Eur. Radiol.* **2024**, *34*, 5320–5330. [CrossRef] [PubMed]
22. Welker, K.; Boxerman, J.; Kalnin, A.; Kaufmann, T.; Shiroishi, M.; Wintermark, M. ASFNR Recommendations for Clinical Performance of MR Dynamic Susceptibility Contrast Perfusion Imaging of the Brain. *Am. J. Neuroradiol.* **2015**, *36*, E41–E51. [CrossRef] [PubMed]
23. Page, M.J.; McKenzie, J.E.; Bossuyt, P.M.; Boutron, I.; Hoffmann, T.C.; Mulrow, C.D.; Shamseer, L.; Tetzlaff, J.M.; Akl, E.A.; Brennan, S.E.; et al. The PRISMA 2020 Statement: An Updated Guideline for Reporting Systematic Reviews. *BMJ* **2021**, *372*, n71. [CrossRef] [PubMed]
24. Láinez Ramos-Bossini, A. Relative Cerebral Blood Volume Derived from Dynamic Contrast Enhancement Perfusion MRI in Predicting IDH Mutation Status of Brain Gliomas. Protocol for a Systematic Review and Meta-Analysis. *Syst. Rev.* **2022**, *16*, 143.
25. Whiting, P.F.; Rutjes, A.W.S.; Westwood, M.E.; Mallett, S.; Deeks, J.J.; Reitsma, J.B.; Leeflang, M.M.G.; Sterne, J.A.C.; Bossuyt, P.M.M. QUADAS-2: A Revised Tool for the Quality Assessment of Diagnostic Accuracy Studies. *Ann. Intern. Med.* **2011**, *155*, 529–536. [CrossRef]
26. Plot Digitizer. Free Online Tool. Available online: https://plotdigitizer.com/app (accessed on 2 February 2025).
27. Deeks, J.J.; Higgins, J.P.T.; Altman, D.G. (Eds.) *Chapter 10: Analysing Data and Undertaking Meta-Analyses*; Cochrane: London, UK, 2023.
28. Higgins, J.P.T.; Li, T.; Deeks, J.J. (Eds.) *Chapter 6: Choosing Effect Measures and Computing Estimates of Effect*; Cochrane: London, UK, 2021.
29. Wan, X.; Wang, W.; Liu, J.; Tong, T. Estimating the Sample Mean and Standard Deviation from the Sample Size, Median, Range and/or Interquartile Range. *BMC Med. Res. Methodol.* **2014**, *14*, 135. [CrossRef]
30. Hanley, J.A.; McNeil, B.J. The Meaning and Use of the Area under a Receiver Operating Characteristic (ROC) Curve. *Radiology* **1982**, *143*, 29–36. [CrossRef]
31. Kawabata, E.; Major-Smith, D.; Clayton, G.L.; Shapland, C.Y.; Morris, T.P.; Carter, A.R.; Fernández-Sanlés, A.; Borges, M.C.; Tilling, K.; Griffith, G.J.; et al. Accounting for Bias Due to Outcome Data Missing Not at Random: Comparison and Illustration of Two Approaches to Probabilistic Bias Analysis: A Simulation Study. *BMC Med. Res. Methodol.* **2024**, *24*, 278. [CrossRef]
32. Hai, Y.; Qin, G. Direct Estimation of the Area under the Receiver Operating Characteristic Curve with Verification Biased Data. *Stat. Med.* **2020**, *39*, 4789–4820. [CrossRef]
33. Zhou, X.; Obuchowski, N.; McClish, D. *Statistical Methods in Diagnostic Medicine*; John Wiley & Sons, Inc.: Hoboken, NJ, USA, 2002; ISBN 9780471347729.
34. Lainez Ramos-Bossini, A.J.; Lopez Zuniga, D.; Ruiz Santiago, F.; Láinez Ramos-Bossini, A.J.; López Zúñiga, D.; Ruiz Santiago, F. Percutaneous Vertebroplasty versus Conservative Treatment and Placebo in Osteoporotic Vertebral Fractures: Meta-Analysis and Critical Review of the Literature. *Eur. Radiol.* **2021**, *31*, 8542–8553. [CrossRef]
35. Láinez Ramos-Bossini, A.J.; Gámez Martínez, A.; Luengo Gómez, D.; Valverde-López, F.; Melguizo, C.; Prados, J. Prevalence of Sarcopenia Determined by Computed Tomography in Pancreatic Cancer: A Systematic Review and Meta-Analysis of Observational Studies. *Cancers* **2024**, *16*, 3356. [CrossRef] [PubMed]
36. Láinez Ramos-Bossini, A.J.; Gámez Martínez, A.; Luengo Gómez, D.; Valverde-López, F.; Morillo Gil, A.J.; González Flores, E.; Salmerón Ruiz, Á.; Jiménez Gutiérrez, P.M.; Melguizo, C.; Prados, J. Computed Tomography-Based Sarcopenia and Pancreatic Cancer Survival-A Comprehensive Meta-Analysis Exploring the Influence of Definition Criteria, Prevalence, and Treatment Intention. *Cancers* **2025**, *17*, 607. [CrossRef] [PubMed]
37. Láinez Ramos-Bossini, A.; Jiménez Gutiérerz, P.; Moraleda Cabrera, B.; Bueno Caravacal, L.; González Díez, M.; Ruiz Santiago, F. Risk of New Vertebral Compression Fractures and Serious Adverse Effects after Vertebroplasty. A Systematic, Critical Review and Meta-Analysis of Randomized Controlled Trials. *Quant. Imaging Med. Surg.* **2024**, *14*, 7848–7861. [CrossRef]
38. Ahn, S.H.; Ahn, S.S.; Park, Y.W.; Park, C.J.; Lee, S.-K. Association of Dynamic Susceptibility Contrast- and Dynamic Contrast-Enhanced Magnetic Resonance Imaging Parameters with Molecular Marker Status in Lower-Grade Gliomas: A Retrospective Study. *Neuroradiol. J.* **2023**, *36*, 49–58. [CrossRef]
39. Brendle, C.; Klose, U.; Hempel, J.-M.; Schittenhelm, J.; Skardelly, M.; Tabatabai, G.; Ernemann, U.; Bender, B. Association of Dynamic Susceptibility Magnetic Resonance Imaging at Initial Tumor Diagnosis with the Prognosis of Different Molecular Glioma Subtypes. *Neurol. Sci.* **2020**, *41*, 3625–3632. [CrossRef]

40. Choi, K.S.; Choi, S.H.; Jeong, B. Prediction of IDH Genotype in Gliomas with Dynamic Susceptibility Contrast Perfusion MR Imaging Using an Explainable Recurrent Neural Network. *Neuro Oncol.* **2019**, *21*, 1197–1209. [CrossRef]
41. Cindil, E.; Sendur, H.N.; Cerit, M.N.; Erdogan, N.; Celebi, F.; Dag, N.; Celtikci, E.; Inan, A.; Oner, Y.; Tali, T. Prediction of IDH Mutation Status in High-Grade Gliomas Using DWI and High T1-Weight DSC-MRI. *Acad. Radiol.* **2022**, *29*, S52–S62. [CrossRef]
42. Guo, L.; Li, X.; Cao, H.; Hua, J.; Mei, Y.; Pillai, J.J.; Wu, Y. Inflow-Based Vascular-Space-Occupancy (IVASO) Might Potentially Predict IDH Mutation Status and Tumor Grade in Diffuse Cerebral Gliomas. *J. Neuroradiol.* **2022**, *49*, 267–274. [CrossRef]
43. Brendle, C.; Hempel, J.-M.; Schittenhelm, J.; Skardelly, M.; Tabatabai, G.; Bender, B.; Ernemann, U.; Klose, U. Glioma Grading and Determination of *IDH* Mutation Status and *ATRX* Loss by DCE and ASL Perfusion. *Clin. Neuroradiol.* **2018**, *28*, 421–428. [CrossRef]
44. Hong, E.K.; Choi, S.H.; Shin, D.J.; Jo, S.W.; Yoo, R.-E.; Kang, K.M.; Yun, T.J.; Kim, J.; Sohn, C.-H.; Park, S.-H.; et al. Comparison of Genetic Profiles and Prognosis of High-Grade Gliomas Using Quantitative and Qualitative MRI Features: A Focus on G3 Gliomas. *Korean J. Radiol.* **2021**, *22*, 233–242. [CrossRef]
45. Kickingereder, P.; Bonekamp, D.; Nowosielski, M.; Kratz, A.; Sill, M.; Burth, S.; Wick, A.; Eidel, O.; Schlemmer, H.-P.; Radbruch, A.; et al. Radiogenomics of Glioblastoma: Machine Learning-Based Classification of Molecular Characteristics by Using Multiparametric and Multiregional MR Imaging Features. *Radiology* **2016**, *281*, 907–918. [CrossRef] [PubMed]
46. Lee, S.; Choi, S.H.; Ryoo, I.; Yoon, T.J.; Kim, T.M.; Lee, S.-H.; Park, C.-K.; Kim, J.-H.; Sohn, C.-H.; Park, S.-H.; et al. Evaluation of the Microenvironmental Heterogeneity in High-Grade Gliomas with IDH1/2 Gene Mutation Using Histogram Analysis of Diffusion-Weighted Imaging and Dynamic-Susceptibility Contrast Perfusion Imaging. *J. Neurooncol.* **2015**, *121*, 141–150. [CrossRef] [PubMed]
47. Lee, M.K.; Park, J.E.; Jo, Y.; Park, S.Y.; Kim, S.J.; Kim, H.S. Advanced Imaging Parameters Improve the Prediction of Diffuse Lower-Grade Gliomas Subtype, IDH Mutant with No 1p19q Codeletion: Added Value to the T2/FLAIR Mismatch Sign. *Eur. Radiol.* **2020**, *30*, 844–854. [CrossRef] [PubMed]
48. Lee, M.H.; Kim, J.; Kim, S.-T.; Shin, H.-M.; You, H.-J.; Choi, J.W.; Seol, H.J.; Nam, D.-H.; Lee, J.-I.; Kong, D.-S. Prediction of IDH1 Mutation Status in Glioblastoma Using Machine Learning Technique Based on Quantitative Radiomic Data. *World Neurosurg.* **2019**, *125*, e688–e696. [CrossRef]
49. Lu, J.; Li, X.; Li, H. Perfusion Parameters Derived from MRI for Preoperative Prediction of IDH Mutation and MGMT Promoter Methylation Status in Glioblastomas. *Magn. Reson. Imaging* **2021**, *83*, 189–195. [CrossRef]
50. Ozturk, K.; Soylu, E.; Tolunay, S.; Narter, S.; Hakyemez, B. Dynamic Contrast-Enhanced T1-Weighted Perfusion Magnetic Resonance Imaging Identifies Glioblastoma Immunohistochemical Biomarkers via Tumoral and Peritumoral Approach: A Pilot Study. *World Neurosurg.* **2019**, *128*, e195–e208. [CrossRef]
51. Pruis, I.J.; Koene, S.R.; van der Voort, S.R.; Incekara, F.; Vincent, A.J.P.E.; van den Bent, M.J.; Lycklama À Nijeholt, G.J.; Nandoe Tewarie, R.D.S.; Veldhuijzen van Zanten, S.E.M.; Smits, M. Noninvasive Differentiation of Molecular Subtypes of Adult Nonenhancing Glioma Using MRI Perfusion and Diffusion Parameters. *Neurooncol. Adv.* **2022**, *4*, vdac023. [CrossRef]
52. Prysiazhniuk, Y.; Server, A.; Leske, H.; Bech-Aase, Ø.; Helseth, E.; Eijgelaar, R.S.; Fuster-García, E.; Brandal, P.; Bjørnerud, A.; Otáhal, J.; et al. Diffuse Glioma Molecular Profiling with Arterial Spin Labeling and Dynamic Susceptibility Contrast Perfusion MRI: A Comparative Study. *Neurooncol. Adv.* **2024**, *6*, vdae113. [CrossRef]
53. Song, S.; Wang, L.; Yang, H.; Shan, Y.; Cheng, Y.; Xu, L.; Dong, C.; Zhao, G.; Lu, J. Static (18)F-FET PET and DSC-PWI Based on Hybrid PET/MR for the Prediction of Gliomas Defined by IDH and 1p/19q Status. *Eur. Radiol.* **2021**, *31*, 4087–4096. [CrossRef]
54. Tan, W.; Xiong, J.; Huang, W.; Wu, J.; Zhan, S.; Geng, D. Noninvasively Detecting Isocitrate Dehydrogenase 1 Gene Status in Astrocytoma by Dynamic Susceptibility Contrast MRI. *J. Magn. Reson. Imaging* **2017**, *45*, 492–499. [CrossRef]
55. Zhang, H.-W.; Lyu, G.-W.; He, W.-J.; Lei, Y.; Lin, F.; Wang, M.-Z.; Zhang, H.; Liang, L.-H.; Feng, Y.-N.; Yang, J.-H. DSC and DCE Histogram Analyses of Glioma Biomarkers, Including IDH, MGMT, and TERT, on Differentiation and Survival. *Acad. Radiol.* **2020**, *27*, e263–e271. [CrossRef] [PubMed]
56. van Santwijk, L.; Kouwenberg, V.; Meijer, F.; Smits, M.; Henssen, D. A Systematic Review and Meta-Analysis on the Differentiation of Glioma Grade and Mutational Status by Use of Perfusion-Based Magnetic Resonance Imaging. *Insights Imaging* **2022**, *13*, 102. [CrossRef] [PubMed]
57. Hilario, A.; Hernandez-Lain, A.; Sepulveda, J.M.; Lagares, A.; Perez-Nuñez, A.; Ramos, A. Perfusion MRI Grading Diffuse Gliomas: Impact of Permeability Parameters on Molecular Biomarkers and Survival. *Neurocirugia (Engl. Ed.)* **2019**, *30*, 11–18. [CrossRef]
58. Siakallis, L.; Topriceanu, C.-C.; Panovska-Griffiths, J.; Bisdas, S. The Role of DSC MR Perfusion in Predicting IDH Mutation and 1p19q Codeletion Status in Gliomas: Meta-Analysis and Technical Considerations. *Neuroradiology* **2023**, *65*, 1111–1126. [CrossRef]

59. Leu, K.; Boxerman, J.L.; Ellingson, B.M. Effects of MRI Protocol Parameters, Preload Injection Dose, Fractionation Strategies, and Leakage Correction Algorithms on the Fidelity of Dynamic-Susceptibility Contrast MRI Estimates of Relative Cerebral Blood Volume in Gliomas. *Am. J. Neuroradiol.* **2017**, *38*, 478–484. [CrossRef]
60. Cha, S.; Knopp, E.A.; Johnson, G.; Wetzel, S.G.; Litt, A.W.; Zagzag, D. Intracranial Mass Lesions: Dynamic Contrast-Enhanced Susceptibility-Weighted Echo-Planar Perfusion MR Imaging. *Radiology* **2002**, *223*, 11–29. [CrossRef]
61. Boxerman, J.L.; Schmainda, K.M.; Weisskoff, R.M. Relative Cerebral Blood Volume Maps Corrected for Contrast Agent Extravasation Significantly Correlate with Glioma Tumor Grade, Whereas Uncorrected Maps Do Not. *Am. J. Neuroradiol.* **2006**, *27*, 859–867.
62. Boxerman, J.L.; Quarles, C.C.; Hu, L.S.; Erickson, B.J.; Gerstner, E.R.; Smits, M.; Kaufmann, T.J.; Barboriak, D.P.; Huang, R.H.; Wick, W.; et al. Consensus Recommendations for a Dynamic Susceptibility Contrast MRI Protocol for Use in High-Grade Gliomas. *Neuro Oncol.* **2020**, *22*, 1262–1275. [CrossRef]
63. Alger, J.R.; Schaewe, T.J.; Lai, T.C.; Frew, A.J.; Vespa, P.M.; Etchepare, M.; Liebeskind, D.S.; Saver, J.L.; Kidwell, S.C. Contrast Agent Dose Effects in Cerebral Dynamic Susceptibility Contrast Magnetic Resonance Perfusion Imaging. *J. Magn. Reson. Imaging* **2009**, *29*, 52–64. [CrossRef]
64. Wang, C.; Liu, F.; Zhang, L.; Song, Y.; Pan, Z.; Li, G.; Bian, H.; Yuan, X. Comparison of Normalized Cerebral Blood Flow between Different Post-Processing Methods of Dynamic Susceptibility Contrast Perfusion-Weighted Imaging and Arterial Spin Labeling in Gliomas with Different Grading. *Quant. Imaging Med. Surg.* **2024**, *14*, 8720–8733. [CrossRef]
65. Yao, Y.; Gu, S.; Liu, J.; Li, J.; Wu, J.; Luo, T.; Li, Y.; Ge, B.; Wang, J. Comparison of Three Algorithms for Predicting Infarct Volume in Patients with Acute Ischemic Stroke by CT Perfusion Software: Bayesian, CSVD, and OSVD. *Diagnostics* **2023**, *13*, 1810. [CrossRef] [PubMed]
66. Vankayalapati, S.; Kulanthaivelu, K.; Lanka, V.; Chakrabarti, D.; Saini, J.; Bhat, M.; Prasad, C.; Pendharkar, H.; Kotwal, A.; Mangla, R.; et al. Quantitative Characterization of Tumoural Leakage Phenomena Using Dynamic Susceptibility Contrast Perfusion Imaging. *Res. Sq.* **2021**. [CrossRef]
67. Kudo, K.; Uwano, I.; Hirai, T.; Murakami, R.; Nakamura, H.; Fujima, N.; Yamashita, F.; Goodwin, J.; Higuchi, S.; Sasaki, M. Comparison of Different Post-Processing Algorithms for Dynamic Susceptibility Contrast Perfusion Imaging of Cerebral Gliomas. *Magn. Reson. Med. Sci.* **2017**, *16*, 129–136. [CrossRef]
68. Chelebian, E.; Fuster-Garcia, E.; Álvarez-Torres, M.D.M.; Juan-Albarracín, J.; García-Gómez, J.M. Higher Vascularity at Infiltrated Peripheral Edema Differentiates Proneural Glioblastoma Subtype. *PLoS ONE* **2020**, *15*, e0232500. [CrossRef]
69. Del Mar Álvarez-Torres, M.; Fuster-García, E.; Juan-Albarracín, J.; Puig, J.; Balaña, C.; Capellades, J.; Emblem, K.E.; García-Gómez, J.M. Differential Effect of MGMT Methylation between Moderate or High Vascular Profile in IDH Wildtype Glioblastoma. *Cancer Res.* **2021**, *81*, 2654. [CrossRef]
70. Del Mar Álvarez-Torres, M.; Juan-Albarracín, J.; Fuster-Garcia, E.; Bellvís-Bataller, F.; Lorente, D.; Reynés, G.; Font de Mora, J.; Aparici-Robles, F.; Botella, C.; Muñoz-Langa, J.; et al. Robust Association between Vascular Habitats and Patient Prognosis in Glioblastoma: An International Multicenter Study. *J. Magn. Reson. Imaging* **2020**, *51*, 1478–1486. [CrossRef]
71. Álvarez-Torres, M.D.M.; López-Cerdán, A.; Andreu, Z.; de la Iglesia Vayá, M.; Fuster-Garcia, E.; García-García, F.; García-Gómez, J.M. Vascular Differences between IDH-Wildtype Glioblastoma and Astrocytoma IDH-Mutant Grade 4 at Imaging and Transcriptomic Levels. *NMR Biomed.* **2023**, *36*, e5004. [CrossRef]
72. Emblem, K.E.; Due-Tonnessen, P.; Hald, J.K.; Bjornerud, A.; Pinho, M.C.; Scheie, D.; Schad, L.R.; Meling, T.R.; Zoellner, F.G. Machine Learning in Preoperative Glioma MRI: Survival Associations by Perfusion-Based Support Vector Machine Outperforms Traditional MRI. *J. Magn. Reson. Imaging* **2014**, *40*, 47–54. [CrossRef]
73. Mayerhoefer, M.E.; Materka, A.; Langs, G.; Häggström, I.; Szczypiński, P.; Gibbs, P.; Cook, G. Introduction to Radiomics. *J. Nucl. Med.* **2020**, *61*, 488–495. [CrossRef]
74. Su, C.-Q.; Chen, X.-T.; Duan, S.-F.; Zhang, J.-X.; You, Y.-P.; Lu, S.-S.; Hong, X.-N. A Radiomics-Based Model to Differentiate Glioblastoma from Solitary Brain Metastases. *Clin. Radiol.* **2021**, *76*, 629.e11–629.e18. [CrossRef]
75. Acquitter, C.; Piram, L.; Sabatini, U.; Gilhodes, J.; Cohen-Jonathan, E.M.; Ken, S.; Lemasson, B. Radiomics-Based Detection of Radionecrosis Using Harmonized Multiparametric MRI. *Cancers* **2022**, *14*, 286. [CrossRef] [PubMed]
76. Foltyn-Dumitru, M.; Schell, M.; Rastogi, A.; Sahm, F.; Kessler, T.; Wick, W.; Bendszus, M.; Brugnara, G.; Vollmuth, P. Impact of Signal Intensity Normalization of MRI on the Generalizability of Radiomic-Based Prediction of Molecular Glioma Subtypes. *Eur. Radiol.* **2024**, *34*, 2782–2790. [CrossRef] [PubMed]
77. Bhandari, A.P.; Liong, R.; Koppen, J.; Murthy, S.V.; Lasocki, A. Noninvasive Determination of IDH and 1p19q Status of Lower-Grade Gliomas Using MRI Radiomics: A Systematic Review. *Am. J. Neuroradiol.* **2021**, *42*, 94–101. [CrossRef] [PubMed]
78. Hashido, T.; Saito, S.; Ishida, T. A Radiomics-Based Comparative Study on Arterial Spin Labeling and Dynamic Susceptibility Contrast Perfusion-Weighted Imaging in Gliomas. *Sci. Rep.* **2020**, *10*, 6121. [CrossRef]

79. Crisi, G.; Filice, S. Predicting MGMT Promoter Methylation of Glioblastoma from Dynamic Susceptibility Contrast Perfusion: A Radiomic Approach. *J. Neuroimaging* **2020**, *30*, 458–462. [CrossRef]
80. Parvaze, S.; Bhattacharjee, R.; Singh, A.; Ahlawat, S.; Patir, R.; Vaishya, S.; Shah, T.J.; Gupta, R.K. Radiomics-Based Evaluation and Possible Characterization of Dynamic Contrast Enhanced (DCE) Perfusion Derived Different Sub-Regions of Glioblastoma. *Eur. J. Radiol.* **2023**, *159*, 110655. [CrossRef]

diagnostics

MDPI

Case Report

Hybrid Positron Emission Tomography and Magnetic Resonance Imaging Guided Microsurgical Management of Glial Tumors: Case Series and Review of the Literature

Yusuf Sukru Caglar [1], Murat Buyuktepe [1,2,*], Emre Yagiz Sayaci [1], Ihsan Dogan [1], Melih Bozkurt [1,3], Elif Peker [4], Cigdem Soydal [5], Elgin Ozkan [5] and Nuriye Ozlem Kucuk [5]

1 Department of Neurosurgery, Ankara University School of Medicine, 06230 Ankara, Turkey; scaglar@ankara.edu.tr (Y.S.C.); emresa89@gmail.com (E.Y.S.); ihsandogan@ankara.edu.tr (I.D.)
2 Department of Neurosurgery, Unye State Hospital, 05230 Ordu, Turkey
3 Department of Neurosurgery, Memorial Bahcelievler Hospital, 34180 Istanbul, Turkey; melihbozkurt@hotmail.com
4 Department of Radiology, Ankara University School of Medicine, 06230 Ankara, Turkey; epeker@ankara.edu.tr
5 Department of Nuclear Medicine, Ankara University School of Medicine, 06230 Ankara, Turkey; csoydal@ankara.edu.tr (C.S.); eozkan@ankara.edu.tr (E.O.); okucuk@medicine.ankara.edu.tr (N.O.K.)
* Correspondence: muratbuyuktepe@hotmail.com; Tel.: +90-535-0581-467

Abstract: In this case series, we aimed to report our clinical experience with hybrid positron emission tomography (PET) and magnetic resonance imaging (MRI) navigation in the management of recurrent glial brain tumors. Consecutive recurrent neuroglial brain tumor patients who underwent PET/MRI at preoperative or intraoperative periods were included, whereas patients with non-glial intracranial tumors including metastasis, lymphoma and meningioma were excluded from the study. A total of eight patients (mean age 50.1 ± 11.0 years) with suspicion of recurrent glioma tumor were evaluated. Gross total tumor resection of the PET/MRI-positive area was achieved in seven patients, whereas one patient was diagnosed with radiation necrosis, and surgery was avoided. All patients survived at 1-year follow-up. Five (71.4%) of the recurrent patients remained free of recurrence for the entire follow-up period. Two patients with glioblastoma had tumor recurrence at the postoperative sixth and eighth months. According to our results, hybrid PET/MRI provides reliable and accurate information to distinguish recurrent glial tumor from radiation necrosis. With the help of this differential diagnosis, hybrid imaging may provide the gross total resection of recurrent tumors without harming eloquent brain areas.

Keywords: hybrid imaging; magnetic resonance imaging; positron emission tomography; radiation necrosis; recurrent glial tumor

1. Introduction

Gliomas are the most common malignant tumors of the brain, accounting for approximately 80% of all cancers in the central nervous system, and the incidence has risen in recent decades with improved diagnostic imaging [1,2]. The main differential diagnoses of gliomas are lymphoma, metastasis and inflammatory/infectious diseases. The standard care of high-grade gliomas comprises early detection and maximum safe surgical resection followed by postoperative chemoradiotherapy [3]. Despite the advancements in diagnosis and treatment, the survival of those with brain tumors still remains poor [4,5]. In addition to patient characteristics including age and Karnofsky score, the histological subtype of tumor, the level of differentiation and extent of tumor removal are important prognostic factors [5–8]. Since the interaction of tumors with eloquent brain areas mainly determines the surgical approach and, thereby, extent of tumor removal, there have been increasing demands on preoperative imaging methods revealing overall extensions of tumor tissue. It is also important to evaluate the presence of residual tumor tissue intraoperatively, as well as to differentiate tumor recurrence from pseudorecurrence and radiation necrosis in the follow-up period.

Magnetic resonance imaging (MRI) and positron emission tomography (PET) are well-established imaging modalities that are widely used in neuro-oncology. However, considering brain tumors with structural, functional or metabolic information only is inadequate for pathologic estimation and treatment planning. As both techniques are complementary and essential for diagnosis and follow-up, hybrid multimodal imaging with integrated PET/MRI might have the potential to improve glioma management [9].

In this preliminary study, we aimed to report our experience with hybrid PET/MRI navigation in the management of recurrent brain tumors.

2. Materials and Methods

This study was approved by the IRB Committee of the Ankara University (Date: 21 May 2021, Number: I5-318-21). Written informed consent was obtained from each patient before enrollment, and this study adhered to the tenets of the Declaration of Helsinki.

In this case series study, consecutive high-grade glioma patients who had been treated with total or gross total resection surgery followed by chemoradiotherapy were evaluated. Patients with a high index of suspicion for glioma recurrence during the follow-up period who also underwent a hybrid PET/MRI scan at our hospital from October 2018 to May 2021 were included in the study. Patients with non-glial intracranial tumors including metastasis, lymphoma and meningioma were excluded from the study. Hybrid images were used for differential diagnosis, treatment planning and intraoperative guidance.

All patients underwent PET/MRI on a fully integrated General Electric system Signa PET/MRI with a head coil (General Electric Healthcare, Chicago, IL, USA). This system is equipped with a 3-T magnet and a high-resolution PET detector, integrated with Time-Of-Flight (TOF) technology, and provides the simultaneous acquisition of PET and MRI data [10]. The PET/MRI scans were performed 45 min after the intravenous administration of ^{18}F-fluorodeoxyglucose (FDG), during which the patients rested in a quiet room. At least 6 h of fasting was required prior to its administration. The patients were placed in the scanner, and contiguous transaxial slices were obtained.

For PET/MRI neuronavigation, all the patients included in the study had T2-weighted propeller axial images (TR: 3570, TE:110, FOV: 240, slice thickness/gap:5/0.5), sagittal 3D FLAIR images (TR > 6000, TE:105, TI: 1500–1800, FOV: 260, slice thickness/gap:1.2/0) and pre- and post-contrast sagittal 3DT1WI BRAVO images (3D, TR:8, TE:3, FOV: 260, slice thickness/gap:1.2/0). For contrast-enhanced imaging, gadobutrol (Gadovist, Bayer Schering Pharma, Berlin, Germany) or gadoterate meglumine (dotarem; Guerbet, Aulnay-sous-Bois, France) was administered at a single dose of 0.1 mmol/kg by intravenous bolus injection at a rate of 2 mL/s.

Data were described as the mean $\pm$ standard deviation for numerical and frequency (percentage) for categorical variables. Statistical analyses were performed with the Statistical Package for Social Sciences (SPSS Version 24.0, Chicago, IL, USA).

3. Results

Eight patients (five males), with a mean age of 50.1 $\pm$ 11.0 years (range, 28–62 years), were included in the study. Table 1 shows the clinical and demographic data of patients.

All patients underwent uneventful neurosurgical procedures and did not encounter any neurological deficit thereafter. Hybrid PET/MRI images were used for surgical planning and intraoperative guidance in tumor resection. Gross total tumor resection of the PET/MRI-positive area was achieved in all patients, except case 1, whose PET/MRI was reported as radiation necrosis. The extent of resection was confirmed with postoperative CT or MRI in all seven patients.

Table 1. Demographical and clinical features of patients.

Case	Age (Years)	Sex	Histological Diagnosis of Primary Tumor	Localization	Size (cm)	Tracer	Surgery
1	59	M	Glioblastoma	L Frontal	2.3 × 3.5 × 2.8	FDG	None
2	48	M	Diffuse Astrocytoma	L Frontal	6.9 × 4.8 × 4.6	FDG	Gross total resection
3	58	F	Glioblastoma	L Frontoparietal	3.0 × 3.2 × 3.4	FDG	Gross total resection
4	45	M	Gemistocytic Astrocytoma	L Frontoparietal	2.5 × 2.0 × 1.9	FDG	Gross total resection
5	53	M	Glioblastoma	L Temporal	2.0 × 2.0 × 2.3	FDG	Gross total resection
6	47	F	Oligodendroglioma	R Temporal	3.3 × 3.4 × 2.6	FDG	Gross total resection
7	28	M	Glioblastoma	R Hippocampus	6.0 × 4.5 × 4.5	FDG	Gross total resection
8	63	F	Glioblastoma	L Frontoparietal	5.4 × 4.7 × 3.7	FDG	Gross total resection

Abbreviations: F: female, FDG: fluorodeoxyglucose, L: left, M: male, R: right.

A postoperative histopathological investigation of the tumors revealed recurrent glioma (Table 1). All patients survived at 1-year follow-up. In case 1, the diameter of the radiation necrosis area was stable, and no new neurological symptoms were encountered at 1-year follow-up. Five (71.4%) patients remained free of recurrence for the entire follow-up period. Two patients with glioblastoma had tumor recurrence at the postoperative sixth and eighth months.

3.1. Illustrative Cases: Case 3

A 58-year-old female patient applied to our hospital with a complaint of dysarthria for 1 week. She had been operated on once for intracranial tumor previously, and the postoperative histologic diagnosis was high-grade glioma, followed by radiochemotherapy and adjuvant chemotherapy with Temozolamide. Cranial MRI revealed an enhancing mass lesion in the left frontoparietal lobe, whereas MR spectroscopy (MRS) suggested radiation necrosis. PET/MRI showed an F-^{18}FDG hot spot suggesting recurrent glioma (Figure 1). The patient underwent gross total resection using hybrid PET/MRI neuronavigation. Hybrid images provided data to delineate tumor margins and resection borders with high accuracy. Histopathological evaluation confirmed the diagnosis of recurrent glioma.

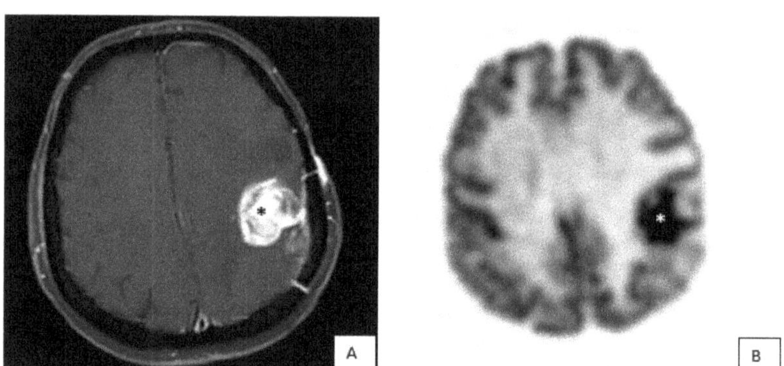

Figure 1. Case 3. Magnetic resonance imaging (MRI) (**A**) revealed an enhancing mass lesion (black asterisk) in the left frontoparietal lobe. A hybrid PET/MRI image (**B**) showed a hot spot (white asterisk), suggesting recurrent glioma.

3.2. Illustrative Cases: Case 5

In a 53-year-old male patient with a complaint of aphasia and orobuccal seizure, a recurrent suspicious contrast-enhancing lesion within his temporal lobe occurred 8 months after GBM resection. T2W MRI showed a hyperintense mass lesion containing cystic and necrotic areas. After contrast administration, the lesion enhanced heterogeneously. PET/MRI images showed focal hot spots within the previously operated area as well as in a different area (Figure 2). Hybrid images helped to distinguish between recurrence and postradiation effects and optimized re-resection. Gross total tumor removal was achieved with hybrid neuronavigation, and histologic examination revealed glioblastoma, which was suggested as postradiation necrosis on MRI images. At postoperative month 6, MRI images revealed a hyperintense mass lesion, suggesting tumor recurrence, but the patient refused re-treatment.

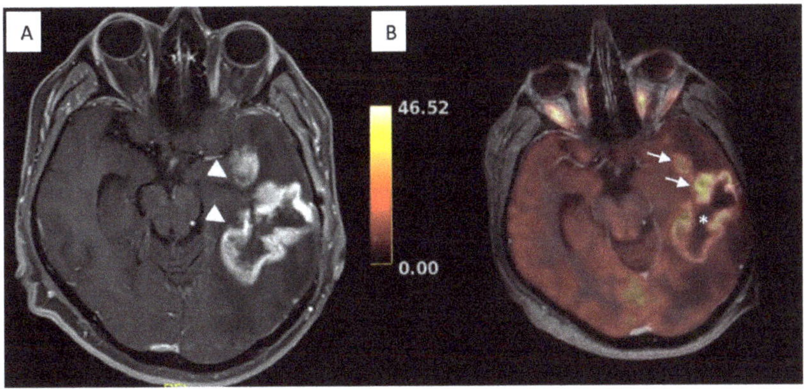

Figure 2. Case 5. T1-weighted magnetic resonance imaging (MRI) (**A**) revealed heterogenous contrasting lesions (arrowheads). Positron emission tomography/MRI images (**B**) showed focal hot spots (arrows) within the previously operated area (asterisk) as well as in a different area.

4. Discussion

According to our results, imaging is very helpful for the differential diagnosis of tumor recurrences from treatment-related changes, as well as the surgical planning of neuroglial brain tumors.

Neurosurgical imaging systems are important in neuro-oncology, and they are continuously improving in diagnostic performance and patient comfort. While MRI is the most widely used tool for the diagnosis and follow-up of high-grade glioma, the reliability of the conventional MRI series is limited in the determination of treatment response or tumor progression due to potential treatment-induced signal changes [11–13]. One of the diagnostic dilemmas in the follow-up period of high-grade glioma cases is pseudoprogression, which is defined as an enlarging or new lesion appearing on MRI after the concurrent administration of radiotherapy and chemotherapy (i.e., temozolamide) but without any true progression. It is attributed to radiation necrosis and inflammatory changes or treatment-related alterations in the blood–brain barrier, leading to increased vascular permeability [14]. It is seen in up to 36% of high-grade glioma [15,16]. There is an increasing demand for definitive radiological criteria for a differential diagnosis of pseudoprogression and true progression to prevent any invasive biopsy or premature cessation of efficacious therapeutic agents. Pseudoresponse, on the other hand, is a rapid resolution of focal enhancement on MRI without a true remission of the tumor and is mostly caused by the anti-angiogenic effect of Bevacizumab [17,18].

In post-treatment high-grade glioma cases, the determination of metabolic activity in enhanced areas on MRI is crucial for the differential diagnosis of true progression or true response. Advanced MRI sequences, including perfusion MRI and MRS, provide more metabolic information and thus better diagnostic accuracy in recurrent glioma cases compared to conventional MRI [18]. Restricted diffusion and an elevated relative cerebral blood volume are indicative for true progression, rather than pseudoprogression [19]. But the cut-off values of PWI are variable in the reported studies, and clinical experience is limited with MRS [18]. As yet, no single technique can be regarded as a gold standard. Nevertheless, more precise information about the metabolic activity of tumor tissue can be obtained by PET imaging. It allows for the combination of multiple diagnostic data, such as tumor blood volume and glucose uptake with the help of radioactive substances. However, it is still limited by low spatial and temporal resolution [20]. There is a need to develop new modalities integrating anatomical, functional and biological information, leading to extremely accurate diagnostic examination and surgical planning. The hybrid PET/MRI scanner is the first implementation of two modalities, in which PET photons and MR signals are co-registered in multimodal images. It allows for the combination of the high contrast and morphological resolution of MRI with the metabolic and physiological information from the integrated PET scan in a single session [21].

There are three different options for combining PET and MRI data: (i) the retrospective fusion of separate PET and MRI images; (ii) sequential/co-planar PET/MRI, during which the patient remains positioned on the same table and travels from PET to MRI; and (iii) integrated hybrid PET/MRI, which provides the simultaneous acquisition of data [22]. There are a number of technical factors limiting the accuracy of images in all combined PET/MRI protocols, but simultaneous PET/MRI provides the best image fusion with a better spatial and temporal resolution. Besides its technical and clinical advantages, obtaining PET and MRI images simultaneously provides decreased examination time and increased comfort for often severely ill patients [23]. Both retrospective fusion and sequential PET/MRI protocols have a longer scanning time compared to hybrid PET/MRI, which may also lead to serious artifacts from patients' voluntary movements due to long-lasting imaging [21].

In the previous literature, Jena et al. prospectively evaluated 26 malignant glioma cases with hybrid PET/MRI to assess glioma recurrence versus radiation necrosis and reported that the highest diagnostic accuracy (96.9%) was achieved by a combined analysis of PET and MRI parameters such as the mean target-to-background ratio and choline-to-creatinine value [24]. Similarly, Sogani et al. conducted a prospective study on 32 consecutive glioma patients with suspicions of recurrence using integrated PET/MRI and again demonstrated that the combination of PET and MRI parameters improved the predictive value for the differentiation of true progression from treatment-related changes, compared to any single parameter. The reported diagnostic accuracy, sensitivity and specificity of integrated analysis were as high as 96.87%, 100% and 85.7%, respectively [25]. Furthermore, Pyka et al. evaluated 63 lesions suggestive of glioma recurrence and performed a dynamic PET scan, as well as morphologic MRI, perfusion MRI and diffusion MRI on the hybrid PET/MRI scanner [26]. They reported that a multiparametric analysis of PET and MRI metrics provided synergistic value for the differential diagnosis of glioma progression, with 76% sensitivity and 100% specificity [26]. In our series, hybrid PET/MRI, morphological MRI, MRS or perfusion MRI images were compared in high-grade glioma patients. While all modalities were to some extent able to discriminate between progression and pseudoprogression, hybrid PET/MRI outcomes were highly correlated with a histopathological diagnosis of glioma recurrences. Indeed, these were more reliable than MRS outcomes. Hybrid PET/MRI and MRI techniques were congruent in terms of tumor size, since both techniques demonstrated an MRI-based structure.

To date, different radiopharmaceuticals for PET scans have been used in neuro-oncology [27]. FDG is well known and the most widely available PET tracer. It indicates glucose uptake and metabolism and thus differentiates low- from high-grade gliomas. Its uptake is increased in high-grade gliomas, whereas well-differentiated neuroepithelial tumors exhibit a low level of accumulation due to a low level of glycolysis [28]. FDG uptake was also evaluated for the assessment of the isocitrate dehydrogenase (IDH) genotype and thereby for the prediction of prognosis in glioma patients [29]. Although it is widely used for tumor grading and biopsy planning, non-specific FDG uptake by normal brain tissue or during inflammation is the main disadvantage. On the other hand, radiolabeled amino acids (i.e., ^{18}F-deoxyphenylalanine; ^{18}F-fluoroethlythyrosine, F-FET; ^{11}C-methionine, C-MET; ^{18}F-fluoro-L3,4-dehydroxyphenylalanine, F-FDOPA) indicate amino acid uptake and protein synthesis. These tracers are recommended by international guidelines to complement MRI in the clinical management of patients with gliomas [30,31]. Several studies investigated the potential of amino acid PET tracers for the diagnosis of molecular markers of gliomas, including the IDH genotype, 1p/19q codeletion and O-methyl guanine methyltransferase (MGMT) promoter methylation status [32–35]. In addition, these tracers are more reliable than FDG in a postradiation assessment of recurrences, due to relatively less uptake by inflammation. F-FET has been shown to differentiate the recurrence of brain metastases from treatment-related changes with high accuracy [36,37], and C-MET PET and structural MRI images were used to develop a reliable model for distinguishing recurrent brain tumor from radiation necrosis [38,39]. Recently, an artificial amino acid tracer, anti-1-amino-3-^{18}F-fluorocyclobutane-1-carboxylic acid (^{18}F-FACBC), was defined in brain tumors; increased FACBC uptake was demonstrated in high-grade gliomas, compared to normal brain tissue [40,41]. In a study conducted on recurrent glioma cases, the tumor uptake of ^{18}F-FACBC was reported to be correlated with C-MET but provide significantly higher image contrast [42]. Another group of tracers are choline-labeled PET tracers (^{11}C-choline, ^{18}F-fluorocholine), which are markers for lipid metabolism and plasma membrane turnover. They have the advantages of better tumor delineation than other tracers due to the very low uptake by normal brain tissue [27,43]. Lastly, prostate-specific membrane antigen (PSMA), which is a transmembrane glycoprotein and highly expressed in prostate cancer, was found to be expressed in high-grade gliomas due to tumor neovascularization [44,45]. In the setting of the suspicious recurrence of high-grade gliomas, PSMA uptake was demonstrated to be significantly higher among tumor recurrences, compared to radiation necrosis [46]. Although there is a strong concordance between FDG and PSMA uptake in the initial diagnosis of high-grade gliomas and evaluation of tumor recurrences, PSMA-targeting radiopharmaceuticals were found to be more accurate than FDG, due to the absence of physiological radiopharmaceutical uptake in normal brain parenchyma [47,48]. Overall, in recent studies using PET/MRI for the assessment of glioma recurrence, the F-FET tracer has been utilized most [49]. However, in our study, we were only able to use the FDG tracer during PET scans due to local availability. Even so, FDG-PET/MRI was found to be effective in terms of the differentiation of radiation necrosis from progression.

In addition to recent advancements in neuroimaging, the use of fluorescence agents such as 5-aminolevulinic acid (5-ALA), indocyanine green (ICG), or sodium fluoresceine allows for a further visualization of tumoral tissue and has been demonstrated to maximize the extent of resection intraoperatively [50]. Furthermore, Barbagallo et al. evaluated the extent of resection in recurrent gliomas using multimodal imaging with intraoperative CT, MRI, PET, ultrasonography and fluoroscopy [51]. They reported increased safety and efficacy with recurrent high-grade glioma and brain alterations secondary to radiochemotherapy [51]. Fluorescence guidance helped to discriminate tumoral and non-tumoral changes during surgery, whereas PET/MRI was used to differentiate recurrences during preoperative surgical planning.

There are several limitations in our study, including a limited number of patients. This limits the generalizability of our findings. Still, a histopathological evaluation of PET/MRI-positive areas was performed in all patients and thereby enhanced the quality of interpretation of hybrid PET/MRI outcomes. We believe the results of our cases may be important to understanding the clinical role of PET/MRI in differential diagnosis as well as surgical planning.

In conclusion, the hybrid PET/MRI of recurrent glial tumors could increase diagnostic accuracy in the prediction of disease progression and play a game-changing role in the management of high-grade glioma patients. Further prospective studies with a larger number of patients may help to establish the diagnostic value and clinical implementation of new hybrid imaging techniques.

Author Contributions: Conceptualization, Y.S.C.; Data curation, M.B. (Murat Buyuktepe); Formal analysis, M.B. (Murat Buyuktepe); Investigation, M.B. (Murat Buyuktepe); Methodology, Y.S.C., M.B. (Murat Buyuktepe), I.D. and M.B. (Melih Bozkurt); Resources, Y.S.C., I.D., M.B. (Melih Bozkurt), E.P., C.S. and E.O.; Supervision, Y.S.C., E.O. and N.O.K.; Writing—original draft, M.B. (Murat Buyuktepe); Writing—review and editing, Y.S.C., M.B. (Murat Buyuktepe), E.Y.S., I.D., M.B. (Melih Bozkurt), E.P., C.S. and E.O. All authors have read and agreed to the published version of the manuscript.

Funding: This research received no external funding.

Institutional Review Board Statement: The study was conducted in accordance with the Declaration of Helsinki, and approved by the Institutional Review Board of Ankara University School of Medicine (protocol code: I5-318-21, date of approval: 21 May 2021).

Informed Consent Statement: Written informed consent has been obtained from the patients to publish this paper.

Data Availability Statement: The data presented in this study are available on request from the corresponding author. The data are not publicly available due to the ethical reasons.

Conflicts of Interest: The authors declare no conflicts of interest.

References

1. Ostrom, Q.T.; Gittleman, H.; Stetson, L.; Virk, S.; Barnholtz-Sloan, J.S. Epidemiology of Intracranial Gliomas. *Prog. Neurol. Surg.* **2018**, *30*, 1–11. [CrossRef] [PubMed]
2. Schwartz, S.M. Epidemiology of Cancer. *Clin. Chem.* **2024**, *70*, 140–149. [CrossRef] [PubMed]
3. Stupp, R.; Mason, W.P.; van den Bent, M.J.; Weller, M.; Fisher, B.; Taphoorn, M.J.B.; Belanger, K.; Brandes, A.A.; Marosi, C.; Bogdahn, U. Radiotherapy plus Concomitant and Adjuvant Temozolomide for Glioblastoma. *N. Engl. J. Med.* **2005**, *352*, 987–996. [CrossRef] [PubMed]
4. McKinney, P.A. Brain tumours: Incidence, survival, and aetiology. *J. Neurol. Neurosurg. Psychiatry* **2004**, *75*, 12–14. [CrossRef] [PubMed]
5. Lacroix, M.; Abi-Said, D.; Fourney, D.R.; Gokaslan, Z.L.; Shi, W.; DeMonte, F.; Lang, F.F.; McCutcheon, I.E.; Hassenbusch, S.J.; Holland, E. A multivariate analysis of 416 patients with glioblastoma multiforme: Prognosis, extent of resection, and survival. *J. Neurosurg.* **2001**, *95*, 190–198. [CrossRef] [PubMed]
6. Stark, A.M.; Nabavi, A.; Mehdorn, H.M.; Blömer, U. Glioblastoma multiforme: Report of 267 cases treated at a single institution. *Surg. Neurol.* **2005**, *63*, 162–169. [CrossRef] [PubMed]
7. Mineo, J.F.; Bordron, A.; Baroncini, M.; Ramirez, C.; Maurage, C.A.; Blond, S.; Dam-Hieu, P. Prognosis factors of survival time in patients with glioblastoma multiforme: A multivariate analysis of 340 patients. *Acta Neurochir.* **2007**, *149*, 245–253. [CrossRef] [PubMed]
8. Luo, C.; Song, K.; Wu, S.; Hameed, N.U.F.; Kudulaiti, N.; Xu, H.; Qin, Z.Y.; Wu, J.S. The prognosis of glioblastoma: A large, multifactorial study. *Br. J. Neurosurg.* **2021**, *35*, 555–561. [CrossRef] [PubMed]
9. Tempany, C.M.C.; Jayender, J.; Kapur, T.; Bueno, R.; Golby, A.; Agar, N.; Jolesz, F.A. Multimodal imaging for improved diagnosis and treatment of cancers. *Cancer* **2015**, *121*, 817–827. [CrossRef]
10. Boellaard, R.; Quick, H.H. Current Image Acquisition Options in PET/MR. *Semin. Nucl. Med.* **2015**, *45*, 192–200. [CrossRef]
11. Smits, M. MRI biomarkers in neuro-oncology. *Nat. Rev. Neurol.* **2021**, *17*, 486–500. [CrossRef] [PubMed]
12. Rao, P. Role of MRI in paediatric neurooncology. *Eur. J. Radiol.* **2008**, *68*, 259–270. [CrossRef] [PubMed]
13. Hu, L.S.; Hawkins-Daarud, A.; Wang, L.; Li, J.; Swanson, K.R. Imaging of intratumoral heterogeneity in high-grade glioma. *Cancer Lett.* **2020**, *477*, 97–106. [CrossRef] [PubMed]
14. Peca, C.; Pacelli, R.; Elefante, A.; Del Basso De Caro, M.L.; Vergara, P.; Mariniello, G.; Giamundo, A.; Maiuri, F. Early clinical and neuroradiological worsening after radiotherapy and concomitant temozolomide in patients with glioblastoma: Tumour progression or radionecrosis? *Clin. Neurol. Neurosurg.* **2009**, *111*, 331–334. [CrossRef] [PubMed]
15. Thust, S.C.; van den Bent, M.J.; Smits, M. Pseudoprogression of brain tumors. *J. Magn. Reson. Imaging* **2018**, *48*, 571–589. [CrossRef] [PubMed]
16. Abbasi, A.W.; Westerlaan, H.E.; Holtman, G.A.; Aden, K.M.; van Laar, P.J.; van der Hoorn, A. Incidence of Tumour Progression and Pseudoprogression in High-Grade Gliomas: A Systematic Review and Meta-Analysis. *Clin. Neuroradiol.* **2018**, *28*, 401–411. [CrossRef] [PubMed]
17. Hughes, K.L.; O'Neal, C.M.; Andrews, B.J.; Westrup, A.M.; Battiste, J.D.; Glenn, C.A. A systematic review of the utility of amino acid PET in assessing treatment response to bevacizumab in recurrent high-grade glioma. *Neuro-Oncology Adv.* **2021**, *3*, vdab003. [CrossRef] [PubMed]
18. van de Weijer, T.; Broen, M.P.G.; Moonen, R.P.M.; Hoeben, A.; Anten, M.; Hovinga, K.; Compter, I.; van der Pol, J.A.J.; Mitea, C.; Lodewick, T.M. The Use of ^{18}F-FET-PET-MRI in Neuro-Oncology: The Best of Both Worlds—A Narrative Review. *Diagnostics* **2022**, *12*, 1202. [CrossRef]
19. Shah, R.; Vattoth, S.; Jacob, R.; Manzil, F.F.P.; O'Malley, J.P.; Borghei, P.; Patel, B.N.; Curé, J.K. Radiation Necrosis in the Brain: Imaging Features and Differentiation from Tumor Recurrence. *RadioGraphics.* **2012**, *32*, 1343–1359. [CrossRef] [PubMed]
20. Puttick, S.; Bell, C.; Dowson, N.; Rose, S.; Fay, M. PET, MRI, and simultaneous PET/MRI in the development of diagnostic and therapeutic strategies for glioma. *Drug. Discov. Today* **2015**, *20*, 306–316. [CrossRef]
21. Aiello, M.; Cavaliere, C.; Marchitelli, R.; D'Albore, A.; De Vita, E.; Salvatore, M. Hybrid PET/MRI Methodology. *Int. Rev. Neurobiol.* **2018**, *141*, 97–128. [CrossRef] [PubMed]

22. Pietrzyk, U.; Herzog, H. Does PET/MR in human brain imaging provide optimal co-registration? A critical reflection. *Magn. Reason. Mater. Phys. Biol. Med.* **2013**, *26*, 137–147. [CrossRef]
23. Preuss, M.; Werner, P.; Barthel, H.; Nestler, U.; Christiansen, H.; Hirsch, F.W.; Fritzsch, D.; Hoffmann, K.T.; Bernhard, M.K.; Sabri, O. Integrated PET/MRI for planning navigated biopsies in pediatric brain tumors. *Child. Nerv. Syst.* **2014**, *30*, 1399–1403. [CrossRef]
24. Jena, A.; Taneja, S.; Gambhir, A.; Mishra, A.K.; D'souza, M.M.; Verma, S.M.; Hazari, P.P.; Negi, P.; Jhadav, G.K.; Sogani, S.K. Glioma Recurrence Versus Radiation Necrosis. *Clin. Nucl. Med.* **2016**, *41*, e228–e236. [CrossRef]
25. Sogani, S.; Jena, A.; Taneja, S.; Gambhir, A.; Mishra, A.; D'Souza, M.; Verma, S.M.; Hazari, P.P.; Negi, P.; Jadhav, G.K. Potential for differentiation of glioma recurrence from radionecrosis using integrated ^{18}F-fluoroethyl-L-tyrosine (FET) positron emission tomography/magnetic resonance imaging: A prospective evaluation. *Neurol. India* **2017**, *65*, 293. [CrossRef]
26. Pyka, T.; Hiob, D.; Preibisch, C.; Gempt, J.; Wiestler, B.; Schlegel, J.; Straube, C.; Zimmer, C. Diagnosis of glioma recurrence using multiparametric dynamic ^{18}F-fluoroethyl-tyrosine PET-MRI. *Eur. J. Radiol.* **2018**, *103*, 32–37. [CrossRef]
27. Almansory, K.O.; Fraioli, F. Combined PET/MRI in brain glioma imaging. *Br. J. Hosp. Med.* **2019**, *80*, 380–386. [CrossRef] [PubMed]
28. Hanahan, D.; Weinberg, R.A. Hallmarks of cancer: The next generation. *Cell* **2011**, *144*, 646–674. [CrossRef]
29. Li, L.; Mu, W.; Wang, Y.; Liu, Z.; Liu, Z.; Wang, Y.; Ma, W.; Kong, Z.; Wang, S.; Zhou, X.; et al. A non-invasive radiomic method using ^{18}F-FDG PET predicts isocitrate dehydrogenase genotype and prognosis in patients with Glioma. *Front. Oncol.* **2019**, *9*, 1183. [CrossRef] [PubMed]
30. Albert, N.L.; Weller, M.; Suchorska, B.; Galldiks, N.; Soffietti, R.; Kim, M.M.; la Fougère, C.; Pope, W.; Law, I.; Arbizu, J.; et al. Response assessment in neuro-oncology working group and European Association for Neuro-Oncology recommendations for the clinical use of PET imaging in gliomas. *Neuro Oncol.* **2016**, *18*, 1199–1208. [CrossRef]
31. Law, I.; Albert, N.L.; Arbizu, J.; Boellaard, R.; Drzezga, A.; Galldiks, N.; la Fougère, C.; Langen, K.J.; Lopci, E.; Lowe, V.; et al. Joint EANM/EANO/RANO practice guidelines/SNMMI procedure standards for imaging of gliomas using PET with radiolabelled amino acids and [^{18}F]FDG: Version 1.0. *Eur. J. Nucl. Med. Mol. Imaging* **2019**, *46*, 540–557. [CrossRef] [PubMed]
32. Lohmann, P.; Meißner, A.K.; Kocher, M.; Bauer, E.K.; Werner, J.M.; Fink, G.R.; Shah, N.J.; Langen, K.J.; Galldiks, N. Feature-based PET/MRI radiomics in patients with brain tumors. *Neurooncol. Adv.* **2021**, *2* (Suppl. S4), iv15–iv21. [CrossRef] [PubMed]
33. Haubold, J.; Demircioglu, A.; Gratz, M.; Glas, M.; Wrede, K.; Sure, U.; Antoch, G.; Keyvani, K.; Nittka, M.; Kannengiesser, S.; et al. Non-invasive tumor decoding and phenotyping of cerebral gliomas utilizing multiparametric ^{18}F-FET PET-MRI and MR Fingerprinting. *Eur. J. Nucl. Med. Mol. Imaging* **2020**, *47*, 1435–1445. [CrossRef] [PubMed]
34. Yu, P.; Ning, J.; Xu, B.; Liu, J.; Dang, H.; Lin, M.; Feng, X.; Grimm, R.; Tian, J. Histogram analysis of 11C-methionine integrated PET/MRI may facilitate to determine the O6-methylguanylmethyltransferase methylation status in gliomas. *Nucl. Med. Commun.* **2019**, *40*, 850–856. [CrossRef] [PubMed]
35. Kong, Z.; Lin, Y.; Jiang, C.; Li, L.; Liu, Z.; Wang, Y.; Dai, C.; Liu, D.; Qin, X.; Wang, Y.; et al. ^{18}F-FDG-PET-based Radiomics signature predicts MGMT promoter methylation status in primary diffuse glioma. *Cancer Imaging* **2019**, *19*, 58. [CrossRef] [PubMed]
36. Galldiks, N.; Stoffels, G.; Filss, C.P.; Piroth, M.D.; Sabel, M.; Ruge, M.I.; Herzog, H.; Shah, N.J.; Fink, G.R.; Coenen, H.H.; et al. Role of *O*-(2-^{18}F-fluoroethyl)-L-tyrosine PET for differentiation of local recurrent brain metastasis from radiation necrosis. *J. Nucl. Med.* **2012**, *53*, 1367–1374. [CrossRef]
37. Lohmann, P.; Kocher, M.; Ceccon, G.; Bauer, E.K.; Stoffels, G.; Viswanathan, S.; Ruge, M.I.; Neumaier, B.; Shah, N.J.; Fink, G.R.; et al. Combined FET PET/MRI radiomics differentiates radiation injury from recurrent brain metastasis. *Neuroimage Clin.* **2018**, *20*, 537–542. [CrossRef]
38. Wang, K.; Qiao, Z.; Zhao, X.; Li, X.; Wang, X.; Wu, T.; Chen, Z.; Fan, D.; Chen, Q.; Ai, L. Individualized discrimination of tumor recurrence from radiation necrosis in glioma patients using an integrated radiomics-based model. *Eur. J. Nucl. Med. Mol. Imaging* **2019**, *47*, 1400–1411. [CrossRef] [PubMed]
39. Hotta, M.; Minamimoto, R.; Miwa, K. 11C-methionine-PET for differentiating recurrent brain tumor from radiation necrosis: Radiomics approach with random forest classifier. *Sci. Rep.* **2019**, *9*, 15666. [CrossRef]
40. Castello, A.; Albano, D.; Muoio, B.; Castellani, M.; Panareo, S.; Rizzo, A.; Treglia, G.; Urso, L. Diagnostic Accuracy of PET with ^{18}F-Fluciclovine ([^{18}F]FACBC) in Detecting High-Grade Gliomas: A Systematic Review and Meta-Analysis. *Diagnostics* **2023**, *13*, 3610. [CrossRef]
41. Karlberg, A.; Pedersen, L.K.; Vindstad, B.E.; Skjulsvik, A.J.; Johansen, H.; Solheim, O.; Skogen, K.; Kvistad, K.A.; Bogsrud, T.V.; Myrmel, K.S.; et al. Diagnostic accuracy of anti-3-[^{18}F]-FACBC PET/MRI in gliomas. *Eur. J. Nucl. Med. Mol. Imaging* **2024**, *51*, 496–509. [CrossRef] [PubMed]
42. Michaud, L.; Beattie, B.J.; Akhurst, T.; Dunphy, M.; Zanzonico, P.; Finn, R.; Mauguen, A.; Schöder, H.; Weber, W.A.; Lassman, A.B.; et al. ^{18}F-Fluciclovine (^{18}F-FACBC) PET imaging of recurrent brain tumors. *Eur. J. Nucl. Med. Mol. Imaging* **2020**, *47*, 1353–1367. [CrossRef] [PubMed]
43. Li, F.-M.; Nie, Q.; Wang, R.-M.; Chang, S.M.; Zhao, W.-R.; Zhu, Q.; Liang, Y.K.; Yang, P.; Zhang, J.; Jia, H.W.; et al. 11C-CHO PET in optimization of target volume delineation and treatment regimens in postoperative radiotherapy for brain gliomas. *Nucl. Med. Biol.* **2012**, *39*, 437–442. [CrossRef]

44. Schwenck, J.; Tabatabai, G.; Skardelly, M.; Reischl, G.; Beschorner, R.; Pichler, B.; la Fougère, C. In vivo visualization of prostate-specific membrane antigen in glioblastoma. *Eur. J. Nucl. Med. Mol. Imaging* **2015**, *42*, 170–171. [CrossRef] [PubMed]
45. Akgun, E.; Akgun, M.Y.; Selçuk, H.H.; Uzan, M.; Sayman, H.B. PSMA PET/MR in the differentiation of low and high grade gliomas: Is ^{68}Ga PSMA PET/MRI useful to detect brain gliomas? *Eur. J. Radiol.* **2020**, *130*, 109199. [CrossRef] [PubMed]
46. Muoio, B.; Albano, D.; Dondi, F.; Bertagna, F.; Garibotto, V.; Kunikowska, J.; Piccardo, A.; Annunziata, S.; Espeli, V.; Migliorini, D.; et al. Diagnostic Accuracy of PET/CT or PET/MRI Using PSMA-Targeting Radiopharmaceuticals in High-Grade Gliomas: A Systematic Review and a Bivariate Meta-Analysis. *Diagnostics* **2022**, *12*, 1665. [CrossRef] [PubMed]
47. Liu, D.; Cheng, G.; Ma, X.; Wang, S.; Zhao, X.; Zhang, W.; Yang, W.; Wang, J. PET/CT using ^{68}Ga-PSMA-617 versus ^{18}F-fluorodeoxyglucose to differentiate low- and high-grade gliomas. *J. Neuroimaging* **2021**, *31*, 733–742. [CrossRef]
48. Brighi, C.; Puttick, S.; Woods, A.; Keall, P.; Tooney, P.A.; Waddington, D.E.J.; Sproule, V.; Rose, S.; Fay, M. Comparison between [^{68}Ga]Ga-PSMA-617 and [^{18}F]FET PET as Imaging Biomarkers in Adult Recurrent Glioblastoma. *Int. J. Mol. Sci.* **2023**, *24*, 16208. [CrossRef] [PubMed]
49. Overcast, W.B.; Davis, K.M.; Ho, C.Y.; Hutchins, G.D.; Green, M.A.; Graner, B.D.; Veronesi, M.C. Advanced imaging techniques for neuro-oncologic tumor diagnosis, with an emphasis on PET-MRI imaging of malignant brain tumors. *Curr. Oncol. Rep.* **2021**, *23*, 34. [CrossRef]
50. Stummer, W.; Pichlmeier, U.; Meinel, T.; Wiestler, O.D.; Zanella, F.; Reulen, H.J. Fluorescence-guided surgery with 5-aminolevulinic acid for resection of malignant glioma, a randomised controlled multicentre phase III trial. *Lancet Oncol.* **2006**, *7*, 392–401. [CrossRef]
51. Vincenzo Barbagallo, G.M.; Certo, F.; Di Gregorio, S.; Maione, M.; Garozzo, M.; Peschillo, S.; Altieri, R. Recurrent high-grade glioma surgery, a multimodal intraoperative protocol to safely increase extent of tumor resection and analysis of its impact on patient outcome. *Neurosurg. Focus.* **2021**, *50*, E20. [CrossRef] [PubMed]

diagnostics

MDPI

Article

Seizures Following Carotid Endarterectomy: A Comprehensive Meta-Analysis of 69,479 Patients and Evidence-Based Recommendations for Perioperative Care

Kruthajn Rajesh [1,2,3], Helen Shen [1,2,3] and Sonu M. M. Bhaskar [1,2,3,4,5,6,*]

1 Global Health Neurology Lab, Sydney, NSW 2150, Australia
2 UNSW Medicine and Health, University of New South Wales (UNSW), South West Sydney Clinical Campuses, Sydney, NSW 2170, Australia
3 Ingham Institute for Applied Medical Research, Clinical Sciences Stream, Sydney, NSW 2170, Australia
4 NSW Brain Clot Bank, NSW Health Pathology, Sydney, NSW 2170, Australia
5 Department of Neurology and Neurophysiology, Liverpool Hospital and South Western Sydney Local Health District (SWSLHD), Sydney, NSW 2170, Australia
6 National Cerebral and Cardiovascular Center (NCVC), Department of Neurology, Division of Cerebrovascular Medicine and Neurology, Suita 564-8565, Osaka, Japan
* Correspondence: sonu.bhaskar@globalhealthneurolab.org or bhaskar.sonu@ncvc.go.jp; Tel.: +81-90-9274-1265

Abstract: Background: Seizures are a rare but potentially serious complication following carotid endarterectomy (CEA). Understanding their prevalence and associated factors is crucial for optimizing perioperative care and improving patient outcomes. This meta-analysis aimed to estimate the pooled prevalence of seizures following CEA and explore clinical and procedural factors contributing to their occurrence. **Methods**: We conducted a systematic review and meta-analysis of studies reporting on seizures following CEA. A systematic search of PubMed, Embase, and Cochrane CENTRAL databases was performed, following PRISMA and MOOSE guidelines. Random-effects meta-analysis was used to calculate the pooled prevalence of postoperative seizures. Heterogeneity was assessed using the I^2 statistic. A total of 20 studies, encompassing 69,479 patients, were included. **Results**: The overall pooled prevalence of seizures following CEA was 1% (95% CI: 0–2%; $p < 0.001$), with significant heterogeneity ($I^2 = 93.52\%$). Prospective studies reported a higher pooled prevalence (2%, 95% CI 0–4%; $I^2 = 76.34\%$) compared to retrospective studies (0%, 95% CI 0–1%; $I^2 = 91.51\%$). Male predominance was noted among patients who experienced seizures, and hypertension was the most common comorbidity. Cerebral hyperperfusion syndrome was identified as a key contributing factor to postoperative seizures. Data on long-term outcomes, including the development of epilepsy, were insufficient for further analysis. The methodological quality of the included studies varied, with most studies demonstrating a moderate risk of bias. **Conclusions**: Seizures occur in approximately 1% of patients following CEA, with higher rates observed in prospective studies. Cerebral hyperperfusion syndrome is an important contributor to this rare complication. We provide evidence-based specific recommendations for seizure management and introduce the SMART-CEA Checklist, a practical framework to guide perioperative care and reduce complications. Future research should focus on long-term outcomes, including epilepsy, and incorporate standardized methodologies to improve data reliability and guide clinical practice.

Keywords: carotid endarterectomy; CEA; seizures; epilepsy; cerebrovascular disorders; cerebral hyperperfusion syndrome; stroke prevention

1. Background

Carotid endarterectomy (CEA) is a widely performed surgical procedure to mitigate the risk of ischemic stroke in patients with significant carotid artery stenosis [1]. By removing atherosclerotic plaques from the carotid artery, CEA improves blood flow and reduces cerebrovascular event recurrence [1]. Despite its proven efficacy in stroke prevention, the procedure is not without risks, with postoperative complications posing significant challenges to patient recovery [2]. Among these, seizures represent a rare but serious neurological complication with the potential to adversely impact patient outcomes and quality of life [3–6].

Seizures following CEA are believed to arise from cerebral hyperperfusion syndrome, a condition characterized by impaired cerebral autoregulation and excessive blood flow to previously hypoperfused brain regions [7]. This abrupt alteration in cerebral hemodynamics can result in neuronal hyperactivity, leading to seizures, cerebral edema, or, in severe cases, intracranial hemorrhage [8]. Hypertensive encephalopathy, another frequently implicated factor, may exacerbate the risk of seizures in the postoperative period. However, the exact mechanisms and risk factors underlying these events remain poorly understood [6]. While individual studies have reported on seizure occurrence post-CEA, no comprehensive synthesis of the available evidence has been conducted to elucidate the prevalence, clinical characteristics, and potential long-term consequences, such as the progression to epilepsy [4,5,9–11].

Understanding the prevalence and clinical burden of seizures following CEA is crucial for improving perioperative management strategies and informing clinical guidelines [12]. Seizures, even when transient, are associated with increased morbidity, longer hospital stays, and higher healthcare costs [13]. Identifying patients at higher risk for postoperative seizures could enable targeted interventions, including closer hemodynamic monitoring and tailored blood pressure management [14].

This study aims to address the existing knowledge gap by conducting a meta-analysis to estimate the pooled prevalence of seizures in patients undergoing CEA [8]. Additionally, we aim to explore the clinical characteristics of seizures, risk factors, and the potential progression to epilepsy. By synthesizing the available evidence, we seek to provide evidence-based insights that may guide therapeutic strategies, improve perioperative care, and inform future research in this critical area of interventional neuroradiology and vascular surgery.

Objectives

This study aims to conduct a comprehensive meta-analysis to:

(1) Investigate the pooled prevalence of seizures following CEA.
(2) Analyze the potential progression of postoperative seizures to epilepsy.

2. Materials and Methods

2.1. Literature Search and Study Selection

A systematic search for relevant studies from 1 January 1980 to December 2024 was conducted using PubMed, Embase, and Cochrane Central Register of Controlled Trials (CENTRAL) databases. The search terms included "carotid endarterectomy", "CEA", "carotid surgery", "endarterectomy", "postoperative seizures", "seizure", "epilepsy", "status epilepticus", "hyperperfusion", "cerebral hyperperfusion", "postoperative hyperperfusion", "cerebral reperfusion injury", "hypertension", "blood pressure", "BP control", "cerebral hypoperfusion", "impaired vasoreactivity", and "cerebral autoregulation". A comprehensive and structured search strategy was implemented, with additional details provided in the Online Supplemental Information (Search Strategy). Studies not written in

English or those not involving human participants were excluded. To identify further relevant studies, a manual review of references from key articles, systematic reviews, and meta-analyses was performed. The organization of studies and various subgroup analyses included in the meta-analysis is illustrated in a flowchart, following the Preferred Reporting Items for Systematic Reviews and Meta-Analyses (PRISMA) guidelines (Figure 1) [15]. Compliance with the 2020 checklist (Supplemental Table S1) [15] and the Meta-analysis of Observational Studies in Epidemiology (MOOSE) checklist (Supplemental Table S2) was ensured, with these documents available in the Online Supplemental Information. This study was registered in Open Science, registration number "hckr3" (https://osf.io/hckr3/ (accessed on 21 June 2024)).

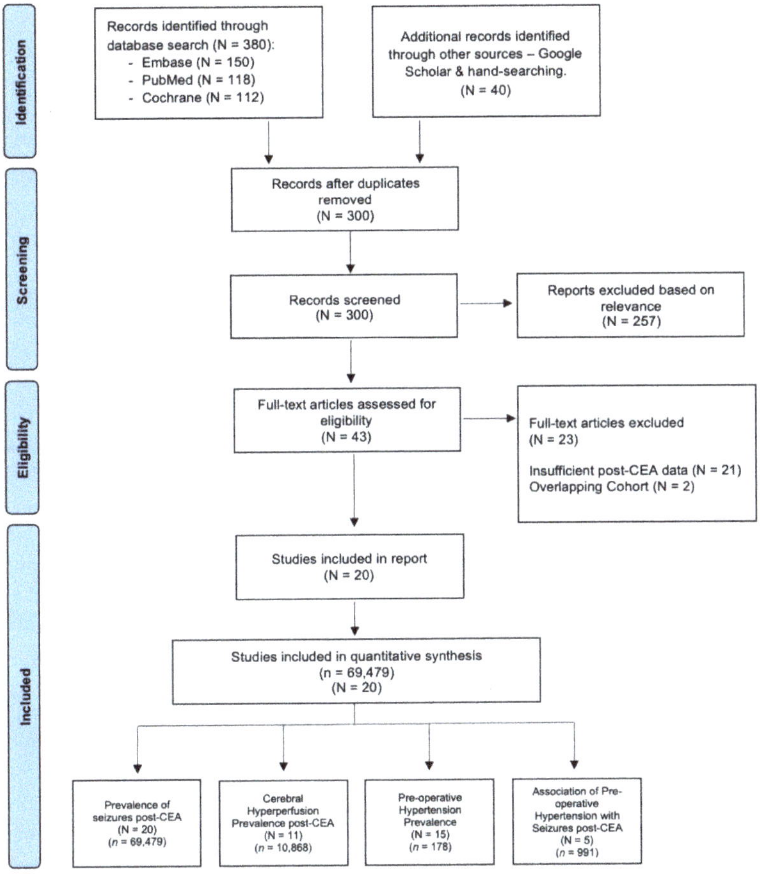

Figure 1. PRISMA flowchart of included studies in the meta-analysis of seizures following carotid endarterectomy (CEA). This figure illustrates the study selection process using the Preferred Reporting Items for Systematic Reviews and Meta-Analyses (PRISMA) framework, offering a clear depiction of the studies incorporated in the meta-analysis. Abbreviations: N—number of studies; *n*—cohort size; CEA—carotid endarterectomy.

2.2. Inclusion and Exclusion Criteria

Studies were eligible for inclusion if they met the following criteria: (a) patients diagnosed with seizures or with a history of epilepsy; (b) patients eligible for CEA; (c) participants aged 18 years or older; (d) reporting on post-CEA seizures or epilepsy or cerebral hyperperfusion syndrome or related complications (e.g., hypertension, hypoperfusion);

reported data on pre-operative or postoperative blood pressure management; (e) employed a robust methodological design, including prospective or retrospective observational studies, randomized controlled trials, or meta-analyses; and (f) included a minimum sample size of 20 patients per group to ensure statistical reliability. Studies were excluded if they met any of the following criteria: (a) non-human or preclinical studies; (b) studies with overlapping datasets or duplicate publications; (c) studies where the full-text article was unavailable; (d) studies presented solely in abstract form without sufficient data on CEA-related outcomes or postoperative complications; (e) studies with anecdotal evidence, case reports, or editorials lacking robust data for meta-analysis; and (f) studies with unclear or inconsistent definitions of seizures or epilepsy. Seizures were defined as excessive hypersynchronous neuronal discharge in the brain, leading to a paroxysmal alteration of neurologic function, consistent with established clinical criteria to ensure uniformity across included studies [16]. Hypertension was defined according to the American Heart Association (AHA) guidelines as a blood pressure of $\geq$130/80 mmHg, providing a standardized threshold for identifying hypertensive patients [17]. Postoperative cerebral hyperperfusion syndrome was characterized as a greater-than-100% increase in cerebral blood flow or middle cerebral artery velocity compared to pre-operative baseline levels, as measured using transcranial Doppler or perfusion imaging [18].

2.3. *Data Extraction and Methodological Quality Assessment*

A meticulous data extraction and methodological quality assessment process was conducted to ensure the reliability and validity of the findings. EndNote v. 21.0 software (Clarivate Analytics, London, UK) was used to manage references and screen titles and abstracts. Articles that did not meet the eligibility criteria were excluded during this initial screening phase. Two authors independently performed the screening, and any discrepancies were resolved through discussion or consultation with a third reviewer. Articles that passed the initial screening were further assessed for inclusion in the systematic review or meta-analysis based on pre-defined eligibility criteria.

A standardized data extraction form was used to systematically collect key information from each included study. The extracted data included: (a) Study characteristics: author, year of publication, country, and study design (prospective or retrospective). (b) Patient demographics: age, gender distribution, sample size, and clinical characteristics of patients' CEA. (c) CEA details: procedural characteristics, perioperative management protocols, and follow-up durations. (d) Seizure outcomes: prevalence of seizures, seizure subtypes (e.g., focal, generalized), severity (e.g., status epilepticus), and progression to epilepsy, if reported. (e) Risk factors and complications: data on cerebral hyperperfusion syndrome, hypertension, and blood pressure control.

The methodological quality of the included studies was assessed using the modified Jadad scale (MJA), which evaluates study design, randomization, blinding, and reporting of withdrawals or dropouts. Each study was assigned a quality score, with higher scores indicating better methodological rigor. The results of the quality assessment are summarized in Supplemental Table S3. Two independent reviewers conducted the quality assessment, and disagreements were resolved through joint discussions to reach consensus.

To address the study objectives, data were collected on the total number of patients undergoing CEA, the proportion who experienced postoperative seizures (prevalence), and those who developed epilepsy over time (incidence). However, during data extraction, it became evident that most studies lacked sufficient longitudinal data to reliably assess the progression from seizures to epilepsy. As a result, the analysis primarily focused on the prevalence of seizures and associated risk factors following CEA. The incidence of epilepsy was identified as an area for future investigation. The data extraction process adhered to the PRISMA guidelines, and compliance with the PRISMA 2020 checklist and the MOOSE guidelines was ensured.

2.4. Statistical Methodology

Statistical analyses were conducted using STATA v. 13.0 (StataCorp, College Station, TX, USA). Baseline data were extracted from all included studies, and descriptive statistics were used to summarize patient demographics, study characteristics, and seizure prevalence. For studies reporting medians and interquartile ranges (IQRs), means and standard deviations (SDs) were estimated using the method proposed by Wan et al. [19]. Adjustments to 95% confidence intervals (95% CIs) were made using the 'cimethod (exact)' and 'ftt' commands in STATA. A random-effects model was employed to pool prevalence estimates of seizures following CEA, accounting for between-study variability. The random-effects model was chosen due to the anticipated heterogeneity across studies in terms of study design, patient populations, and diagnostic criteria for seizures. The pooled prevalence was reported as a percentage with 95% CIs.

Four types of subgroup analyses were conducted to explore the prevalence and associations related to seizures following CEA: (1) the pooled prevalence of seizures post-CEA; (2) the prevalence of pre-operative hypertension among patients who experienced seizures post-CEA; (3) the prevalence of cerebral hyperperfusion post-CEA; and (4) the association between pre-operative hypertension and seizures post-CEA. The organization of these subgroup analyses and the study selection process is illustrated in Figure 1. Heterogeneity across studies was assessed using the I^2 statistic, which quantifies the proportion of total variation in effect estimates due to between-study heterogeneity rather than chance. Heterogeneity was categorized as follows: low: $I^2 < 40\%$; moderate: $I^2 = 30–60\%$; substantial: $I^2 = 50–90\%$; considerable: $I^2 = 75–100\%$. To explore potential sources of heterogeneity, subgroup analyses and sensitivity analyses were performed.

Subgroup analyses were conducted to investigate differences in seizure prevalence based on the following: *study design*: prospective vs. retrospective studies; *follow-up duration*: short-term (≤7 days) vs. longer-term (>7 days) follow-up; and *geographic region*: studies conducted in different regions to account for variations in clinical practice and patient populations.

Sensitivity analyses were performed by excluding studies with high risk of bias (as determined by the modified Jadad scale) to assess the robustness of the pooled prevalence estimate. Additionally, a leave-one-out analysis was conducted to evaluate the influence of individual studies on the overall results.

Publication bias was assessed using funnel plots and Egger's test for small-study effects. Asymmetry in the funnel plot would suggest potential publication bias, which was further quantified using Egger's regression test. A p-value < 0.05 was considered indicative of significant publication bias.

All statistical tests were two-tailed, and a p-value < 0.05 was considered statistically significant. Confidence intervals were reported at the 95% level.

3. Results

3.1. Description of Included Studies

A total of 20 studies [4–6,8–11,20–32], encompassing 69,479 patients, were included in this meta-analysis. The cohort sizes varied widely, ranging from 25 to 51,001 patients. The incidence of seizures post-CEA was low, with reported rates ranging from 0.01% to 13%. The mean age of patients was 67.7 years, with SDs reported between 8.7 and 15 years across studies. Male predominance was noted in most studies where gender data were available, particularly among patients who experienced seizures. Hypertension was the most common comorbidity, affecting 71.9% of patients, followed by coronary artery disease (23%). The prevalence of previous stroke or transient ischemic attack (TIA) varied significantly, with some studies reporting rates as high as 70%. Smoking was prevalent in 8 cohorts [8,9,11,22,23,28,31,32], while diabetes was reported in 10 cohorts [4,5,8,9,11,22,23,28,31,32].

Follow-up durations for seizure detection post-CEA ranged from 1 to 8 days, reflecting variability in study designs and monitoring protocols. Detailed clinical characteristics of the included studies are presented in Table 1. The methodological quality of the studies, assessed using the modified Jadad scale, revealed variable quality and risk of bias, as summarized in Supplemental Table S3. Funding bias was identified in only one study (Buczek et al. [5]). These findings highlight the heterogeneity in study designs, patient populations, and reporting practices, underscoring the need for standardized methodologies in future research.

3.2. Overall Prevalence of Seizures in Patients Undergoing CEA

The meta-analysis presented in Figure 2, comprising 69,479 patients within 20 studies [4–6,8–11,20–32], evaluates the prevalence of seizures in patients undergoing CEA. The findings indicate that the overall prevalence of seizures post-CEA is low, with prospective studies reporting slightly higher rates compared to retrospective studies. Specifically, seizure prevalence in prospective studies ranged from 0% to 13%, with a pooled prevalence of 2% (95% CI 0–4) and considerable heterogeneity (I^2 = 76.34). Retrospective studies reported seizure rates between 0% and 1%, with a pooled prevalence of 0% (95% CI 0–1) and considerable heterogeneity (I^2 = 91.51). When data from all included studies were combined, the overall pooled prevalence of seizures post-CEA was 1% (95% CI 0–2; $p < 0.001$), with significant heterogeneity (I^2 = 93.52). The pooled prevalence of seizures following CEA, stratified by study design, revealed slightly higher rates in prospective studies compared to retrospective studies. This stratified analysis is presented in Supplemental Figure S3.

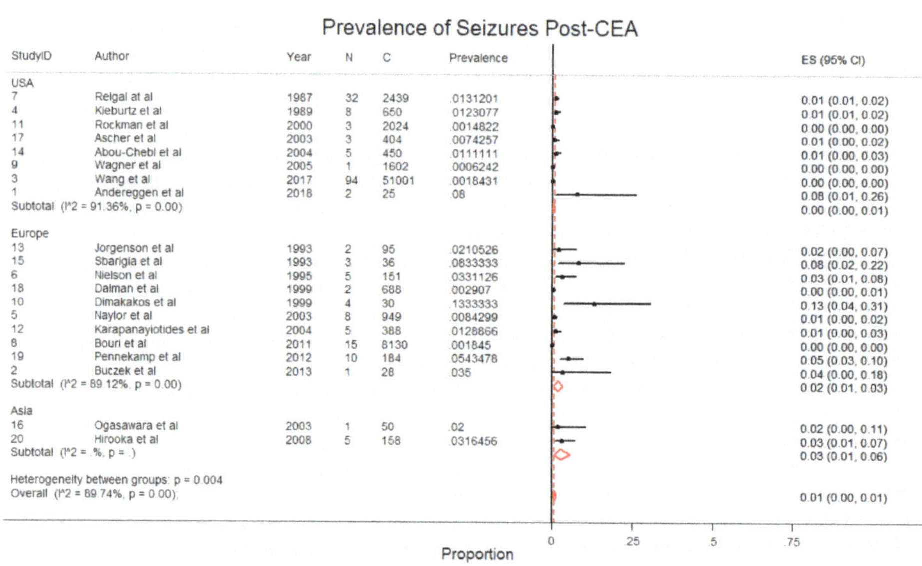

Figure 2. Pooled prevalence of seizures following carotid endarterectomy (CEA) across included studies [4–6,8–11,20–32]. This figure displays the prevalence of seizures in patients after receiving carotid endarterectomy. Abbreviations: CEA—carotid endarterectomy; N—number of patients with seizures; C—overall cohort; ES—effect size; CI—confidence interval; I^2—the proportion of total variation in effect estimate due to between-study heterogeneit.

Table 1. Characteristics of included studies in the meta-analysis of seizures following carotid endarterectomy.

Study ID	Author	Year	Region	Study Type	Sample Size (*n*)	Seizure Prevalence (*n*, %)	Follow-Up Duration (Days)	Age (Years ± SD)	Male (*n*, %) *	AF (*n*, %)	HL (*n*, %)	HTN (n, %)	CAD (*n*, %)	Previous stroke/TIA (*n*, %)	Smoking (*n*, %)	Diabetes (*n*, %)
1	Andereggen et al. [11]	2018	USA	Prospective	25	2 (8.0)	1–5	71.0 ± 8.7	18 (72.0)	-	20 (80.0)	20 (80.0)	9 (36.0)	17 (68.0)	17 (68.0)	8 (32.0)
2	Buczek et al. [5]	2013	Europe	Prospective	28	1 (3.6)	2–5	70.2 ± 9.4	23 (82.1)	-	-	22 (78.6)	-	11 (39.3)	-	8 (28.6)
3	Wang et al. [9]	2017	USA	Retrospective	51,001	94 (0.2)	3–6	70.2 ± 9.4	30,804 (60.4)	-	-	45,238 (88.7)	14,586 (28.6)	15,096 (29.6)	24,276 (47.6)	17,697 (34.7)
4	Kieburtz et al. [8]	1989	USA	Retrospective	650	8 (1.2)	7	69.5 ± 10.0	-	-	-	488 (75.1)	-	81 (12.5)	569 (87.5)	81 (12.5)
5	Naylor et al. [6]	2003	Europe	Prospective	949	8 (0.8)	2–8	65.8 ± 10.4	4 (0.4) œ	-	-	-	-	-	-	-
6	Nielson et al. [4]	1995	Europe	Prospective	151	5 (3.3)	5–7	62.0	97 (64.2)	-	-	-	40 (26.0)	59 (39.0)	-	17 (11.0)
7	Reigal et al. [10]	1987	USA	Retrospective	2439	32 (1.3)	1–7	-	-	-	-	-	-	-	-	-
8	Bouri et al. [30]	2011	Europe	Retrospective	8130	15 (0.2)	3–6	66.0 ± 9.5	-	-	-	1545 (19.0)	-	-	-	-
9	Wagner et al. [20]	2005	USA	Retrospective	1602	1 (0.1)	1–7		-	-	-	-	-	224 (14.0)		
10	Dimakakos et al. [28]	1999	Europe	Prospective	30	4 (13.3)	1–7	66.6 ± 15.0	22 (73.0)	-	18 (60.0)	17 (57.0)	17 (57.0)		15 (50.0)	5 (17.0)
11	Rockman et al. [22]	2000	USA	Retrospective	2024	3 (0.1)	1–7	68.7 ± 9.4	1295 (64.0)	-	-	1416 (70.0)	951 (47.0)	850 (42.0)	971 (48.0)	506 (25.0)
12	Karapanayiotides et al. [25]	2004	Europe	Prospective	388	5 (1.3)	2–7	70.4 ± 6.2	77 (20.0)	-	-	230 (59.0)	-			
13	Jorgenson et al. [26]	1993	Europe	Prospective	95	2 (2.1)	1–14	59.0 ±12.0	62 (65.0)	-	-	44 (46.0)	-	48 (51.0)		
14	Abou-Chebl et al. [32]	2004	USA	Retrospective	450	5 (1.1)	1–4	72.7 ± 10.9	-	-	197 (44.0)	339 (75.0)	255 (57.0)		225 (50.0)	176 (39.0)
15	Sbarigia et al. [21]	1993	Europe	Prospective	36	3 (8.3)	1–2	67.0 ± 6.0	32 (89.0)	-	-	27 (75.0)	-			
16	Ogasawara et al. [24]	2003	Asia	Prospective	50	1 (2.0)	1–6	68.6 ± 5.8	44 (88.0)	-	-	-	-			
17	Ascher et al. [31]	2003	USA	Prospective	404	3 (0.7)	1–8	69.0 ± 8.0	221 (55.0)	-	-	275 (68.0)	98 (24.0)	129 (32.0)	176 (44.0)	122 (30.0)
18	Dalman et al. [29]	1999	Europe	Prospective	688	2 (0.3)	1–7	69.0 ± 10.3	447 (65.0)	-	-	-	-			
19	Pennekamp et al. [23]	2012	Europe	Prospective	184	10 (5.4)	1–7	68.8 ± 10.9	141 (77.0)	-	164 (89.0)	135 (73.0)	50 (27.0)		61 (33.0)	36 (20.0)
20	Hirooka et al. [27]	2008	Asia	Prospective	158	5 (3.2)	1–7	67.2 ± 6.5	150 (95.0)	-	-	128 (81.0)	-	111 (70.0)	-	-

Abbreviations: *n*—number of patients; SD—standard deviation; AF—atrial fibrillation; HL—hyperlipidaemia; HTN—hypertension; CAD—coronary artery disease; TIA—transient ischemic attack. * Note: Demographics are based on the entire cohort. Clinical demographics (e.g., 'Male') are based on the subset of patients who experienced a seizure post-CEA).

3.3. Prevalence of Pre-Operative Hypertension Among Patients Who Experienced Seizures Post-CEA

This subgroup comprised 178 patients drawn from 15 studies [4,6,8–11,21,22,25–28,30–32]. Figure 3 depicts the prevalence of pre-operative hypertension among patients who experienced seizures following CEA. The findings reveal that pre-operative hypertension is a highly prevalent comorbidity in this patient population, underscoring its potential role as a significant risk factor for postoperative seizures. In studies conducted in the USA, the prevalence of pre-operative hypertension ranged from 67% to 100%, with a pooled prevalence of 95% (95% CI: 85% to 100%) and low heterogeneity (I^2 = 17.5%). Similarly, European studies reported prevalence rates between 50% and 100%, with a pooled prevalence of 90% (95% CI: 76% to 99%) and no observed heterogeneity (I^2 = 0%). In contrast, studies conducted in Asia reported a lower prevalence of 60% (95% CI: 15% to 95%), although this estimate was based on a smaller number of studies, limiting its generalizability. The overall pooled prevalence of pre-operative hypertension among patients with post-CEA seizures was 93% (95% CI: 85% to 98%), with low heterogeneity (I^2 = 13.37%), indicating consistency across most included studies. The pooled prevalence of pre-operative hypertension among patients who experienced seizures following CEA, stratified by study design, demonstrated consistent findings across both prospective [91%, 95% CI 77–100%; I^2 = 0%] and retrospective [89%, 95% CI 76–99%; I^2 = 43.95%] studies. These results are detailed in Supplemental Figure S4.

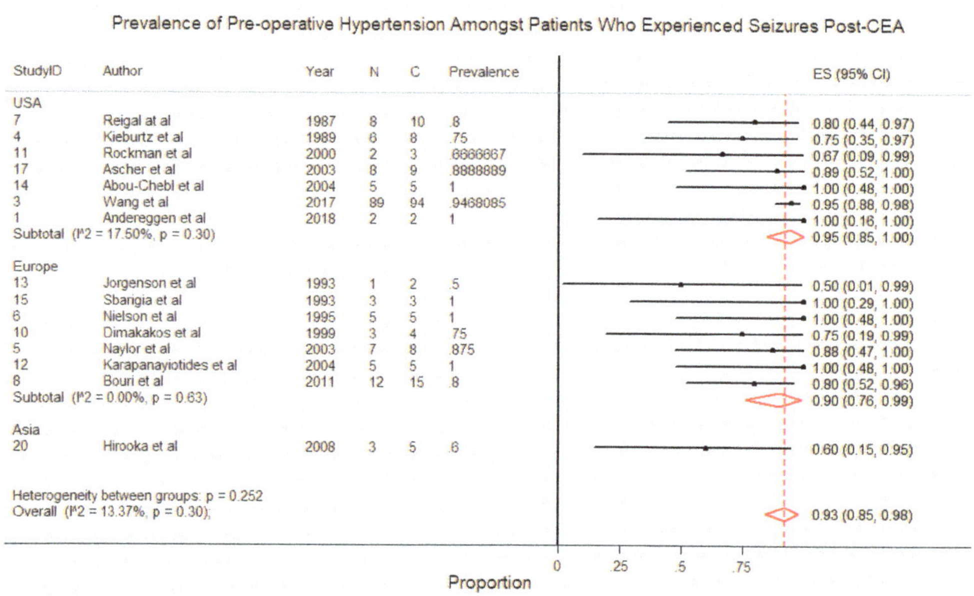

Figure 3. Prevalence of pre-operative hypertension among patients who experienced seizures following carotid endarterectomy (CEA) [4,6,8–11,21,22,25–28,30–32]. Abbreviations: CEA—carotid endarterectomy; N—number of patients with seizures; C—overall cohort; ES—effect size; CI—confidence interval; I^2—the proportion of total variation in effect estimate due to between-study heterogeneity.

3.4. Prevalence of Cerebral Hyperperfusion Post-CEA

The meta-analysis presented in Figure 4 comprises 10,868 patients from 11 studies [4,5,20,21,23,24,26–28,30,31], evaluating the prevalence of cerebral hyperperfusion among patients following CEA. The findings reveal notable regional variations in the reported prevalence of cerebral hyperperfusion, with higher rates observed in European studies compared to those from other regions. Specifically, European studies reported prevalence rates ranging from 2% to 70%, with a pooled prevalence of 14% (95% CI: 3% to 33%) and considerable heterogeneity (I^2 = 98.16%), reflecting variability in study populations and methodologies. In Asia, the pooled prevalence was 10% (95% CI: 7% to 15%) with no observed heterogeneity, suggesting more consistent findings across studies in this region. Conversely, studies conducted in the USA reported significantly lower prevalence rates, with a pooled prevalence of 1% (95% CI: 0% to 1%) with no heterogeneity reported. Overall, the pooled prevalence of cerebral hyperperfusion post-CEA across all studies was 10% (95% CI: 5% to 16%), with considerable heterogeneity (I^2 = 97.43%). The pooled prevalence of cerebral hyperperfusion syndrome following CEA, stratified by study design, highlighted significant variability between prospective [14%, 95% CI 5–26%; I^2 = 95.6%] and retrospective [1%, 95% CI 1–1%; I^2 = 0%] studies. This analysis is illustrated in Supplemental Figure S5.

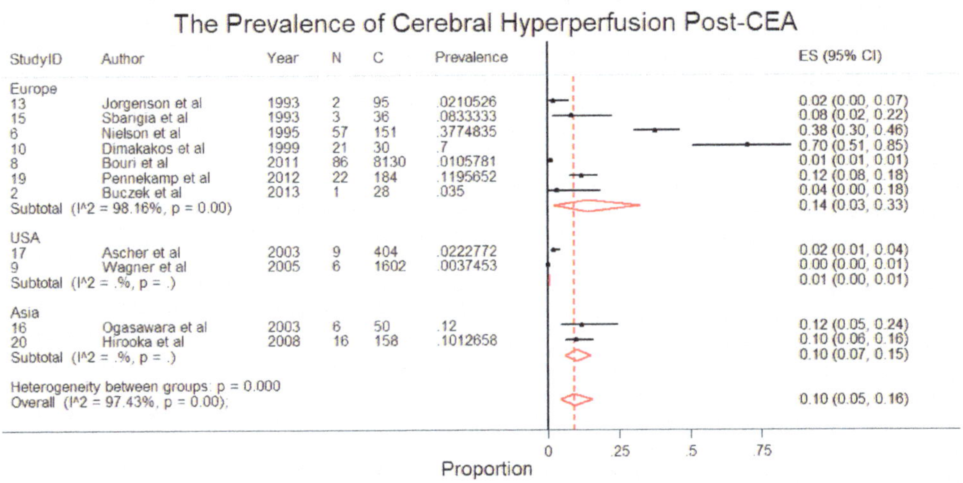

Figure 4. Prevalence of cerebral hyperperfusion syndrome following carotid endarterectomy (CEA) [4,5,20,21,23,24,26–28,30,31]. Abbreviations: CEA—carotid endarterectomy; N—number of patients with seizures; C—overall cohort; ES—effect size; CI—confidence interval; I^2—the proportion of total variation in effect estimate due to between-study heterogeneity.

3.5. Association Between Pre-Operative Hypertension and Seizures Post-CEA

Figure 5, consisting of 19 patients from five studies [21,25,26,28,32], portrays the findings of the meta-analysis on the association between pre-operative hypertension and the odds of developing seizures after CEA. The analysis suggests that pre-operative hypertension may be associated with an increased risk of seizures post-CEA, although the association was not statistically significant. The pooled odds ratio (OR) was 2.71 (95% CI: 0.78–9.41, $p > 0.05$), indicating a potential trend toward increased risk. However, the wide confidence intervals reflect variability in sample sizes and effect estimates across the included studies. Importantly, no heterogeneity was observed among the studies (I^2 = 0%, $p = 0.921$), suggesting consistency in the reported findings despite the lack of statistical significance. The influence of a single study on the meta-analysis for the association between pre-operative hypertension and seizures post-CEA is illustrated in Supplemental Figure S1. The funnel plot with pseudo 95% confidence limits for the meta-analysis is presented in Supplemental Figure S2.

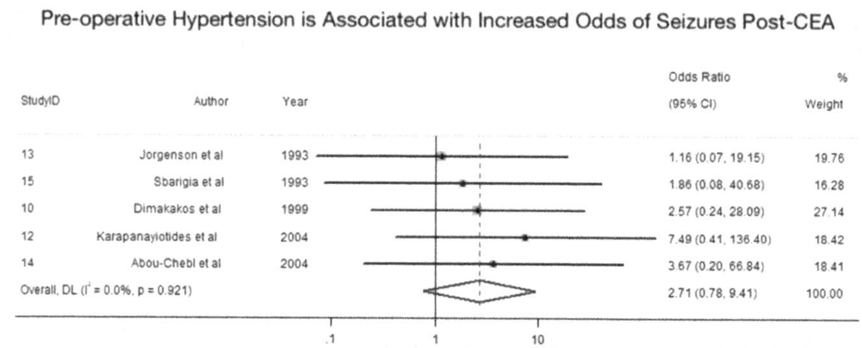

Figure 5. Association between pre-operative hypertension and seizures following carotid endarterectomy (CEA) [21,25,26,28,32]. Abbreviations: CEA—carotid endarterectomy; CI—confidence interval; DL—DerSimonian and Laird method; I^2—the proportion of total variation in effect estimate due to between-study heterogeneity.

4. Discussion

Our study is the first to provide evidence-based insights into the prevalence of seizures following CEA, identifying this rare but clinically significant complication in approximately 1% of patients. These findings underscore the necessity of personalized treatment strategies for a small albeit high-risk subgroup. Pre-operative hypertension, with a pooled prevalence of 93% among patients who experienced seizures, emerged as a key predisposing factor, further associated with elevated odds of postoperative seizures. This association suggests a potential mechanistic link between hypertension-related cerebral dysregulation and adverse perioperative neurological outcomes.

Cerebral hyperperfusion syndrome (CHS), identified in 10% of patients, displayed substantial geographic variability, likely reflecting differences in diagnostic definitions and criteria across studies. The high heterogeneity in European studies particularly underscores the need for standardized diagnostic approaches and consistent monitoring protocols. These findings collectively emphasize the critical importance of stringent perioperative blood pressure control and the implementation of tailored risk mitigation strategies in vulnerable patients.

The observed differences in seizure prevalence between study designs may reflect variations in monitoring intensity, follow-up durations, and diagnostic rigor. Prospective studies, with standardized protocols, reported a broader range of seizure events compared to retrospective analyses, which may be limited by incomplete or underreported data. Despite the low overall prevalence, the significant heterogeneity observed calls for further investigation into the interplay between CHS, perioperative hypertension, and patient-specific risk factors.

The geographic differences in CHS prevalence likely stem from variations in surgical techniques, patient selection, and perioperative management protocols. Tailored approaches—including strict perioperative blood pressure control, routine use of transcranial Doppler, and advanced imaging—may reduce CHS incidence and its associated complications, including seizures and intracranial hemorrhage. While the evidence supporting pre-operative hypertension as a predictor of postoperative seizures remains inconclusive, its high prevalence in this cohort underscores the need for aggressive yet cautious management. Gradual management may be more appropriate in cases of severe symptomatic carotid stenosis to mitigate the risk of stroke progression [33]. These findings reinforce the critical need for optimizing blood pressure management in the perioperative period to improve outcomes and minimize complications. Standardized reporting practices and extended follow-up protocols are essential for future research to refine our understanding of this rare complication. This will enhance our ability to stratify risk, develop targeted interventions, and ensure optimal perioperative care for patients undergoing CEA.

The pathophysiology of seizures following CEA is multifactorial and complex. Cerebral hyperperfusion syndrome has been identified as a primary contributor, leading to complications such as cerebral edema and dysregulation of the brain's autoregulatory capacity [7,34]. This syndrome results from an abrupt increase in cerebral blood flow that the brain's vascular system fails to modulate, causing increased intracranial pressure and subsequent neuronal damage [33]. Hypertension, particularly hypertensive encephalopathy, may also play a role [6], as it is characterized by a rapid onset of neurological symptoms, including seizures, due to severely elevated blood pressure. Elevated middle cerebral artery velocities (MCAVs) further complicate the clinical picture, blurring the lines between cause and effect. Both hyperperfusion and hypertension must be carefully managed post-CEA to reduce the risk of seizures and other complications [6,35].

Our study presents evidence-based insights into real-world prevalence data compared to previous reports, with an estimated pooled prevalence of 1% (range: 0–2%). While prior studies have broadly addressed cognitive decline and hyperperfusion syndrome, they have not specifically focused on seizure prevalence, highlighting a critical gap in the literature [36–39]. There is a substantial lack of data on the prevalence and management of epilepsy following CEA. Current AHA guidelines do not address protocols for managing patients at greater risk of postoperative seizures, underscoring the need for further research in this area [39].

Cerebral hyperperfusion syndrome, although rare, can lead to high mortality due to its association with intracranial hemorrhages. It typically presents as a unilateral headache, confusion, seizures, or focal neurological signs [40]. Treating physicians must remain vigilant for seizure development and implement appropriate management strategies.

Current management includes pre-operative assessments, peri-operative monitoring, and postoperative care. Pre-operative assessments should focus on identifying and managing uncontrolled hypertension, particularly in patients with systolic blood pressures above 180 mmHg [6]. Perioperative management involves maintaining normotension and normocarbia, adhering to anesthesia guidelines, and utilizing TCD monitoring to detect hyperperfusion [6]. Despite these measures, some patients may still develop seizures post-CEA, requiring prompt treatment with diazepam for seizures, labetalol for severe hypertension, and dexamethasone for cerebral edema [6]. CT imaging is essential to exclude intracranial hemorrhage in these cases [6,41]. Emerging evidence suggests that perioperative use of TCD monitoring can improve outcomes by identifying patients at risk of hyperperfusion and intracerebral hemorrhage [29].

In the broader context of carotid revascularization, alternative techniques such as carotid artery stenting (CAS) and transcarotid artery revascularization (TCAR) have emerged as viable options, particularly for high-risk patients [42]. While CAS is associated with a higher risk of stroke and embolization, it may have a lower incidence of cranial nerve injuries compared to CEA [43]. TCAR, a newer technique, combines aspects of both CEA and CAS, utilizing flow reversal to reduce embolic risk during stenting [44]. Early data suggest that TCAR may offer better outcomes in terms of stroke prevention, with fewer complications in high-risk patients [45].

However, data on seizure prevalence specific to CAS and TCAR remain sparse [46]. Given the role of hyperperfusion and embolic phenomena in seizure pathophysiology, these techniques may carry differential risks, warranting further investigation [47]. Future studies should systematically evaluate these differences to inform patient-specific treatment strategies.

4.1. Limitations

This study has several limitations. First, data on symptom severity, diagnostic duration, and seizure phenotype (e.g., epilepsy or status epilepticus) were insufficient across multiple studies, preventing a comprehensive meta-analysis. Discrepancies in sample sizes and demographic data across studies compromised the validity and accuracy of our pooled prevalence estimates. The lack of detailed information on patients' past medical history of seizures, which could increase their risk, further limits the generalizability of our findings.

Considerable heterogeneity was observed among the included studies, suggesting they may have been estimating different quantities due to variations in study design, patient populations, and methodologies. The high heterogeneity observed in the meta-analyses, particularly for pooled prevalence estimates of seizures and cerebral hyperperfusion syndrome, suggests significant variability in study designs, patient populations, and diagnostic criteria, which may have impacted the reliability of the findings. Furthermore, the inclusion of studies spanning a wide time period introduces the possibility that advancements in surgical techniques, anesthesia protocols, and perioperative care processes may have influenced the reported prevalence of seizures. These temporal variations, along with individual patient differences, were not accounted for in the analysis, potentially impacting the consistency of the findings.

Another notable limitation is the lack of available data on pre-operative cerebral hypoperfusion or impaired vasoreactivity and their association with postoperative seizures following CEA. Despite their potential relevance, insufficient research has explored these variables comprehensively, leaving a significant gap in understanding their role as risk factors. Future studies should prioritize investigating cerebral hypoperfusion using advanced imaging modalities, such as MRI and CT perfusion, alongside other emerging biomarkers, to better identify patients at risk and develop targeted preventative strategies.

Systems-level factors, such as variations in treatment protocols, anesthesia techniques, and diagnostic procedures, also differed across studies. Previous evidence suggests that the type of anesthesia can impact clinical outcomes post-CEA [48], indicating the need for further research on the effects of anesthesia techniques on seizure risk [49]. Variations in the rigor of pre- and intra-operative assessments may also affect the reported prevalence of seizures. Additionally, the inconsistent reporting of long-term monitoring and follow-up durations for seizure detection post-CEA likely led to missed incidental seizures, further complicating the interpretation of results. The inconsistent reporting of key variables, such as follow-up durations, seizure detection methods, and regional differences in clinical practices, further complicates the interpretation and generalizability of the results. Since seizures are not commonly anticipated during CEA, the lack of consistent data collection and reporting practices may have introduced potential confounding effects.

4.2. Recommendations

Table 2 provides a comprehensive summary of specific recommendations for managing seizures and related complications following CEA, based on evidence and expert consensus. These recommendations address critical aspects of care, such as optimizing pre-operative blood pressure control (graded 1a for strong evidence) [30,38,50,51] and implementing smoking cessation programs pre-operatively (graded 2b for conditional evidence) [52–55]. The grading system highlights the strength and quality of evidence supporting each recommendation, ensuring clarity for clinical application.

Table 2. Evidence-based recommendations for the management of seizures and related complications following carotid endarterectomy (CEA).

Specific Recommendation	Explanation	Grading	Grading Justification
Optimize pre-operative blood pressure (BP) control	Pre-operative BP control should be optimized, particularly in patients with hypertension, to reduce the risk of cerebral hyperperfusion syndrome and seizures post-CEA.	1b	Strong recommendation supported by good-quality evidence from observational studies and clinical guidelines showing hypertension as a significant risk factor for postoperative complications [38,56].
Routine use of transcranial Doppler (TCD) monitoring	Routine use of TCD monitoring during and after CEA to identify patients at risk of cerebral hyperperfusion syndrome.	2a	Moderate-quality evidence from observational studies and clinical practice guidelines demonstrating the utility of TCD in detecting hyperperfusion and preventing complications [29,57,58].
Monitor patients with history of stroke or transient ischemic attack (TIA) postoperatively	Patients with a history of stroke or TIA should be closely monitored postoperatively for seizures, as they represent a high-risk subgroup.	2b	Moderate-quality evidence from observational studies indicates that prior cerebrovascular events increase the risk of seizures post-CEA, though further research is needed to confirm causality [59].
Implement smoking cessation programs pre-operatively	Smoking cessation programs should be implemented pre-operatively for patients undergoing CEA to reduce overall vascular risk and potential postoperative complications.	2b	Weaker recommendation based on lower-quality evidence from observational studies linking smoking to worse vascular outcomes, though direct evidence for seizure prevention is limited [52–55].
Standardize long-term follow-up for seizure development post-CEA	Long-term follow-up and monitoring for seizure development post-CEA should be standardized, extending beyond the immediate postoperative period to capture delayed events.	2c	Conditional recommendation based on emerging evidence and expert consensus, as current studies lack consistent long-term follow-up data to assess seizure progression or epilepsy development [60].
Use perioperative anesthetic protocols to maintain normotension and normocarbia	Use of perioperative anesthetic protocols that maintain normotension and normocarbia to minimize the risk of cerebral hyperperfusion syndrome and associated seizures.	2a	Moderate-quality evidence from observational studies and clinical practice guidelines regarding perioperative management studies showing that maintaining stable hemodynamics reduces the risk of hyperperfusion and seizures [61,62].
Treat cerebral hyperperfusion syndrome with antihypertensive agents and sedatives	Patients with cerebral hyperperfusion syndrome should be promptly treated with antihypertensive agents (e.g., labetalol) or sedatives (e.g., Dexmedetomidine) to manage symptoms and prevent seizures.	2b	Moderate-quality evidence from observational studies and clinical practice guidelines supports the use of these interventions, though randomized controlled trials are lacking [47,63].
Future studies should focus on identifying biomarkers or imaging predictors	Future studies should focus on identifying biomarkers or imaging predictors (e.g., quantitative MRI or TCD) for seizure risk stratification in patients undergoing CEA.	Not graded	No specific grade assigned due to the lack of direct evidence; this recommendation reflects the need for further research to improve risk prediction and patient outcomes [57,64,65].
Early identification and management of cerebral hyperperfusion syndrome (CHS)	Implement early identification protocols for CHS using TCD or advanced imaging modalities (e.g., MRI, CT perfusion) to detect hyperperfusion and prevent complications such as seizures.	2a	Moderate-quality evidence supports the use of TCD and imaging for identifying CHS, though further research is needed to standardize protocols and validate their effectiveness [29,58,66].
Gradual blood pressure reduction in severe symptomatic carotid stenosis	Gradually reduce blood pressure in patients with severe symptomatic carotid stenosis to minimize the risk of stroke progression and hyperperfusion syndrome.	2a	Observational studies and expert consensus suggest that gradual blood pressure management reduces complications, though high-quality RCTs are lacking [61].
Use of anticonvulsants in high-risk patients	Consider prophylactic use of anticonvulsants in high-risk patients (e.g., those with prior seizures, CHS, or severe hypertension) undergoing CEA.	2c	Conditional recommendation based on limited evidence and expert consensus, with a need for further research to establish efficacy and safety [61].
Tailored perioperative anesthesia protocols	Tailor anesthesia protocols to individual patient risk profiles, including the use of regional anesthesia where appropriate, to reduce hemodynamic fluctuations and seizure risk.	2b	Moderate-quality evidence supports the benefits of regional anesthesia, though its applicability may vary based on patient and procedural factors [6,48,49].
Patient education on postoperative symptoms	Educate patients and caregivers on recognizing early symptoms of CHS and seizures (e.g., severe headache, confusion, focal neurological deficits) to ensure prompt medical attention.	2c	Conditional recommendation based on expert consensus, as evidence on the impact of patient education on outcomes is limited [67,68].
Standardized use of advanced imaging for risk stratification	Incorporate advanced imaging techniques (e.g., quantitative MRI, CT perfusion) preoperatively to assess cerebral vasoreactivity and identify patients at high risk for postoperative seizures.	2c	Emerging evidence supports the utility of advanced imaging, but further studies are needed to validate its role in routine clinical practice [64,69].
Multidisciplinary approach to perioperative care	Adopt a multidisciplinary approach involving neurologists, vascular surgeons, anesthesiologists, and radiologists to optimize perioperative care and reduce seizure risk.	Not graded	No specific evidence available to grade this recommendation, but it reflects expert consensus and best practices in perioperative care.
Long-term monitoring for cognitive decline	Implement long-term monitoring for cognitive decline and neurological complications in patients undergoing CEA, particularly those with postoperative seizures.	2c	Conditional recommendation based on limited evidence linking seizures and CHS to cognitive decline, with a need for further research [70].

Recommendations are based on the findings of the meta-analysis, published evidence and expert consensus. Implement long-term monitoring for cognitive decline and neurological complications in patients undergoing CEA, particularly those with postoperative seizures. Grading reflects the strength of the recommendation and the quality of supporting evidence, as outlined in the grading system. Emerging evidence and further research may refine these recommendations. Explanation of Grading: 1a: Strong recommendation with robust evidence from multiple randomized controlled trials (RCTs) or systematic reviews; 1b: Strong recommendation with good-quality evidence but some variability or limitations in study design or population; 2a: Weaker recommendation based on moderate-quality evidence, acknowledging certain limitations in the data; 2b: Weaker recommendation with lower-quality evidence, often from observational studies or less rigorous trials; 2c: Conditional recommendation based on emerging evidence or expert consensus, reflecting the need for further research; Not graded: Recommendations based on inconclusive or emerging evidence, often highlighting areas for future investigation. Abbreviations: TIA—transient ischemic attack; CEA—carotid endarterectomy; CHS—cerebral hyperperfusion syndrome; TCD—transcranial Doppler; BP—blood pressure; MRI—magnetic resonance imaging.

To improve outcomes and address current gaps, future studies should focus on establishing standardized follow-up periods and implementing long-term monitoring protocols to capture delayed seizure events. Consistent reporting guidelines, including detailed documentation of follow-up timeframes and seizure occurrences, are essential for improving data reliability. Multi-center collaborations can help validate findings across diverse populations, while advanced monitoring techniques, such as TCD and quantitative MRI, may enhance risk stratification. Additionally, educating patients on self-monitoring and clearly defining seizure types across studies will improve comparability and guide clinical decision making. By addressing these limitations, future research can refine management strategies and optimize patient care following CEA.

SMART-CEA Checklist: A Practical Framework for Preventing and Managing Postoperative Seizures Following Carotid Endarterectomy

To bridge existing gaps and build upon evidence-based recommendations, we present the SMART-CEA Checklist (Figure 6; also available as Supplemental S2) as a practical framework for clinicians to optimize the screening and management of seizures and associated complications following CEA. This tool integrates key findings from our meta-analysis and the existing literature, focusing on pre-operative risk assessment, perioperative monitoring, and postoperative care.

SMART-CEA Checklist for Screening and Management of Seizures and Associated Complications Post-Carotid Endarterectomy

Step	Action	Description	Tick/Check
Preoperative Screening			
1. Assess patient history	Evaluate for prior seizures, epilepsy, stroke, transient ischemic attack (TIA), or uncontrolled hypertension.	Identify high-risk patients based on medical history.	☐
2. Optimize blood pressure (BP)	Ensure preoperative BP control, targeting <130/80 mmHg.	Optimize BP to reduce the risk of cerebral hyperperfusion syndrome and seizures.	☐
3. Smoking cessation counseling	Advise and support smoking cessation prior to surgery.	Implement smoking cessation programs to reduce vascular risk and postoperative complications.	☐
4. Evaluate comorbidities	Screen for hypertension, coronary artery disease (CAD), diabetes, and hyperlipidemia.	Identify and manage comorbidities that may increase perioperative risk.	☐
5. Preoperative imaging	Perform transcranial Doppler (TCD) or other imaging to assess cerebral autoregulation and perfusion status.	Use advanced imaging (e.g., TCD, MRI, CT perfusion) to assess cerebral vasoreactivity and identify high-risk patients.	☐
Intraoperative Management			
6. Maintain hemodynamic stability	Use anesthetic protocols to maintain normotension and normocarbia during surgery.	Tailor anesthesia protocols to individual patient risk profiles to reduce hemodynamic fluctuations and seizure risk.	☐
7. Monitor cerebral perfusion	Use TCD monitoring intraoperatively to detect hyperperfusion or impaired autoregulation.	Routine use of TCD monitoring during surgery to identify patients at risk of cerebral hyperperfusion syndrome.	☐
Postoperative Monitoring			
8. Monitor for seizures	Observe for seizures or neurological changes during the first 1–8 days postoperatively.	Closely monitor high-risk patients, particularly those with a history of stroke or TIA.	☐
9. Monitor BP closely	Maintain BP within target range (<140/90 mmHg) using antihypertensive agents as needed.	Gradual BP reduction is recommended in patients with severe symptomatic carotid stenosis to minimize complications.	☐
10. Assess for hyperperfusion syndrome	Monitor for symptoms such as unilateral headache, confusion, focal neurological deficits, or seizures.	Early identification of cerebral hyperperfusion syndrome (CHS) is critical to prevent seizures and other complications.	☐
Management of Seizures and Complications			
11. Treat seizures promptly	Administer benzodiazepines (e.g., diazepam) for acute seizures.	Prompt treatment of seizures is essential to prevent further complications.	☐
12. Manage cerebral hyperperfusion syndrome	Use antihypertensive agents (e.g., labetalol) and corticosteroids (e.g., dexamethasone) as needed.	Treat CHS promptly to manage symptoms and prevent seizures.	☐
13. Perform imaging if seizures occur	Conduct CT or MRI to rule out intracranial hemorrhage or other complications.	Imaging is critical to identify underlying causes of seizures, such as hemorrhage or ischemia.	☐
14. Consider anticonvulsants in high-risk patients	Prophylactic use of anticonvulsants in patients with prior seizures, CHS, or severe hypertension.	Conditional recommendation based on limited evidence; consider for high-risk patients.	☐
Long-Term Follow-Up			
15. Standardize follow-up	Schedule regular follow-ups to monitor for delayed seizures or neurological complications.	Long-term follow-up is essential to capture delayed events and assess progression to epilepsy or cognitive decline.	☐
16. Educate patients	Provide education on recognizing seizure symptoms and when to seek medical attention.	Educate patients and caregivers on early symptoms of CHS and seizures to ensure timely intervention.	☐
17. Consider advanced monitoring	Use advanced imaging (e.g., quantitative MRI) or biomarkers for high-risk patients.	Emerging evidence supports the use of advanced imaging and biomarkers for risk stratification and monitoring.	☐
18. Monitor for cognitive decline	Implement long-term monitoring for cognitive decline and neurological complications, particularly in patients with postoperative seizures.	Conditional recommendation based on limited evidence linking seizures and CHS to cognitive decline.	☐
Multidisciplinary Approach			
19. Adopt a multidisciplinary approach	Involve neurologists, vascular surgeons, anesthesiologists, and radiologists to optimize perioperative care.	Collaboration among specialists ensures comprehensive risk assessment, monitoring, and management of complications.	☐

Figure 6. SMART-CEA Checklist: a practical guide for screening and management of seizures and

associated complications post-carotid endarterectomy. SMART-CEA stands for: S—**Screening:** Assess risk factors such as hypertension, prior seizures, TIA, and smoking; M—**Monitoring:** Monitor cerebral perfusion and blood pressure intraoperatively and postoperatively; A—**Assessing:** Assess for hyperperfusion syndrome and seizure symptoms; R—**Responding:** Respond promptly to seizures and complications with appropriate interventions; T—**Tailoring:** Tailor long-term follow-up and patient education for seizure prevention and management; and CEA—carotid endarterectomy. The SMART-CEA checklist provides a practical, step-by-step guide for clinicians to ensure comprehensive screening, monitoring, and management of seizures and associated complications in patients undergoing CEA. Each step includes a tick/check option for easy tracking and implementation in clinical workflows. Abbreviations: AF—atrial fibrillation; HL—hyperlipidaemia; HTN—hypertension; CAD—coronary artery disease; TIA—transient ischaemic attack; CEA—carotid endarterectomy; TCD—transcranial Doppler; BP—blood pressure; CT—computed tomography; MRI—magnetic resonance imaging.

The acronym "SMART" encapsulates five critical steps: screening for risk factors, monitoring cerebral perfusion and blood pressure, assessing for hyperperfusion syndrome and seizure symptoms, responding promptly to complications with appropriate interventions, and tailoring long-term follow-up and education. By offering clear, actionable steps, the checklist aims to standardize care processes, facilitate early detection of complications such as CHS, and ensure timely and effective management of seizures.

Designed to be user-friendly and easily incorporated into routine clinical workflows, the SMART-CEA Checklist has the potential to improve patient outcomes significantly. However, its implementation requires further validation across diverse clinical settings to assess its broader applicability and ensure its effectiveness in optimizing perioperative care.

5. Conclusions

In conclusion, seizures following CEA are rare but clinically significant, with an overall pooled prevalence of 1%, as demonstrated in this meta-analysis of 69,479 patients. The slightly higher prevalence observed in prospective studies and the identification of cerebral hyperperfusion syndrome as a key contributing factor emphasize the need for diligent perioperative blood pressure management and close neurological monitoring. To address these risks, we provide evidence-based specific recommendations and introduce the SMART-CEA Checklist, a practical framework designed to guide clinicians in optimizing perioperative care and reducing complications. However, significant heterogeneity across studies and limited data on long-term outcomes, such as progression to epilepsy, highlight the need for standardized diagnostic criteria, consistent follow-up protocols, and multi-center collaborations. Future research should focus on improving data reliability, identifying reliable predictors, and exploring long-term outcomes to enhance personalized care and optimize patient outcomes.

Supplementary Materials: The following supporting information can be downloaded at: https://www.mdpi.com/article/10.3390/diagnostics15010006/s1, Table S1: PRISMA checklist for the meta-analysis of seizures following carotid endarterectomy; Table S2: MOOSE checklist for meta-analyses of observational studies included in the study on seizures post-carotid endarterectomy; Table S3: Jaded analysis for methodological quality, risk of bias, and test for funding bias in the meta-analysis; Figure S1: Influence of a single study on the meta-analysis of the association between pre-operative hypertension and seizures following carotid endarterectomy; Figure S2: Funnel plot with pseudo 95% confidence limits for the meta-analysis of seizures post-carotid endarterectomy; Figure S3. Meta-analysis of pooled prevalence of seizures following carotid endarterectomy stratified by study design (prospective vs. retrospective); Figure S4. Meta-analysis of pooled prevalence of pre-operative hypertension among patients who experienced seizures following carotid endarterectomy stratified by study design (prospective vs. retrospective); Figure S5. Meta-analysis of pooled prevalence of cerebral hyperperfusion syndrome following carotid endarterectomy stratified by study design (prospective vs. retrospective); www.mdpi.com/xxx/s2, Supplemental SI2 SMART-CEA Checklist.

Author Contributions: S.M.M.B. conceived the study, contributed to the planning, drafting, and revision of the manuscript, and supervised the members of the Global Health Neurology Lab (K.R. and H.S.). S.M.M.B. encouraged K.R. and H.S. to investigate and supervised the findings of this work. K.R. and S.M.M.B. wrote the first draft of this paper. S.M.M.B. conceived and developed the SMART-CEA checklist introduced in this study. All authors have read and agreed to the published version of the manuscript.

Funding: The financial support for a separate project was received through the Grant-in-Aid for Scientific Research (KAKENHI) (PI: S.M.M.B.), funded by the Japan Society for the Promotion of Science (JSPS), Japanese Ministry of Education, Culture, Sports, Science and Technology (MEXT), Japan (Grant ID: 23KF0126). S.M.M.B. was awarded the JSPS International Fellowship, supported by MEXT and the Australian Academy of Science, for the period 2023–2025 (Grant ID: P23712).

Institutional Review Board Statement: Not applicable. All analyses were based on previously published studies; thus, no ethical approval or patient consent was required.

Informed Consent Statement: Not applicable.

Data Availability Statement: The original contributions presented in the study are included in the article and Online Supplemental Information, and further inquiries can be directed to the corresponding author.

Acknowledgments: We acknowledge the JSPS International Fellowship (Grant ID: P23712) and the Grant-in-Aid for Scientific Research (KAKENHI) (Grant ID: 23KF0126) for their financial support.

Conflicts of Interest: S.M.M.B. reports leadership or fiduciary roles in various organizations, including the *National Cerebral and Cardiovascular Center (Osaka, Japan)* as Visiting Director (2023–2025); *Rotary District 9675 (Sydney, Australia)* as District Chair for Diversity, Equity, and Inclusion; the *Global Health and Migration Hub Community, Global Health Hub Germany (Berlin, Germany)* as Chair, Founding Member, and Manager; and editorial board memberships at *PLOS One, BMC Neurology, Frontiers in Neurology, Frontiers in Stroke, Frontiers in Public Health, Journal of Aging Research, Neurology International, Diagnostics, and BMC Medical Research Methodology*. Additionally, SMMB serves as a Member of the College of Reviewers for the *Canadian Institutes of Health Research (CIHR), Government of Canada;* Director of Research for the *World Headache Society (Bengaluru, India)*; a member of the Scientific Review Committee at *Cardiff University Biobank (Cardiff, UK)*; and as an Expert Adviser/Reviewer for the Cariplo Foundation (Milan, Italy). These roles are unrelated to the submitted work. Other authors (K.R. and H.S.) report no conflicts of interest. The funding body had no influence on this study design, data collection, analysis, interpretation of findings, or manuscript preparation. The content is solely the responsibility of the authors and does not necessarily represent the official views of the affiliated or funding organizations.

References

1. Rerkasem, A.; Orrapin, S.; Howard, D.P.; Rerkasem, K. Carotid endarterectomy for symptomatic carotid stenosis. *Cochrane Database Syst. Rev.* **2020**, *9*, CD001081. [CrossRef]
2. Morris, D.R.; Ayabe, K.; Inoue, T.; Sakai, N.; Bulbulia, R.; Halliday, A.; Goto, S. Evidence-Based Carotid Interventions for Stroke Prevention: State-of-the-art Review. *J. Atheroscler. Thromb.* **2017**, *24*, 373–387. [CrossRef] [PubMed]
3. Manole, A.M.; Sirbu, C.A.; Mititelu, M.R.; Vasiliu, O.; Lorusso, L.; Sirbu, O.M.; Ionita Radu, F. State of the Art and Challenges in Epilepsy-A Narrative Review. *J. Pers. Med.* **2023**, *13*, 623. [CrossRef]
4. Nielsen, T.G.; Sillesen, H.; Schroeder, T.V. Seizures following carotid endarterectomy in patients with severely compromised cerebral circulation. *Eur. J. Vasc. Endovasc. Surg.* **1995**, *9*, 53–57. [CrossRef]
5. Buczek, J.; Karlinski, M.; Kobayashi, A.; Bialek, P.; Czlonkowska, A. Hyperperfusion syndrome after carotid endarterectomy and carotid stenting. *Cerebrovasc. Dis.* **2013**, *35*, 531–537. [CrossRef]
6. Naylor, A.R.; Evans, J.; Thompson, M.M.; London, N.J.; Abbott, R.J.; Cherryman, G.; Bell, P.R. Seizures after carotid endarterectomy: Hyperperfusion, dysautoregulation or hypertensive encephalopathy? *Eur. J. Vasc. Endovasc. Surg.* **2003**, *26*, 39–44. [CrossRef] [PubMed]

7. Biller, J.; Feinberg, W.M.; Castaldo, J.E.; Whittemore, A.D.; Harbaugh, R.E.; Dempsey, R.J.; Caplan, L.R.; Kresowik, T.F.; Matchar, D.B.; Toole, J.; et al. Guidelines for carotid endarterectomy: A statement for healthcare professionals from a special writing group of the Stroke Council, American Heart Association. *Stroke* **1998**, *29*, 554–562. [CrossRef] [PubMed]
8. Kieburtz, K.; Ricotta, J.J.; Moxley, R.T., 3rd. Seizures following carotid endarterectomy. *Arch. Neurol.* **1990**, *47*, 568–570. [CrossRef] [PubMed]
9. Wang, G.J.; Beck, A.W.; DeMartino, R.R.; Goodney, P.P.; Rockman, C.B.; Fairman, R.M. Insight into the cerebral hyperperfusion syndrome following carotid endarterectomy from the national Vascular Quality Initiative. *J. Vasc. Surg.* **2017**, *65*, 381–389 e382. [CrossRef] [PubMed]
10. Reigel, M.M.; Hollier, L.H.; Sundt, T.M., Jr.; Piepgras, D.G.; Sharbrough, F.W.; Cherry, K.J. Cerebral hyperperfusion syndrome: A cause of neurologic dysfunction after carotid endarterectomy. *J. Vasc. Surg.* **1987**, *5*, 628–634. [CrossRef] [PubMed]
11. Andereggen, L.; Amin-Hanjani, S.; El-Koussy, M.; Verma, R.K.; Yuki, K.; Schoeni, D.; Hsieh, K.; Gralla, J.; Schroth, G.; Beck, J.; et al. Quantitative magnetic resonance angiography as a potential predictor for cerebral hyperperfusion syndrome: A preliminary study. *J. Neurosurg.* **2018**, *128*, 1006–1014. [CrossRef] [PubMed]
12. Di Gennaro, G.; Casciato, S.; Quarato, P.P.; Mascia, A.; D'Aniello, A.; Grammaldo, L.G.; De Risi, M.; Meldolesi, G.N.; Romigi, A.; Esposito, V.; et al. Acute postoperative seizures and long-term seizure outcome after surgery for hippocampal sclerosis. *Seizure* **2015**, *24*, 59–62. [CrossRef] [PubMed]
13. Fiest, K.M.; Sauro, K.M.; Wiebe, S.; Patten, S.B.; Kwon, C.S.; Dykeman, J.; Pringsheim, T.; Lorenzetti, D.L.; Jette, N. Prevalence and incidence of epilepsy: A systematic review and meta-analysis of international studies. *Neurology* **2017**, *88*, 296–303. [CrossRef]
14. Stavem, K.; Bjornaes, H.; Langmoen, I.A. Long-term seizures and quality of life after epilepsy surgery compared with matched controls. *Neurosurgery* **2008**, *62*, 326–334; discussion 334-325. [CrossRef] [PubMed]
15. Page, M.J.; McKenzie, J.E.; Bossuyt, P.M.; Boutron, I.; Hoffmann, T.C.; Mulrow, C.D.; Shamseer, L.; Tetzlaff, J.M.; Akl, E.A.; Brennan, S.E.; et al. The PRISMA 2020 statement: An updated guideline for reporting systematic reviews. *BMJ* **2021**, *372*, n71. [CrossRef] [PubMed]
16. Stafstrom, C.E.; Carmant, L. Seizures and epilepsy: An overview for neuroscientists. *Cold Spring Harb. Perspect. Med.* **2015**, *5*. [CrossRef] [PubMed]
17. Carey, R.M.; Whelton, P.K. Evidence for the Universal Blood Pressure Goal of <130/80 mm Hg Is Strong: Controversies in Hypertension—Pro Side of the Argument. *Hypertension* **2020**, *76*, 1384–1390. [CrossRef]
18. Pennekamp, C.W.; Moll, F.L.; De Borst, G.J. Role of transcranial Doppler in cerebral hyperperfusion syndrome. *J. Cardiovasc. Surg.* **2012**, *53*, 765–771.
19. Wan, X.; Wang, W.; Liu, J.; Tong, T. Estimating the sample mean and standard deviation from the sample size, median, range and/or interquartile range. *BMC Med. Res. Methodol.* **2014**, *14*, 135. [CrossRef] [PubMed]
20. Wagner, W.H.; Cossman, D.V.; Farber, A.; Levin, P.M.; Cohen, J.L. Hyperperfusion syndrome after carotid endarterectomy. *Ann. Vasc. Surg.* **2005**, *19*, 479–486. [CrossRef] [PubMed]
21. Sbarigia, E.; Speziale, F.; Giannoni, M.F.; Colonna, M.; Panico, M.A.; Fiorani, P. Post-carotid endarterectomy hyperperfusion syndrome: Preliminary observations for identifying at risk patients by transcranial Doppler sonography and the acetazolamide test. *Eur. J. Vasc. Surg.* **1993**, *7*, 252–256. [CrossRef] [PubMed]
22. Rockman, C.B.; Jacobowitz, G.R.; Lamparello, P.J.; Adelman, M.A.; Woo, D.; Schanzer, A.; Gagne, P.J.; Landis, R.; Riles, T.S. Immediate reexploration for the perioperative neurologic event after carotid endarterectomy: Is it worthwhile? *J. Vasc. Surg.* **2000**, *32*, 1062–1070. [CrossRef]
23. Pennekamp, C.W.; Tromp, S.C.; Ackerstaff, R.G.; Bots, M.L.; Immink, R.V.; Spiering, W.; de Vries, J.P.; Kappelle, L.J.; Moll, F.L.; Buhre, W.F.; et al. Prediction of cerebral hyperperfusion after carotid endarterectomy with transcranial Doppler. *Eur. J. Vasc. Endovasc. Surg.* **2012**, *43*, 371–376. [CrossRef] [PubMed]
24. Ogasawara, K.; Konno, H.; Yukawa, H.; Endo, H.; Inoue, T.; Ogawa, A. Transcranial regional cerebral oxygen saturation monitoring during carotid endarterectomy as a predictor of postoperative hyperperfusion. *Neurosurgery* **2003**, *53*, 309–314; discussion 314-305. [CrossRef] [PubMed]
25. Karapanayiotides, T.; Meuli, R.; Devuyst, G.; Piechowski-Jozwiak, B.; Dewarrat, A.; Ruchat, P.; Von Segesser, L.; Bogousslavsky, J. Postcarotid endarterectomy hyperperfusion or reperfusion syndrome. *Stroke* **2005**, *36*, 21–26. [CrossRef] [PubMed]
26. Jorgensen, L.G.; Schroeder, T.V. Defective cerebrovascular autoregulation after carotid endarterectomy. *Eur. J. Vasc. Surg.* **1993**, *7*, 370–379. [CrossRef]
27. Hirooka, R.; Ogasawara, K.; Sasaki, M.; Yamadate, K.; Kobayashi, M.; Suga, Y.; Yoshida, K.; Otawara, Y.; Inoue, T.; Ogawa, A. Magnetic resonance imaging in patients with cerebral hyperperfusion and cognitive impairment after carotid endarterectomy. *J. Neurosurg.* **2008**, *108*, 1178–1183. [CrossRef]
28. Dimakakos, P.B.; Tsiligiris, V.; Gouliamos, A.; Kotsis, T.E.; Katsaros, G. Postcarotid endarterectomy symptoms. Pre- and postoperative clinical and MRI findings. *Int. Angiol.* **1999**, *18*, 277–286.

29. Dalman, J.E.; Beenakkers, I.C.; Moll, F.L.; Leusink, J.A.; Ackerstaff, R.G. Transcranial Doppler monitoring during carotid endarterectomy helps to identify patients at risk of postoperative hyperperfusion. *Eur. J. Vasc. Endovasc. Surg.* **1999**, *18*, 222–227. [CrossRef] [PubMed]
30. Bouri, S.; Thapar, A.; Shalhoub, J.; Jayasooriya, G.; Fernando, A.; Franklin, I.J.; Davies, A.H. Hypertension and the post-carotid endarterectomy cerebral hyperperfusion syndrome. *Eur. J. Vasc. Endovasc. Surg.* **2011**, *41*, 229–237. [CrossRef]
31. Ascher, E.; Markevich, N.; Schutzer, R.W.; Kallakuri, S.; Jacob, T.; Hingorani, A.P. Cerebral hyperperfusion syndrome after carotid endarterectomy: Predictive factors and hemodynamic changes. *J. Vasc. Surg.* **2003**, *37*, 769–777. [CrossRef] [PubMed]
32. Abou-Chebl, A.; Yadav, J.S.; Reginelli, J.P.; Bajzer, C.; Bhatt, D.; Krieger, D.W. Intracranial hemorrhage and hyperperfusion syndrome following carotid artery stenting: Risk factors, prevention, and treatment. *J. Am. Coll. Cardiol.* **2004**, *43*, 1596–1601. [CrossRef] [PubMed]
33. van Mook, W.N.; Rennenberg, R.J.; Schurink, G.W.; van Oostenbrugge, R.J.; Mess, W.H.; Hofman, P.A.; de Leeuw, P.W. Cerebral hyperperfusion syndrome. *Lancet Neurol.* **2005**, *4*, 877–888. [CrossRef]
34. Edwards, A.M.; Birchler, C.R.; Park, S.; Baker, J.M.; Molnar, R.G. Cerebral Hyperperfusion Syndrome Presenting As Status Epilepticus Following Carotid Endarterectomy. *Cureus* **2021**, *13*, e20551. [CrossRef]
35. Sharifian, M. Hypertensive encephalopathy. *Iran. J. Child. Neurol.* **2012**, *6*, 1–7. [PubMed]
36. Aceto, P.; Lai, C.; De Crescenzo, F.; Crea, M.A.; Di Franco, V.; Pellicano, G.R.; Perilli, V.; Lai, S.; Papanice, D.; Sollazzi, L. Cognitive decline after carotid endarterectomy: Systematic review and meta-analysis. *Eur. J. Anaesthesiol.* **2020**, *37*, 1066–1074. [CrossRef]
37. Galyfos, G.; Sianou, A.; Filis, K. Cerebral hyperperfusion syndrome and intracranial hemorrhage after carotid endarterectomy or carotid stenting: A meta-analysis. *J. Neurol. Sci.* **2017**, *381*, 74–82. [CrossRef] [PubMed]
38. Huibers, A.E.; Westerink, J.; de Vries, E.E.; Hoskam, A.; den Ruijter, H.M.; Moll, F.L.; de Borst, G.J. Editor's Choice—Cerebral Hyperperfusion Syndrome After Carotid Artery Stenting: A Systematic Review and Meta-analysis. *Eur. J. Vasc. Endovasc. Surg.* **2018**, *56*, 322–333. [CrossRef] [PubMed]
39. Goldstein, L.B.; Hasselblad, V.; Matchar, D.B.; McCrory, D.C. Comparison and meta-analysis of randomized trials of endarterectomy for symptomatic carotid artery stenosis. *Neurology* **1995**, *45*, 1965–1970. [CrossRef]
40. Magee, T.R.; Davies, A.H.; Horrocks, M. Transcranial Doppler evaluation of cerebral hyperperfusion syndrome after carotid endarterectomy. *Eur. J. Vasc. Surg.* **1994**, *8*, 104–106. [CrossRef]
41. Katyal, A.; Bhaskar, S.M.M. Value of pre-intervention CT perfusion imaging in acute ischemic stroke prognosis. *Diagn. Interv. Radiol.* **2021**, *27*, 774–785. [CrossRef] [PubMed]
42. Bagley, J.H.; Priest, R. Carotid Revascularization: Current Practice and Future Directions. *Semin. Intervent Radiol.* **2020**, *37*, 132–139. [CrossRef] [PubMed]
43. Gurm, H.S.; Yadav, J.S.; Fayad, P.; Katzen, B.T.; Mishkel, G.J.; Bajwa, T.K.; Ansel, G.; Strickman, N.E.; Wang, H.; Cohen, S.A.; et al. Long-term results of carotid stenting versus endarterectomy in high-risk patients. *N. Engl. J. Med.* **2008**, *358*, 1572–1579. [CrossRef] [PubMed]
44. Trystula, M.; Musialek, P. Transient flow reversal combined with sustained embolic prevention in transcervical revascularization of symptomatic and highly-emboligenic carotid stenoses for optimized endovascular lumen reconstruction and improved peri- and post-procedural outcomes. *Postep. Kardiol. Interwencyjnej* **2020**, *16*, 495–506. [CrossRef]
45. Zhang, G.Q.; Bose, S.; Stonko, D.P.; Abularrage, C.J.; Zarkowsky, D.S.; Hicks, C.W. Transcarotid artery revascularization is associated with similar outcomes to carotid endarterectomy regardless of patient risk status. *J. Vasc. Surg.* **2022**, *76*, 474–481 e473. [CrossRef]
46. Ezzeldin, M.; Hassan, A.E.; Kerro, A.; Martucci, M.; Hussain, M.S.; Mir, O.; Sheriff, F.G.; Kan, P.; Ezepue, C.; Janjua, N.A.; et al. Carotid Artery Stenting Outcomes by Neurointerventional Surgeons (CASONI). *Stroke Vasc. Interv. Neurol.* **2024**, *0*, e001459. [CrossRef]
47. Farooq, M.U.; Goshgarian, C.; Min, J.; Gorelick, P.B. Pathophysiology and management of reperfusion injury and hyperperfusion syndrome after carotid endarterectomy and carotid artery stenting. *Exp. Transl. Stroke Med.* **2016**, *8*, 7. [CrossRef] [PubMed]
48. McCleary, A.J.; Maritati, G.; Gough, M.J. Carotid endarterectomy; local or general anaesthesia? *Eur. J. Vasc. Endovasc. Surg.* **2001**, *22*, 1–12. [CrossRef]
49. Stoneham, M.D.; Stamou, D.; Mason, J. Regional anaesthesia for carotid endarterectomy. *Br. J. Anaesth.* **2015**, *114*, 372–383. [CrossRef]
50. Sultan, S.; Acharya, Y.; Dulai, M.; Tawfick, W.; Hynes, N.; Wijns, W.; Soliman, O. Redefining postoperative hypertension management in carotid surgery: A comprehensive analysis of blood pressure homeostasis and hyperperfusion syndrome in unilateral vs. bilateral carotid surgeries and implications for clinical practice. *Front. Surg.* **2024**, *11*, 1361963. [CrossRef]
51. Kim, K.H.; Lee, C.H.; Son, Y.J.; Yang, H.J.; Chung, Y.S.; Lee, S.H. Post-carotid endarterectomy cerebral hyperperfusion syndrome: Is it preventable by strict blood pressure control? *J. Korean Neurosurg. Soc.* **2013**, *54*, 159–163. [CrossRef] [PubMed]
52. Hoel, A.W.; Nolan, B.W.; Goodney, P.P.; Zhao, Y.; Schanzer, A.; Stanley, A.C.; Eldrup-Jorgensen, J.; Cronenwett, J.L.; Vascular Study Group of New, E. Variation in smoking cessation after vascular operations. *J. Vasc. Surg.* **2013**, *57*, 1338–1344.e1. [CrossRef] [PubMed]
53. Kim, T.I.; Zhang, Y.; Amin, H.P.; Ochoa Chaar, C.I. Presentation and outcomes of carotid endarterectomy in active smokers. *J. Vasc. Surg.* **2020**, *72*, 1720–1727.e1. [CrossRef] [PubMed]

54. Straus, S.; Vootukuru, N.; Willie-Permor, D.; Elsayed, N.; Ross, E.; Malas, M. The Effect of Preoperative Smoking Status on Carotid Endarterectomy Outcomes in Asymptomatic Patients. *J. Vasc. Surg.* **2024**. [CrossRef] [PubMed]
55. Chamseddine, H.; Shepard, A.; Constantinou, C.; Nypaver, T.; Weaver, M.; Boules, T.; Kavousi, Y.; Onofrey, K.; Peshkepija, A.; Halabi, M.; et al. Pre-operative Smoking Cessation Improves Carotid Endarterectomy Outcomes in Asymptomatic Carotid Stenosis Patients. *J. Vasc. Surg.* **2024**. [CrossRef]
56. Eckstein, H.H. European Society for Vascular Surgery Guidelines on the Management of Atherosclerotic Carotid and Vertebral Artery Disease. *Eur. J. Vasc. Endovasc. Surg.* **2018**, *55*, 1–2. [CrossRef]
57. Fassaert, L.M.M.; Immink, R.V.; van Vriesland, D.J.; de Vries, J.P.M.; Toorop, R.J.; Kappelle, L.J.; Westerink, J.; Tromp, S.C.; de Borst, G.J. Transcranial Doppler 24 Hours after Carotid Endarterectomy Accurately Identifies Patients Not at Risk of Cerebral Hyperperfusion Syndrome. *Eur. J. Vasc. Endovasc. Surg.* **2019**, *58*, 320–327. [CrossRef] [PubMed]
58. Li, Q.; Hua, Y.; Liu, J.; Zhou, F.; Du, L.; Li, J.; Li, Q.; Jiao, L. Intraoperative Transcranial Doppler Monitoring Predicts the Risk of Cerebral Hyperperfusion Syndrome After Carotid Endarterectomy. *World Neurosurg.* **2022**, *165*, e571–e580. [CrossRef] [PubMed]
59. Mehdi, Z.; Birns, J.; Partridge, J.; Bhalla, A.; Dhesi, J. Perioperative management of adult patients with a history of stroke or transient ischaemic attack undergoing elective non-cardiac surgery. *Clin. Med.* **2016**, *16*, 535–540. [CrossRef]
60. Yokoyama, T.; Sunaga, S.; Onuki, H.; Otsuka, K.; Jimbo, H. Nonconvulsive Status Epilepticus Associated with Cerebral Hyperperfusion Syndrome after Carotid Endarterectomy: A Case Report. *NMC Case Rep. J.* **2023**, *10*, 197–202. [CrossRef]
61. Lin, Y.H.; Liu, H.M. Update on cerebral hyperperfusion syndrome. *J. Neurointerv. Surg.* **2020**, *12*, 788–793. [CrossRef]
62. Bevilacqua, S.; Ticozzelli, G.; Orso, M.; Alba, G.; Capoccia, L.; Cappelli, A.; Cernetti, C.; Diomedi, M.; Dorigo, W.; Faggioli, G.; et al. Anesthetic management of carotid endarterectomy: An update from Italian guidelines. *J. Anesth. Analg. Crit. Care* **2022**, *2*, 24. [CrossRef]
63. Chang, E.; Wu, L.; Li, X.; Zhou, J.; Zhi, H.; Sun, M.; Chen, G.; Bi, J.; Li, L.; Li, T.; et al. Dexmedetomidine decreases cerebral hyperperfusion incidence following carotid stenting: A double-blind, randomized controlled trial. *Med.* **2024**. [CrossRef]
64. Fan, X.; Lai, Z.; Lin, T.; You, H.; Wei, J.; Li, M.; Liu, C.; Feng, F. Pre-operative Cerebral Small Vessel Disease on MR Imaging Is Associated With Cerebral Hyperperfusion After Carotid Endarterectomy. *Front. Cardiovasc. Med.* **2021**, *8*, 734392. [CrossRef] [PubMed]
65. Fujimoto, S.; Toyoda, K.; Inoue, T.; Hirai, Y.; Uwatoko, T.; Kishikawa, K.; Yasumori, K.; Ibayashi, S.; Iida, M.; Okada, Y. Diagnostic impact of transcranial color-coded real-time sonography with echo contrast agents for hyperperfusion syndrome after carotid endarterectomy. *Stroke* **2004**, *35*, 1852–1856. [CrossRef]
66. Bender, M.; Malojčić, B. The utility of transcranial color Doppler in cerebral hyperperfusion syndrome. *Front. Neurol.* **2023**, *14*, 1223016. [CrossRef]
67. Hu, M.; Zhang, C.; Xiao, X.; Guo, J.; Sun, H. Effect of intensive self-management education on seizure frequency and quality of life in epilepsy patients with prodromes or precipitating factors. *Seizure—Eur. J. Epilepsy* **2020**, *78*, 38–42. [CrossRef]
68. Aliasgharpour, M.; Dehgahn Nayeri, N.; Yadegary, M.A.; Haghani, H. Effects of an educational program on self-management in patients with epilepsy. *Seizure* **2013**, *22*, 48–52. [CrossRef]
69. Chang, C.H.; Chang, T.Y.; Chang, Y.J.; Huang, K.L.; Chin, S.C.; Ryu, S.J.; Yang, T.C.; Lee, T.H. The role of perfusion computed tomography in the prediction of cerebral hyperperfusion syndrome. *PLoS ONE* **2011**, *6*, e19886. [CrossRef]
70. Araya, S.; Akamatsu, Y.; Ono, Y.; Yamazaki, R.; Fujiwara, S.; Chida, K.; Kobayashi, M.; Koji, T.; Ogasawara, K. Impact of postoperative cerebral hyperperfusion on 2-year cognitive outcomes of patients undergoing carotid endarterectomy. *J. Neurosurg.* **2024**, 1–8. [CrossRef] [PubMed]

diagnostics

MDPI

Brief Report

Captive Bolt Gun-Related Vascular Injury: A Single Center Experience

Jure Pešak *, Andrej Porčnik and Borut Prestor

Department of Neurosurgery, University Medical Centre Ljubljana, 1000 Ljubljana, Slovenia; andrej.porcnik@kclj.si (A.P.); borut.prestor@kclj.si (B.P.)
* Correspondence: jure.pesak@gmail.com

Abstract: This article investigates the clinical and radiological characteristics of captive bolt gun head injuries, a rare form of low-velocity penetrating brain injury. Eleven consecutive patients were included in the study. Vascular injuries and the rate of infection were systematically analyzed. Radiological findings reveal common bolt trajectories in the anterior cranial fossa, with identified risk factors for a poor outcome including trajectory crossing midline, hematocephalus, and paranasal sinus involvement. Only one patient had a good outcome. Despite meticulous microsurgical techniques, this study highlights often unfavorable clinical outcomes in captive bolt gun injuries, with vascular injury identified as a potential contributing risk factor for a poor outcome. Knowledge of variant vascular tree anatomy and corresponding vascular territory is important. To avoid potential vascular injuries, a complete removal of bone fragments was not always performed and it did not increase the rate of infection, challenging the conventional wisdom advocating for the complete removal of bone fragments. These findings contribute novel insights into captive bolt gun-related injuries, paving the way for further research.

Keywords: captive bolt gun; vascular injury; low-velocity penetrating brain injury; skin–bone imprimatum; incomplete bone fragment debridement; frontopolar artery territory; anterior cranial fossa bolt trajectory

1. Introduction

Captive bolt gun (CBG) head injuries represent a rare form of penetrating brain injuries with only a few documented cases in the literature [1–7]. This is a device that is commonly employed in the meat industry to stun animals before slaughter [1,2]. A bolt penetrates the scull, causing direct and indirect injures to the brain parenchyma through bone fragments [1,2]. The bolt length varies among different tool brands, ranging from 60 to 90 mm in various series [1,3,4]. CBG head injuries are classified as low-velocity penetrating brain injuries, given that the bolt's peak velocity ranges between 30 and 60 m per second [1,3,4]. In the rural areas of Middle and Eastern European countries, where the GBG is the most prevalent stun device in the meat industry, it can be utilized in suicide attempts [2,4]. CBG injuries resulting from suicide attempts are usually anticipated in the anterior and middle cranial fossa. The trajectory depth does generally not exceed the bolt length, as the punched-out skin and bone fragments do not act as a secondary projectile due to the low velocity [1]. Moreover, there are typically no exit wounds. Despite being considered low-velocity brain injuries, these patients often have unfavorable outcome [1]. The reason may be due to the additional vascular injuries that are caused directly by bolt or bone fragments. Vascular injuries can result in ischemic lesion in the corresponding vascular territories. These lesions are highly variable, especially in the anterior cerebral artery territory [8,9]. Variations are greater in the smaller branches of the vascular tree [8]. The anatomic distribution of vascular territories can be radiologically assesed despite anatomical variations in the vascular tree [8,9]. There are three known radiological factors of a poor outcome in penetrating head injury: trajectory crossing midline, hematocephalus, and vascular injury [2,7].

The first case studies of CBG head injury were published in 1960 [10]. Sparse clinical case reports, mostly featuring 1–3 case studies per paper, shed light on early clinical findings of the pathology [5,10–12]. Following these initial 13 cases on PubMed written in the English language, the first miniseries of 12 clinical cases was published in 2002, augmented by supplementary experimental data in the field of forensic medicine [4]. The ongoing period of forensic medicine research has advanced to the most developed stage in CBG head injury research to date, expanding the knowledge of specific mechanisms of CBG head injuries through experiments and reports with complicated cases of CBG head injuries [13–20]. Our clinical study presents a single-center experience with CBG head injuries. Potential clinical and radiological prognostic factors were analyzed. It is the first report where CBG-related vascular injuries have been systematically analyzed.

2. Materials and Methods

The clinical study was conducted at the Department of Neurosurgery of the University Medical Centre Ljubljana, Slovenia. All patients with CBG head injury who received either conservative or operative neurosurgical care were included. From December 2016 to December 2023, eleven consecutive patients with CBG head injuries were studied. Medical records were retrospectively analyzed for clinical and radiological factors. Additional telephone interviews with patient relatives were conducted on 13 December 2023, for further clarification of treatment outcomes. General patient data and the time of the incident were recorded. Initial neurological status was evaluated based on the Glasgow coma scale (GCS) at the scene of the incident and on the GCS with pupillary status at the time of admission. Radiological factors of CBG head injury were evaluated using the initial computed tomography (CT) scan at admission. Localization of the entry wound, trajectory length, localization of parenchymal damage, paranasal sinus involvement, hematocephalus occurrence, and midline crossing were recorded. Treatment strategy was tailored according to the clinical status at admission and to the initial CT scan. The surgical technique was noted, considering the degree of bone fragment removal and the effectiveness of paranasal sinus reconstruction. Postoperative ischemic lesions were evaluated within the first 24 h using a CT scan. The radiological signs of secondary ischemic lesion, infection-related injuries, and shunt-dependent hydrocephalus were evaluated by utilizing diagnostic imaging during the postoperative period. The clinical outcome was evaluated based on the Glasgow outcome score (GOS). A favorable outcome was determined as a GOS of 4 or 5, an unfavorable outcome was determined as a GOS of 2 or 3, and death was determined as a GOS of 1. Data are presented along with descriptive statistics.

3. Results

3.1. Patient Characteristics

All of the 11 patients were men (Table 1). The mean age was 59 $\pm$ 12 years (with an interval of 36–94 years). Six patients had a psychiatric history and two patients had major comorbidities—carcinoma. While seven patients had an initial Glasgow coma scale (GCS) score of 14 or above at the scene, only three patients maintained a GCS score of 14 or higher at the time of hospital admission. Three patients presented with a GCS of 3 at the scene and with dilated and unresponsive pupils at admission. The time from the injury to hospital admission could not be reliably established. The mean GCS score at hospital admission was 7 $\pm$ 5.

Table 1. Clinical and radiological characteristics of patients.

Patient	1	2	3	4	5	6	7	8	9	10	11
Gender	male	male	male	male	male	male	male	male	male	male	male
Age	58	65	68	36	94	67	65	43	40	52	67
GCS at scene	15	15	11	3 *	15	14	10	15	3 *	3 *	14
GCS at admission	3	15	3	3	15	3 *	6	15	3 *	3 *	3
Latest GOS	3	3	3	1 *	1	1 *	3	5	1 *	1 *	3
Comorbidities	bipolar	depression	depression	depression	carcinoma	none	none	carcinoma, depression	none	none	depression
PBI entry wound location and side	parasagittal (R)	pterional (R)	pterional (R)	parasagittal (R)	parasagittal (L)	parasagittal (R)	pterional (R)	pterional (R)	temporal (R)	pterional (R)	parasagittal (L)
Trajectory length	82 mm	83 mm	90 mm	82 mm	48 mm	86 mm	83 mm	68 mm	93 mm	95 mm	81 mm
Parenchymal damage	CS + CC	CS	CS + CC	CS + CC	CS	CS + CC + deep structures	CS	CS + CC	CS + deep structures	CS + deep structures	CS + CC + deep structures
Sinuses involvement	frontal	no	no	no	no	frontal	ethmoidal	no	no	no	frontal
Hematocephalus	yes	no	yes	yes	no	yes	no	yes	yes	yes	yes
Midline crossing	no	no	yes	yes	no	no	no	no	yes	yes	yes
Secondary ischemic lesion	frontopolar territory	no	no	no	no	no	no	no	no	no	frontopolar territory
Secondary infection	yes	no	no	x	x	x	no	no	x	x	no
Shunt-dependent hydro-cephalus	yes	no	no	x	x	x	no	no	x	x	no

* Treatment stage when the patient was categorized for palliative care—conservative symptomatic treatment. GCS—Glasgow coma scale. GOS—Glasgow outcome scale. PBI—penetrating brain injury. R—right side. L—left side. CS—cortico-subcortical. CC—corpus callosum. x—Not applicable because the patient died before secondary endpoints could be measured.

3.2. Radiological Characteristics

The entry wounds were located in the pterional region in five patients, in the parasagittal region in five patients, and in the temporal region in one patient (Figure 1). The mean penetrating trajectory length was 80 ± 15 mm (an interval of 48–95 mm). The brand of the CBG could not be determined. All patients exhibited cortico-subcortical parenchymal injury while seven patients had corpus callosum involvement and four patients displayed involvement in the deep structures or in the brainstem. Nine patients developed intracerebral hemorrhage.

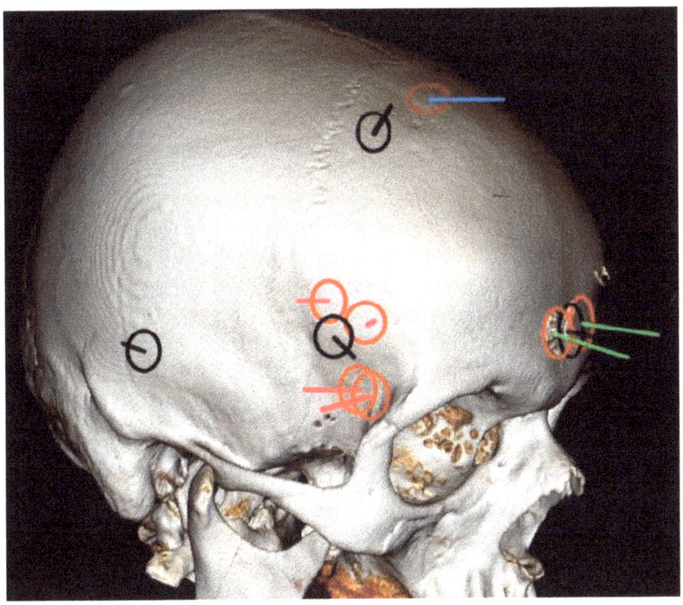

Figure 1. Schematic representation of the points of bone entry wound location and trajectory course.

Three patients had paranasal sinuses involvement, eight patients developed hematocephalus, and the CBG trajectory crossed midline in five patients. Two patients had one proposed radiological factor for a poor outcome while six patients had two factors for a poor outcome and a single patient had all three factors for a poor outcome (Table 1).

The head computed tomography model depicts entry bone wounds marked by circles and corresponding trajectories marked by lines within the circles for all patients. Nine injuries were on the right side and two were on the left side of the head. Trajectories only show their approximate direction and not their depth. For the ease of visualization, all injuries on the left side were symmetrically translocated to the right side. Surgically treated cases are denoted by red circles. Cases treated with only palliative conservative care are represented by black circles and black trajectories. Two of the surgically treated patients with ischemic areas due to the vascular injury of the anterior circulation are presented by green trajectories. Red trajectories indicate surgically treated cases without major vascular injury. The blue trajectory shows the case with the injury of the superior sagittal sinus.

3.3. Primary Treatment and Surgical Technique

Out of the eleven patients, seven underwent surgical treatment (64%). The treatment was performed within 4 h from hospital admission. In cases involving paranasal sinuses, a cranialization of the frontal sinus was performed in all surgical cases, accompanied by additional reconstruction of the galea aponeurotica. A craniotomy was the primary surgical approach in six cases while craniectomy was performed in only one case. Full debridement of intraparenchymal bone fragments was achieved in only two patients, considering the potential for additional iatrogenic brain or vascular injury, prompting caution for complete removal in other cases. Four patients in poor initial condition at admission received only palliative conservative care. Indications for conservative palliative care included a poor clinical condition with symptoms of brain death and/or irreversible neural injuries incompatible with a functional outcome based on the initial head CT scan. All patients who underwent surgical treatment received prophylactic antibiotic treatment for six weeks.

3.4. Radiological and Clinical Outcome

Four patients developed diffuse brain edema without brain perfusion in the first 24 h—all of whom were under palliative conservative care. In those four patients, vascular injury could not be determined. Two out of seven surgically treated patients developed incomplete ischemic lesion in a named small branching artery territory in anterior circulation. Both lesions were in the vascular territory of the frontopolar artery (Figure 2). Notably, five surgically treated patients did not develop an ischemic lesion, as outlined in Table 1.

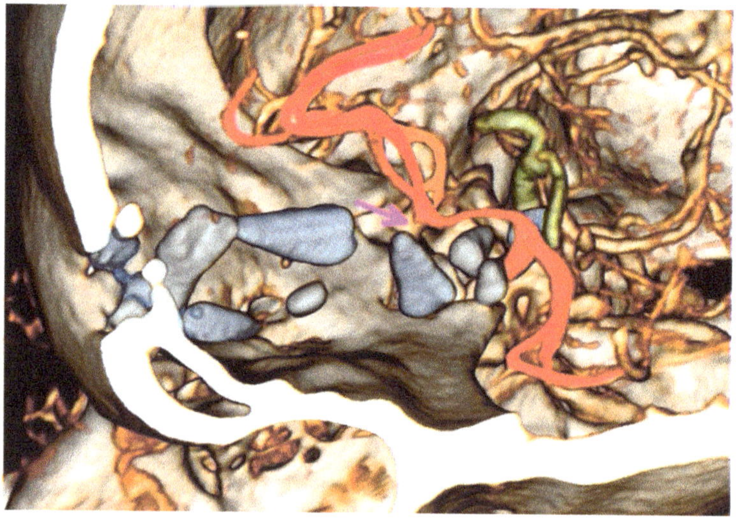

Figure 2. Three-dimensional head computed tomographic angiography reconstruction of patient 10.

One patient developed an intracranial abscess with secondary infection-related parenchymal injury necessitating secondary surgery. One patient developed shunt-dependent hydrocephalus.

The computed tomographic angiography of patient 10 reveals a typical captive bolt gun trajectory in the anterior cranial fossa. Blue-marked bone fragments caused significant direct injury to the brain parenchyma and the left frontopolar artery, as indicated by the purple arrow highlighting the branching stem of the artery with an absence of distal blood flow. Bone fragments located under the circle of Willis pose a potential risk to both the anterior and posterior groups of the perforators. Arteries susceptible to injury include the supraclinoid carotid artery segments, the left middle cerebral artery, and the anterior cerebral artery (marked in red), along with the contralateral middle cerebral artery perforators (the parent artery marked in orange). Injury of the vertebrobasilar system (marked in green) occurs when the trajectories are deeper.

4. Discussion

Head injuries with CBG represent a rare form of low-velocity penetrating brain injury characterized by specific clinical and radiological features. All of our case studies were instances of self-inflicted harm and all were men as described by other researchers [4]; therefore, all injuries were found in the anterior and middle cranial fossa and mostly on the right side. The age range varied significantly, from 36 to 94 years. More than half of the patients exhibited diagnosed depression, which is consistent with the literature [1,2,4,5], and two patients had significant comorbidities.

Prompt intervention in patients with good initial neurological status may spare a substantial portion of brain parenchyma and its vasculature from a secondary injury. However, an initial GCS score of 3 at the scene with unresponsive and dilated pupils at admission significantly correlates with poor outcomes [2]. In our series, despite the absence of three proposed radiological risk factors and of a postoperative ischemic lesion, one surgically treated patient with good initial performance status succumbed to injury, emphasizing the impact of serious comorbidities in the very elderly (a 94-year-old man). A larger series reported mortality rates between 60 and 90% [4–6]. Despite CBG head injuries being categorized as low-velocity penetrating brain injuries, a high mortality is expected due to the self-inflicted mechanism, the high probability of vascular injury, and the high rate of infection.

Similar to the findings in the literature, common entry points were in the right pterional and frontobasal midline areas [4]. Projections of bolt trajectories often include vascular structures. One of the three proposed radiological factors for a poor outcome includes vascular injury such as injury of superior sagittal sinus and its bridging veins and/or anterior cerebral artery branches in the midline, which were injured in two cases in our series. With a mean trajectory length of 80 mm, bolt and/or bone fragments usually do not cause significant direct injury to the brainstem but often reach the anterior and posterior groups of the perforators (Table 1, Figure 2) [8]. Gnjidić et al. reported that the cause of death in five out of seven successful suicides was an injury to blood vessels in the Sylvian fissure and in one out of seven successful suicides, the injury was on the internal carotid artery [4].

The complete removal of all bone fragments with meticulous debridement is advocated to reduce the risk of intracranial infection [4,6]. However, contrary to these authors, our series experienced incomplete debridement of intraparenchymal bone fragments in all but one surgical case, without late postoperative intracranial infection. An intracranial abscess in one case that necessitated secondary surgery, despite complete removal of all bone fragments during the primary surgery, was likely due to latent cerebrospinal fluid leakage through a paranasal sinus fistula. Shunt-dependent hydrocephalus developed in this case because severe ventriculitis occurred. Also, this was a case where craniotomy was performed. In our series, only one out of seven surgically treated cases involved craniectomy. Described are cases with either craniotomy or craniectomy with mixed results [2,4–7]. We consistently employed galea reconstruction and sinus cranialization to separate cranial spaces in cases of paranasal sinus communication, mitigating cerebrospinal fluid-related ascending infections. Complete removal of bone fragments does not seem crucial, especially if iatrogenic injury to the perforators or small branching arteries could occur. Due to the colonization of skin flora at the end of the trajectory in their series, the importance of prolonged antibiotic prophylactic treatment in our surgical cases is emphasized [4]. Geisenberger et al. further showed that almost all cases had skin–bone imprimatum that can explain cutaneous bacterial flora [1]. In our series, the only case requiring secondary surgery due to cerebral abscess had mixed bacterial flora, including non-skin-related Enterococcus casseliflavus and Enterococcus durans. Unusual microbes causing infection might explain this complication leading to secondary surgery.

Even though there was no delayed cerebral ischemia in any named artery's territory or in the anterior or posterior perforator group territory, according to vascular territories described by Vogels et al. [8], two of our surgically treated patients developed an ischemic lesion in the frontopolar artery territory. In both cases, this led to an unfavorable clinical outcome (Table 1).

5. Conclusions

Captive bolt gun head injuries present as low-velocity penetrating brain injuries. This study is the first to shed light from the perspective of vascular injury. Despite a comprehensive understanding of variant anatomy, mechanism of injury, microsurgical techniques, appropriate antibiotic treatment, and intensive care, these injuries often result in unfavorable clinical outcomes. The type of surgical treatment depends on the entry wound location, paranasal sinus involvement, and bolt trajectory. Our study indicates that incomplete removal of deep bone fragments and craniotomy do not elevate infection rates, necessitating secondary surgery. This is important because additional iatrogenic vascular injury due to fragment removal can lead to a worse outcome.

Author Contributions: Conceptualization, J.P. and A.P.; methodology, J.P.; software, J.P. and A.P.; validation, J.P., A.P. and B.P.; formal analysis, J.P and A.P.; investigation, J.P. and A.P.; resources, J.P. and A.P.; data curation, J.P. and A.P.; writing—original draft preparation, J.P. and A.P.; writing—review and editing, J.P., A.P. and B.P.; visualization, J.P.; supervision, B.P.; project administration, B.P. All authors have read and agreed to the published version of the manuscript.

Funding: This research received no external funding.

Institutional Review Board Statement: The study was conducted in accordance with the Declaration of Helsinki. Ethical review and approval were waived for this study due to the retrospective design of the study.

Informed Consent Statement: Informed consent was obtained from all patients involved in the study that can be identified. Additionally, written informed consent to publish this paper was obtained from all patients.

Data Availability Statement: The raw data supporting the conclusions of this article will be made available by the authors on request.

Conflicts of Interest: The authors declare no conflicts of interest. The funders had no role in the design of the study; in the collection, analyses, or interpretation of the data; in the writing of the manuscript; or in the decision to publish the results.

References

1. Geisenberger, D.; Giorgetti, A.; Glardon, M.; Perdekamp, M.G.; Pollak, S.; Pircher, R. The punched-out tissue complex (skin-bone "imprimatum") in shots from captive-bolt guns: Does it act as a secondary projectile? *Int. J. Leg. Med.* **2020**, *134*, 1095–1102. [CrossRef]
2. Marhold, F.; Scheichel, F.; Ladisich, B.; Pruckner, P.; Strasser, E.; Themesl, M.; Ungersboeck, K.; Popadic, B. Surviving the Scene in Civilian Penetrating Brain Injury: Injury Type, Cause and Outcome in a Consecutive Patient Series in Austria. *Front. Surg.* **2022**, *9*, 923949. [CrossRef] [PubMed]
3. Gibson, T.J.; Mason, C.W.; Spence, J.Y.; Barker, H.; Gregory, N.G. Factors Affecting Penetrating Captive Bolt Gun Performance. *J. Appl. Anim. Welf. Sci.* **2015**, *18*, 222–238. [CrossRef] [PubMed]
4. Gnjidić, Z.; Kubat, M.; Malenica, M.; Sajko, T.; Radić, I.; Rumboldt, Z. Epidemiological, forensic, clinical, and imaging characteristics of head injuries acquired in the suicide attempt with captive bolt gun. *Acta Neurochir.* **2002**, *144*, 1271–1277. [CrossRef] [PubMed]
5. Caird, G.R.J. Self-inflicted head trauma using a captive bolt pistol: Report of three cases. *Br. J. Neurosurg.* **2000**, *14*, 349–351. [CrossRef] [PubMed]
6. Oikonomou, A.; Astrinakis, M.; Birbilis, T.; Pavlidis, P.; Prassopoulos, P. Head trauma by captive bolt gun. *BMJ Case Rep.* **2011**, *2011*, bcr0920114809. [CrossRef] [PubMed]
7. Schlag, H.; Neuhoff, J.; Castein, J.; Hoffmann, C.; Kandziora, F. Rupture of the Superior Sagittal Sinus in Penetrating Head Injury—Management of a Rare Trauma Mechanism. *J. Neurol. Surg. Rep.* **2022**, *83*, e3–e7. [CrossRef] [PubMed]
8. Vogels, V.; Dammers, R.; van Bilsen, M.; Volovici, V. Deep Cerebral Perforators: Anatomical Distribution and Clinical Symptoms. *Stroke* **2021**, *52*, E660–E674. [CrossRef] [PubMed]
9. van der Zwan, A.; Hillen, B.; Tulleken, C.A.F.; Dujovny, M.; Dragovic, L. Variability of the territories of the major cerebral arteries. *J. Neurosurg.* **1992**, *77*, 927–940. [CrossRef] [PubMed]
10. Gund, A. Über Bolzenschußverletzungen; zugleich ein Beitrag zur Versorgung offener frontobasaler Impressionen. *Acta Neurochir.* **1960**, *8*, 444–448. [CrossRef] [PubMed]
11. Tordrup, P.; Kjeldsen, S. Accidental injuries from captive-bolt guns (slaughterer's gun). *Injury* **1994**, *25*, 497–499. [CrossRef] [PubMed]

12. Mosdal, C. Cranio-cerebral injuries from Slaughterer's gun. *Acta Neurochir.* **1985**, *74*, 31–34. [CrossRef] [PubMed]
13. Ventura, F.; Blasi, C.; Celesti, R. Suicide with the latest type of slaughterer's gun. *Am. J. Forensic Med. Pathol.* **2002**, *23*, 326–328. [CrossRef] [PubMed]
14. Simic, M.; Draskovic, D.; Stojiljkovic, G.; Vukovic, R.; Budimlija, Z.M. The characteristics of head wounds inflicted by "humane killer" (captive-bolt gun)—A 15-year study. *J. Forensic Sci.* **2007**, *52*, 1182–1185. [CrossRef] [PubMed]
15. Viel, G.; Schröder, A.S.; Püschel, K.; Braun, C. Planned complex suicide by penetrating captive-bolt gunshot and hanging: Case study and review of the literature. *Forensic Sci. Int.* **2009**, *187*, e7–e11. [CrossRef] [PubMed]
16. Perdekamp, M.G.; Kneubuehl, B.P.; Ishikawa, T.; Nadjem, H.; Kromeier, J.; Pollak, S.; Thierauf, A. Secondary skull fractures in head wounds inflicted by captive bolt guns: Autopsy findings and experimental simulation. *Int. J. Leg. Med.* **2010**, *124*, 605–612. [CrossRef]
17. Fanton, L.; Karger, B. Suicide with two shots to the head inflicted by a captive-bolt gun. *J. Forensic Leg. Med.* **2012**, *19*, 90–93. [CrossRef] [PubMed]
18. Pircher, R.; Geisenberger, D.; Perdekamp, M.G.; Neukamm, M.; Pollak, S.; Schmidt, U.; Thierauf-Emberger, A. Suicide with two makes of captive-bolt guns (livestock stunners) fired simultaneously to the forehead. *Int. J. Leg. Med.* **2017**, *131*, 1557–1564. [CrossRef]
19. Veselinović, I.; Žigić, S.; Vapa, D. Suicide with an unusual home-manufactured firearm. *Forensic Sci. Med. Pathol.* **2019**, *15*, 288–291. [CrossRef] [PubMed]
20. Nikolić, S.; Atanasijević, T.; Živković, V. Unusual suicidal penetrating heart injury by captive-bolt gunshot. *Forensic Sci. Med. Pathol.* **2022**, *18*, 260–263. [CrossRef] [PubMed]

diagnostics

MDPI

Case Report

The Impact of Class III Obesity on Outcomes for Vestibular Schwannoma Surgery: A Case Report

Tomaž Šmigoc, Hojka Rowbottom and Janez Ravnik *

Department of Neurosurgery, University Medical Centre Maribor, 2000 Maribor, Slovenia; tomaz.smigoc@ukc-mb.si (T.Š.); hojka.rowbottom@ukc-mb.si (H.R.)

* Correspondence: janez.ravnik@ukc-mb.si

Abstract: Background and Clinical Significance: Vestibular schwannomas (VS) are benign tumors arising from Schwann cells of the eighth cranial nerve. They represent approximately 8% of all intracranial tumors and have an increasing incidence. Larger VS can cause brainstem compression and hydrocephalus, and magnetic resonance imaging (MRI) is the diagnostic modality of choice. Individuals with VS and an elevated body mass index (BMI) can have more postoperative complications due to their weight, which can also negatively impact the preoperative diagnostic process and planning, as well as the surgery itself, as compromises must be made since optimal positioning of the patient is often not feasible. Increased BMI is a recognized risk factor for cerebrospinal fluid (CSF) leak after microscopic resection of a VS. **Case Presentation**: This report presents a case of a patient with class III obesity who had to undergo a right VS resection with preexisting hydrocephalus and the obstacles encountered by the surgical team throughout the diagnostics process since MRI could not be performed and preoperative planning had to be based on computed tomography (CT) scan; operative treatment, where suboptimal patient placement was achieved for a planned retrosigmoid approach to the pontocerebellar angle (PCA) and postoperative rehabilitation, which was hindered by his high BMI (55 kg/m^2) with several complications, such as CSF leak, due to his extreme weight. **Conclusions**: Despite barriers, optimal tumor resection was obtained with a long neurorehabilitation process, with a favorable outcome, emphasizing the role of a multidisciplinary team.

Keywords: vestibular schwannoma; severe obesity; postoperative complications; CSF leak

1. Introduction

Schwannomas represent benign tumors consisting of a clonal population of Schwann cells that have undergone cystic and degenerative changes and are typically attached to peripheral nerves, with most cases being sporadic [1,2]. Vestibular schwannomas (VSs) are tumors arising from Schwann cells of the eighth cranial nerve, which lies next to the seventh cranial nerve, with both nerves leaving the brainstem just below the pons and entering the internal auditory canal with the eighth cranial nerve being responsible for hearing and balance and VSs represent around 8% of all intracranial tumors [3–9]. The majority of VSs are in the posterior fossa, which extends from tentorium cerebelli superiorly to foramen magnum inferiorly, specifically in the angle between the pons and the cerebellar hemisphere (pontocerebellar angle) [10]. Epidemiological research conducted thus far has demonstrated an increase in the incidence [4,9]. VS are equally common in men and women [11]. The median age of VS presentation is 50 years, and it is unilateral in more than 90% of patients [7]. Clinical symptoms of VS vary, including asymmetrical hearing loss, tinnitus, vertigo, ataxia, loss of balance, and headaches [5,6]. Larger tumors can cause hydrocephalus and brainstem compression [12]. The diagnostic modality of choice is magnetic resonance imagining (MRI) with contrast-enhanced T1-weighted scans considered to be the gold standard for the initial evaluation and postoperative assessment of recurrence or residual tumors with computed tomography (CT) playing a complementary role in the evaluation of VS [13]. An audiogram, which in cases of VS shows an asymmetric sensorineural hearing loss, should also be performed in the diagnostic process [14–16]. Treatment options include surgery, observation with serial imaging, and stereotactic radiosurgery [6].

The population of overweight and obese individuals has reached epidemic levels and continues to rise [17]. Body mass index (BMI), based on an individual's height and weight, has been used as a simple tool to classify people into different groups with those whose BMI ranges between 25 kg/m^2 and 29.9 kg/m^2 being classified as overweight and those with BMI 30 kg/m^2 or over as obese, which can be subdivided into class I obesity (30 to less than 35 kg/m^2), class II obesity (35 to less than 40 kg/m^2), and class III obesity or severe obesity (40 kg/m^2 and more) [18,19]. Elevated BMI negatively impacts postoperative outcomes in several surgical specialties, including neurosurgery [20]. Obesity can also negatively impact the diagnostic process, which cannot be performed optimally as diagnostic machines often have maximal weight allowance; hence, adjustments and compromises must be made [21]. Outcomes of a neurological examination can also be impaired by obesity, especially when assessing coordination and gait disturbances [22]. Increased BMI has been recognized as a risk factor for postoperative cerebrospinal fluid (CSF) leak, as well as longer rehabilitation and recovery, with patients often being readmitted or even discharged to a facility other than their home [20,23].

In this case report, we present our unique experience with pontocerebellar schwannoma resection in a patient with class III obesity with the immense obstacles encountered throughout the whole process and compromises we had to make as well as postoperative complications. Additionally, with the literature review, we attempted to compare our experience with the existing body of knowledge and emphasize the issues of severe obesity in neurosurgery, especially when dealing with posterior fossa lesions.

2. Case Report

2.1. History and Diagnostic Process

A 48-year-old man presented to the neurosurgical outpatient clinic at the University Hospital in Maribor, Slovenia, with hearing loss in his right ear that had been worsening for 4 years. An ENT consultant had previously examined him and found signs of sensorineural hearing loss on the right side. The neurological examination revealed hearing loss in the right ear, and on the Romberg test, he swayed to the right but did not fall. The patient also presented with gait ataxia, limiting his daily activities, and mild signs of intracranial hypertension. He suffered from diabetes mellitus type 2, arterial hypertension, dyslipidemia, and obstructive sleep apnea. Before the patient came to the neurosurgical outpatient clinic, a CT scan of his head (Figure 1) was performed, which showed a 4 $\times$ 3 cm tumor in the right cerebellopontine angle, Koos grade IV, which was pushing the right cerebellar hemisphere and the fourth ventricle to one side, closing the Luschka foramen and causing mild obstructive hydrocephalus. As the patient was claustrophobic and his BMI was 55 kg/m^2, MRI could not be performed.

In cases of claustrophobia, an MRI can be performed under general anesthesia; however, this was not an option with our patient. Due to the weight limit of the MRI patient table and the size of the bore, which was too small for the patient's upper body, a suboptimal diagnostic modality, a CT scan, had to be utilized for presurgical planning. Based on the lesion's location and relative isolation from the surrounding tissues, as well as the patient's neurologic status, a VS was suspected; however, our surgical team was extremely limited with information about the relations between the tumor and surrounding structures, such as the brainstem, cerebellar hemisphere, arteries, veins, and cranial nerves.

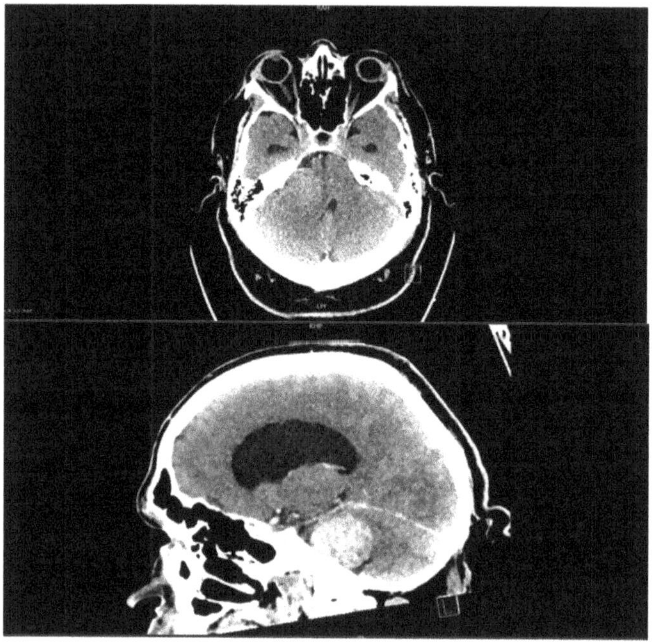

Figure 1. Preoperative CT scan (axial and sagittal view after contrast enhancement) showing a lesion (VS) in the right CPA measuring 4 × 3 cm with obstructive hydrocephalus due to compression of the 4th ventricle.

2.2. Surgery

The patient was presented at a multidisciplinary meeting where different treatment options were discussed. Due to the tumor size with an already existing hydrocephalus and the patient's age, surgery was suggested, and he signed the consent form after being informed of the risk of surgery and additional complications due to his class III obesity. Before the operation, the patient was thoroughly examined by the attending anesthetist, as intubation and ventilation problems were to be expected. Additionally, a chest X-ray was performed before surgery, which, due to the patient's obesity and preexisting sleep apnea, showed signs of poor ventilation and a wider mediastinum. On the day of the operation, he was taken to the operating theatre and, despite the patient exceeding the recommended weight limitations, was placed on the regular operating table. The first obstacle was mask ventilation before induction of general anesthesia, which required two people: one to hold the mask and the other to ventilate manually. During orotracheal intubation, the anesthetist had to stand on a set of steps and use a video laryngoscope at the same time. Once the airway was secured, the surgical team, with the help of the anesthesia team, began to place the patient in a "park bench" position, as a tumor resection was planned through a retrosigmoid approach. Due to the extreme weight, he could not be properly positioned on his left side but was simply tilted onto his left side, strapped down with several Velcro straps above his hips, knees, and legs. The head, which was in the Mayfield skull clamp, was rotated 90 degrees to the left to gain access. Correct positioning of the head for the desired retrosigmoid approach was impossible due to the weight of the head, a short neck, and excessive adipose tissue. As the "park bench" position was not achieved, the approach was obstructed by the patient's shoulder and chest. Additionally, a surgical navigation system could not be used. Before the operation began, the electrodes for intraoperative neuromonitoring of the facial nerve were inserted into the right side of the face, but the signal was weak due to a thick layer of subcutaneous fat tissue. After positioning the patient, a retrosigmoid approach was attempted to remove the tumor. During surgery, part of the right cerebellar hemisphere had to be removed; otherwise, visualization of the cerebellopontine angle (CPA), where the tumor was located, would have been impossible. Due to the suboptimal patient positioning owing to his extreme weight, the surgical trajectory was incorrect, and despite basal cisternostomy and edema reduction, there was still not enough space to visualize the tumor in the CPA; hence, part of the right cerebellar hemisphere had to be sacrificed. A surgical ultrasound aspiration device was used to remove the lesion. During surgery, the posterior inferior cerebellar artery and cranial nerves V to XI were visualized, and it transpired that the tumor was firmly attached to the brainstem. Intraoperative neuromonitoring for the facial nerve was performed throughout the time of tumor removal, but the signal was extremely weak and, therefore, unreliable as the electrodes were not long enough to ensure adequate monitoring. When most of the tumor was removed, a dural substitute was used for closure, and the previously removed bone was not returned as the flap was small and for fear of brain edema. Due to the patient's weight, the preoperative preparation took 80 min, and the surgery took 9 hours and 40 min. Straight after surgery, a CT scan was performed, which showed a postoperative condition with a removed tumor and without a significant hematoma. The patient was transferred to the intensive care unit while still on mechanical ventilation. On the first postoperative day, the patient was extubated. His cardiorespiratory condition was stable, but there was peripheral facial nerve palsy on the right side of his face. On the second postoperative day, he was transferred back to the Department of Neurosurgery, where early postoperative neurorehabilitation was started, but it was extremely difficult due to his weight and right limb ataxia. After one week, he was able to walk with a roller walker. Due to the paralysis of the peripheral facial nerve, a moist chamber was used at night, and artificial tears were administered regularly during the day. Despite great efforts by the physiotherapist, the patient was unable to walk independently. Due to the swelling of the right lower extremity, an ultrasound scan was performed to rule out deep vein thrombosis or thrombophlebitis; low-molecular-weight heparin was administered prophylactically. The dressing of the surgical wound was changed regularly, and there were no signs of inflammation or cerebrospinal fluid leakage. 11 days after surgery, the patient was transferred to a regional hospital for further rehabilitation. The pathohistological report stated that the removed tumor was a VS, a benign tumor, and, therefore, no oncological treatment was required, but complex rehabilitation was planned.

2.3. Postoperative Follow-Up and Complications

At the regional hospital, physiotherapy and rehabilitation continued as planned, and the patient was mobile with the aid of a roller walker. After a week in the regional hospital, the patient developed severe headaches and confusion. A CT scan was performed, which showed postoperative changes but no dynamics compared to the previous scan after surgery. The blood tests showed high inflammatory markers, and a urinary tract infection was also diagnosed. As a central nervous system infection was suspected, a course of antibiotics (metronidazole, ampicillin, ceftriaxone) was prescribed, which was administered for 6 days and exchanged for flucloxacillin when the inflammatory markers decreased. A lumbar puncture was also performed, but the microbiological tests showed no microorganisms in the cerebrospinal fluid. Approximately one month after surgery, a

CSF leak occurred through the surgical wound, and the patient was transferred back to the tertiary center. A further CT scan showed a large soft tissue edema around the craniectomy. Flucloxacillin was replaced by vancomycin and meropenem. During his hospitalization at the Department of Neurosurgery, a lumbar drain was inserted to control the leakage of cerebrospinal fluid through the surgical wound. The placement of the drainage was challenging since the needle was barely long enough to reach the spinal canal. During his 20-day readmission to the tertiary center, the CSF leakage stopped, and it did not reoccur after the removal of the lumbar drainage. The wound healed completely, the inflammatory markers were low, and he was discharged home, equipped with a roller walker and a wheelchair, both of which he learned to use unaided. On discharge, he was prescribed linezolid for 14 days as an extension of the previous intravenous antibiotic treatment. As planned during his hospitalization, he underwent complex rehabilitation in a tertiary healthcare facility and slowly regained his independence in daily activities. Four months after his discharge from the neurosurgery department, he returned to the outpatient clinic. The follow-up CT scan showed postoperative changes with no tumor residue or recurrence. He was able to walk at home without the roller, but the peripheral facial nerve palsy persisted, and he was regularly examined by an ophthalmologist and a plastic surgeon. He continued the use of artificial tears in the day and the moister chamber at night. Two years after the initial surgery, the control CT scan (Figure 2) showed no signs of residual tumor or recurrence. At his last appointment in the neurosurgical outpatient clinic, the patient was mobile with no aid, and due to a persistent facial nerve palsy to the right side, facial reanimation surgery was performed to restore symmetry.

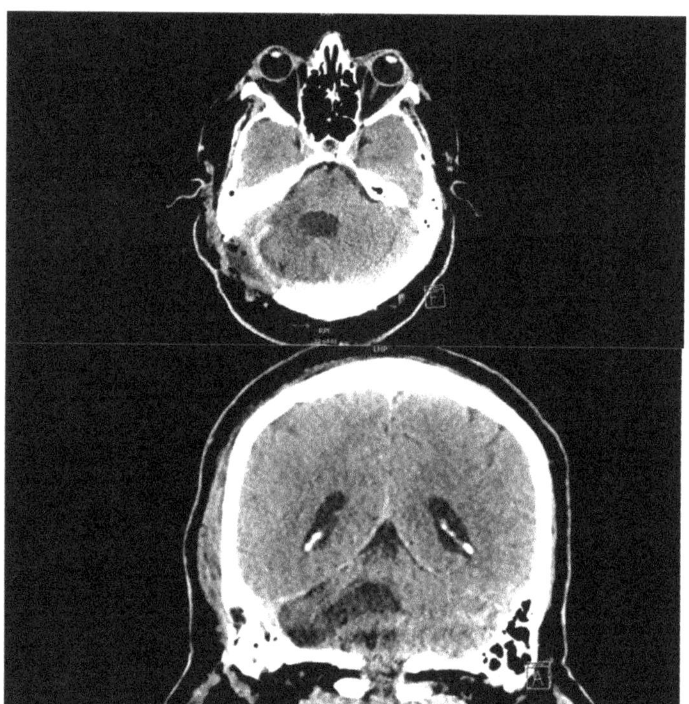

Figure 2. CT scan performed 2 years following the initial surgery, showing no signs of residual tumor or reoccurrence with encephalomalacic changes in the right cerebellar hemisphere. The hypodense subcutaneous inclusions represent the residue of bone wax and fatty tissue used to close the mastoid air cells to prevent rhinorrhea/otorrhea.

3. Discussion

3.1. Vestibular Schwannomas

The first successful VS surgery was performed in 1894 with an initial mortality of almost 80%, however, with the development of the operating microscope, refinement of surgical techniques as well as improvements in antibiotics, the current mortality is approximately 0.2%. Despite advances in surgery, the number of patients treated surgically has been slowly declining, especially for smaller tumors, with an increase in patients being observed with serial imaging or treated with stereotactic radiosurgery [6].

Observation is an option for smaller tumors, older patients, and those with major comorbidities. MR imagining is the preferred technique that provides incomparable tumor characteristics, whereas contrast-enhanced CT of the temporal bones can be utilized as an alternative when the patient cannot undergo MR imagining [7]. In obese individuals with VS, stereotactic radiosurgery might be a superior treatment modality, depending on the size of the lesion and degree of hearing loss as well as the presence of other symptoms [5]; however, that was not an option in our case due to tumor's size, mass effect, and existing hydrocephalus. Additionally, targeted biological therapies, such as bevacizumab, are currently emerging as options for the treatment of VS; however, at the moment, that is only applicable to patients with neurofibromatosis type 2 that have a VS [12].

Surgical excision remains the definitive treatment for larger lesions and younger individuals [6]. VS may be approached by a translabyrinthine, retrosigmoid, or middle fossa craniotomy [7]. Serious complications after surgery, such as stroke, CSF leak, wound infection, intracranial bleeding, and meningitis, are infrequent [6]. Nowadays, the aim of surgery has moved from total resection to functional preservation, especially in cases where the entire tumor mass cannot be safely removed concerning cranial nerves [7].

Being a benign tumor with a slow-growing nature, VS allows a postponement of surgical treatment to mitigate lifestyle factors, such as obesity, before deciding to operate [5]. A perioperative loss of weight is associated with a reduction in deep surgical site infections, abscess formation, and minor wound complications [20]. Weight reduction was proposed to our patient; however, cooperation was not great. Additionally, limited by his diabetes and due to evolving hydrocephalus, there was not enough time for him to lose the required weight, and surgery had to be performed despite the increased risk of complications.

3.2. Obesity in Neurosurgery

The population of overweight and obese people is rising, and in places like the United States of America as well as Europe, it has reached epidemic levels with an estimated prevalence of 42% [17] and has increased by around 50% per decade over the past 20 years. This has been seen among both sexes, all age groups, and races [23,24]. In Slovenia in 2020, 39% of inhabitants were overweight, and 20% were obese, with males and poorly educated individuals being the most affected. The patient presented in this case also comes from a region of Slovenia that has the highest percentage of obese individuals (25.7%), which could be due to cultural differences and mainly rural households with predominantly meat-based diets, processed meat products, and lard used in cooking [25].

Elevated BMI negatively impacts postoperative outcomes in several surgical specialties, including neurosurgery, and it is proven that a BMI above 40 kg/m^2 represents an independent risk factor for perioperative complications [20,26]; these individuals have a higher incidence of obstructive sleep apnea, idiopathic hypertension and even spontaneous CSF leaks [17]. Individuals with class III obesity (BMI above 40 kg/m^2) have a higher risk of surgical site infections, which can be a consequence of longer operating time with greater risk of wound contamination as well as prolonged retraction-related ischemia. Additionally, chronic inflammation and dysfunction of the immune system that is present in obesity and metabolic syndrome can increase the chances of surgical site infection [20,27].

CSF leak remains a common postoperative complication following the microscopic resection of a VS [5,28], which leads to extended hospitalization as well as higher patient morbidity and mortality. Elevated BMI has been recognized as a modifiable risk factor for surgical site infections [28]. Additionally, there is a 22% chance of developing a CSF leak in individuals with class III obesity [20]. Postoperative CSF leak increases the risk of meningitis and reoperation and prolongs hospital stay [17].

It has been proven that obese individuals have elevated intraabdominal pressure, which leads to a higher intrathoracic and cardiac filling pressure, thereby leading to an increase in the baseline intracranial pressure (ICP), which can lead to a postoperative CSF leak [28]. An increase in the baseline ICP could also be due to the fat pannus and its negative effects on venous return, increased levels of serum estrogens, and hypercapnia from obstructive sleep apnea that leads to cerebral vasodilatation, hence further increasing the ICP [20,28].

Additionally, obese patients are likely to experience longer operative times since obesity is linked with a difficult airway, which can prolong the induction of anesthesia. Also, positioning for the surgical procedure can present numerous challenges, thereby prolonging surgical duration [17,29]. Intubation of obese patients is challenging due to the excessive facial, palatal, and pharyngeal soft tissue and impaired jaw, atlantoaxial, and cervical mobility. Pharmacokinetics and pharmacodynamics of medications are altered in obese individuals. Increased positive end-expiratory pressure, a higher fraction of inspired oxygen, and inotropes are often required in obese individuals [20]. An obese patient requires a greater diaphragmatic excursion to provide the same degree of ventilation, their functional residual capacity, expiratory reserve volume and total lung capacity all being decreased [30].

Proper positioning of the patient is vital for a successful neurosurgical procedure, both for a trajectory to the lesion as well as to avoid complications to non-operated-upon tissues. The park bench position, which allows access to the lesion of the cerebellopontine angle, represents a modification of the lateral position with at least one arm positioned outside of the operating table, providing a greater manipulation of the head and neck [30]. A lumbar drain, placed at the time of surgery, can aid and allow better access to a posterior fossa in cases of elevated baseline ICP, and if it remains in place postoperatively for a short period, it can decrease the risk of developing a CSF leak [28].

The recovery time in obese patients tends to be longer [20]. Also, in park bench position, axillary misplacement can lead to limb ischemia, whereas excessive flexion of the torso can lead to brachial plexus injuries when using rigid head fixation. Obese patients are at an increased risk of ulceration during surgery as well as position-related peripheral nerve injury, especially ulnar and lateral femoral cutaneous nerve [30].

3.3. *Our Experience with Severe Obesity and VS Surgery*

Due to his class III obesity, the patient in our case report could not undergo MR imaging, which would have been a preferable and superior technique to the CT scan performed. As the diagnostic imaging revealed obstructive hydrocephalus, he had to be treated despite his obesity and anticipated complications, as there was no time for preoperative weight loss. Due to his age and the size of the neoplasm, surgical treatment was proposed. His obesity was a major problem for both the anesthetic and surgical teams throughout the operation. The preoperative preparation time was prolonged to 80 min, and several issues with ventilation were encountered by the anesthetists, with two consultants present in case of airway or breathing issues. The positioning was suboptimal, as he was only tilted because his extreme weight prevented him from being placed in a correct park bench position, which is required for a retrosigmoid approach. As the position of the body and the head were substandard, the resection was hindered by poor visibility and a lack of maneuvering space for surgical instruments, which was also affected by the position of the patient's shoulder and chest. During surgery, longer instruments had to be utilized. When comparing our surgical time with other cases of CPA VS resection, it took us almost twice as long to resect it. In addition, the electrodes used for intraoperative neuromonitoring of the facial nerve were not long enough due to a thick layer of subcutaneous adipose tissue, so neuromonitoring was unreliable and could not be used as an aid during surgery, which further complicated the resection, as we were also unable to utilize the navigation system.

His class III obesity was also a major obstacle to his postoperative neurorehabilitation, as he required four physiotherapists to assist him with a rollator to prevent him from falling. The nursing team also had issues with taking daily care of the patient due to his severe obesity, as the department did not have specific hoists to help move the patient; therefore, several nurses had to attend to him. In cases of poorly mobile obese individuals, surgical wounds can be subject to less-than-optimal medical care, dehiscence, and consecutive surgical site infection. A cerebrospinal fluid leak, which occurred due to a combination of substandard conditions during resection surgery, increased intracranial and intraabdominal pressure, diabetes, wound dehiscence, and infection, was successfully treated conservatively with antibiotics and the insertion of a lumbar drain. However, the condition significantly prolonged his hospitalization. Had we not been successful with the lumbar drainage, the team planned to revise surgery with another attempt at duroplasty or to try and insert ventriculoperitoneal drainage, which would have been challenging in his case and associated with additional risks and complications, such as migration of the peritoneal catheter and infections.

Obese patients, after surgical treatment, are readmitted more often than nonobese individuals [20,23]. Obese patients are more often discharged to a facility other than their home compared to their normal-weight counterparts [20]. The same was true in our case since the patient had to be hospitalized for 14 days after the first surgery, and he also required additional rehospitalization at our tertiary institute as well as prolonged hospitalization at his community hospital. His recovery was lengthy, with early rehabilitation orientated towards basic everyday activities, which took him 6 months to accomplish and another year to become unaided when walking and further surgery for his right-sided peripheral facial nerve palsy to be corrected.

4. Conclusions

Obesity represents an important risk factor for brain tumor resection surgery as it can mask clinical symptoms and signs typical of brain neoplasms. Due to severe obesity, preoperative diagnostic work-up is often limited. In cases of benign brain lesions, it is vital to preoperatively provide patients with good locomotor and respiratory physiotherapy, an appropriate nutritional regime, and to provide good control over their comorbidities. It is vital that preoperatively and postoperatively anesthetists are prepared for possible complications with intubation and timely extubation. Surgical preoperative preparation in cases of severely obese patients consists of adjustments to the placement of the patient, careful preoperative planning of the resection, and application of additional safety nets, such as intraoperative neuromonitoring; however, the surgical team must be prepared for sudden and unexpected rearrangements. The patient must be made aware of the increased risk of surgery due to their obesity. When a patient is severely obese, the operating times are longer, postoperative neurorehabilitation is longer, and those patients tend to be hospitalized more often than their counterparts with normal BMI. When considering the risk factors, required adaptations, good teamwork, and patient cooperation, the result of resection of benign brain lesions in severely obese individuals can have good results.

Author Contributions: Conceptualization, T.Š., H.R. and J.R.; writing—original draft preparation, T.Š. and H.R.; writing—review and editing, T.Š.; visualization, T.Š. and H.R.; supervision, T.Š. and J.R. All authors have read and agreed to the published version of the manuscript.

Funding: This research received no external funding.

Institutional Review Board Statement: Ethical review and approval were waived for this report due to its retrospective nature and the inability to recognize the patient and their medical data used.

Informed Consent Statement: Informed consent was obtained from all subjects involved in the study. Written informed consent has been obtained from the patient(s) to publish this paper.

Data Availability Statement: The raw data supporting the conclusions of this article will be made available by the authors upon request.

Conflicts of Interest: The authors declare no conflicts of interest.

Abbreviations

The following abbreviations are used in this manuscript:

VS	Vestibular schwannoma
MRI	Magneti resonance imaging
CT	Computed tomography
BMI	Body mass index
CSF	Cerebrospinal fluid
CPA	Cerebellopontine angle
AN	Acoustic neuroma
ICP	Intracranial pressure

References

1. Hilton, D.A.; Hanemann, C.O. Schwannomas and Their Pathogenesis. *Brain Pathol.* **2014**, *24*, 205–220. [CrossRef] [PubMed]
2. MacCollin, M.; Woodfin, W.; Kronn, D.; Short, M.P. Schwannomatosis. *Neurology* **1996**, *46*, 1072–1079. [CrossRef]
3. Goshtasbi, K.; Abouzari, M.; Soltanzadeh-Zarandi, S.; Sarna, B.; Lee, A.; Hsu, F.P.K.; Djalilian, H.R. The Association of Age, Body Mass Index, and Frailty with Vestibular Schwannoma Surgical Morbidity. *Clin. Neurol. Neurosurg.* **2020**, *197*, 106192. [CrossRef]
4. Marinelli, J.P.; Lohse, C.M.; Carlson, M.L. Incidence of Vestibular Schwannoma over the Past Half-Century: A Population-Based Study of Olmsted County, Minnesota. *Otolaryngol. Head Neck Surg.* **2018**, *159*, 717–723. [CrossRef] [PubMed]
5. Nasrollahi, T.S.; Shahrestani, S.; Borrelli, M.; Hopp, M.L.; Wu, A.W.; Tang, D.M.; Yu, J.S. The Influence of Modifiable Risk Factors on Postoperative Outcomes in Patients Receiving Surgery for Resection for Acoustic Neuroma. *Ear Nose Throat J.* 2023, *online ahead of print*. [CrossRef]
6. Hatch, J.L.; Bauschard, M.J.; Nguyen, S.A.; Lambert, P.R.; Meyer, T.A.; McRackan, T.R. National Trends in Vestibular Schwannoma Surgery: Influence of Patient Characteristics on Outcomes. *Otolaryngol. Head Neck Surg.* **2018**, *159*, 102–109. [CrossRef] [PubMed]
7. Lin, E.P.; Crane, B.T. The Management and Imaging of Vestibular Schwannomas. *AJNR Am. J. Neuroradiol.* **2017**, *38*, 2034–2043. [CrossRef]
8. Benoudiba, F.; Toulgoat, F.; Sarrazin, J.-L. The Vestibulocochlear Nerve (VIII). *Diagn. Interv. Imaging* **2013**, *94*, 1043–1050. [CrossRef]
9. Nernekli, K.; Persad, A.R.; Hori, Y.S.; Yener, U.; Celtikci, E.; Sahin, M.C.; Sozer, A.; Sozer, B.; Park, D.J.; Chang, S.D. Automatic Segmentation of Vestibular Schwannomas: A Systematic Review. *World Neurosurg.* **2024**, *188*, 35–44. [CrossRef]
10. Bray, H.N.; Sappington, J.M. A Review of Posterior Fossa Lesions. *Mo. Med.* **2022**, *119*, 553–558.
11. Machetanz, K.; Wang, S.S.; Oberle, L.; Tatagiba, M.; Naros, G. Sex Differences in Vestibular Schwannoma. *Cancers* **2023**, *15*, 4365. [CrossRef]
12. Gupta, V.K.; Thakker, A.; Gupta, K.K. Vestibular Schwannoma: What We Know and Where We Are Heading. *Head Neck Pathol.* **2020**, *14*, 1058–1066. [CrossRef]
13. Goldbrunner, R.; Weller, M.; Regis, J.; Lund-Johansen, M.; Stavrinou, P.; Reuss, D.; Evans, D.G.; Lefranc, F.; Sallabanda, K.; Falini, A.; et al. EANO Guideline on the Diagnosis and Treatment of Vestibular Schwannoma. *Neuro-Oncol.* **2020**, *22*, 31–45. [CrossRef]

14. Vnencak, M.; Huttunen, E.; Aarnisalo, A.A.; Jero, J.; Liukkonen, K.; Sinkkonen, S.T. Evaluation of Pure-Tone Audiometric Protocols in Vestibular Schwannoma Screening. *J. Otol.* **2021**, *16*, 138–143. [CrossRef]
15. Tsuzuki, N.; Kitama, T.; Wasano, K.; Wakabayashi, T.; Hosoya, M.; Nishiyama, T.; Ozawa, H.; Oishi, N. Characteristics of Pure Tone Audiogram in Patients with Untreated Sporadic Vestibular Schwannoma: Analysis of Audiometric Shape and Interaural Differences Stratified by Age and Mode of Onset. *Auris Nasus Larynx* **2024**, *51*, 347–355. [CrossRef] [PubMed]
16. Ruiz-García, C.; Lassaletta, L.; López-Larrubia, P.; Varela-Nieto, I.; Murillo-Cuesta, S. Tumors of the Nervous System and Hearing Loss: Beyond Vestibular Schwannomas. *Hear. Res.* **2024**, *447*, 109012. [CrossRef] [PubMed]
17. Bridgham, K.; Shikara, M.; Ludeman, E.; Eisenman, D.J. Impact of Obesity on Postoperative Complications after Lateral Skull Base Surgery: A Systematic Review. *ORL* **2023**, *85*, 264–274. [CrossRef] [PubMed]
18. Khanna, D.; Peltzer, C.; Kahar, P.; Parmar, M.S. Body Mass Index (BMI): A Screening Tool Analysis. *Cureus* **2022**, *14*, e22119. [CrossRef]
19. Barte, J.C.M.; Veldwijk, J.; Teixeira, P.J.; Sacks, F.M.; Bemelmans, W.J.E. Differences in Weight Loss Across Different BMI Classes: A Meta-Analysis of the Effects of Interventions with Diet and Exercise. *Int.J. Behav. Med.* **2014**, *21*, 784–793. [CrossRef]
20. Castle-Kirszbaum, M.D.; Tee, J.W.; Chan, P.; Hunn, M.K. Obesity in Neurosurgery: A Narrative Review of the Literature. *World Neurosurg.* **2017**, *106*, 790–805. [CrossRef]
21. Ginde, A.A.; Foianini, A.; Renner, D.M.; Valley, M.; Camargo, C.A. The Challenge of CT and MRI Imaging of Obese Individuals Who Present to the Emergency Department: A National Survey. *Obesity* **2008**, *16*, 2549–2551. [CrossRef]
22. Meng, H.; O'Connor, D.P.; Lee, B.-C.; Layne, C.S.; Gorniak, S.L. Alterations in Over-Ground Walking Patterns in Obese and Overweight Adults. *Gait Posture* **2017**, *53*, 145–150. [CrossRef] [PubMed]
23. Aghi, M.K.; Eskandar, E.N.; Carter, B.S.; Curry, W.T.; Barker, F.G. Increased Prevalence of Obesity and Obesity-Related Postoperative Complications in Male Patients with Meningiomas. *Neurosurgery* **2007**, *61*, 754–761. [CrossRef] [PubMed]
24. Ri, M.; Aikou, S.; Seto, Y. Obesity as a Surgical Risk Factor. *Ann. Gastroent. Surg.* **2018**, *2*, 13–21. [CrossRef]
25. Zaletel, M.; Vardič, D.; Hladnik, M. 3.2 Čezmerna Hranjenost in Debelost. Zdravstveni Statistični Letopis Slovenije 2021. Available online: https://nijz.si/publikacije/zdravstveni-statisticni-letopis-2021/ (accessed on 27 March 2025).
26. Madsen, H.J.; Gillette, R.A.; Colborn, K.L.; Henderson, W.G.; Dyas, A.R.; Bronsert, M.R.; Lambert-Kerzner, A.; Meguid, R.A. The Association between Obesity and Postoperative Outcomes in a Broad Surgical Population: A 7-Year American College of Surgeons National Surgical Quality Improvement Analysis. *Surgery* **2023**, *173*, 1213–1219. [CrossRef] [PubMed]
27. Plassmeier, L.; Hankir, M.K.; Seyfried, F. Impact of Excess Body Weight on Postsurgical Complications. *Visc. Med.* **2021**, *37*, 287–297. [CrossRef]
28. Copeland, W.R.; Mallory, G.W.; Neff, B.A.; Driscoll, C.L.W.; Link, M.J. Are There Modifiable Risk Factors to Prevent a Cerebrospinal Fluid Leak Following Vestibular Schwannoma Surgery? *J. Neurosurg.* **2015**, *122*, 312–316. [CrossRef]
29. McHayle, A.; Pertsch, N.J.; Toms, S.A.; Weil, R.J. Operative Duration and Early Outcomes in Patients Having a Supratentorial Craniotomy for Brain Tumor: A Propensity Matched Analysis. *J. Clin. Neurosci.* **2021**, *92*, 207–214. [CrossRef]
30. Marotta, D.A.; Brazdzionis, J.; Fiani, B.; Duong, J.; Noel, J.; Siddiqi, J. Perioperative Positioning in Neurosurgery: A Technical Note on Park Bench Positioning for the Obese Patient Using the "Arrowhead" Technique. *Cureus* **2021**, *13*, e16932. [CrossRef]

diagnostics

MDPI

Case Report

Neck Schwannoma Masking as Thyroid Tumour: Into the Deep of Diagnostics and Anatomy

Serghei Covantsev [1,*], Anna Bumbu [2], Anna Sukhotko [2], Evghenii Zakurdaev [3], Ivan Kuts [2] and Andrey Evsikov [2]

[1] Department of Clinical Research and Development, Botkin Hospital, 125284 Moscow, Russia
[2] Department of Oncology, Botkin Hospital, 125284 Moscow, Russia
[3] Department of Pathology, Botkin Hospital, 125284 Moscow, Russia
* Correspondence: kovantsev.s.d@gmail.com

Abstract: Schwannomas are benign nerve sheath tumours that exhibit a slow rate of growth. In the vast majority of cases, schwannomas manifest as asymptomatic masses. The presence of symptomatic lesions may necessitate surgical removal. The incidence of schwannomas ranges from 4.4 to 5.23 cases per 100,000 population, accounting for approximately 7% of all primary tumours in the central nervous system. There is a limited number of case reports describing schwannomas outside the central nervous system. In rare instances, schwannomas may originate at the level of the thyroid gland. In such cases, incidental neck schwannomas may be mistaken for thyroid or parathyroid tumours. The increasing incidence of thyroid cancer draws more attention to all thyroid nodules, both benign and malignant. Thyroid nodules are detected in up to 65% of autopsies, with only 4–6.5% being malignant. Thyroid tumours are typically diagnosed by USG; however, they are often revealed incidentally during neck CT or MRI for other conditions. To rule out malignancy, tumour verification is required. The modern diagnosis of thyroid cancer is based on fine-needle aspiration (FNA) biopsy and cytology, which is classified according to the Bethesda classification system. However, not all FNAs are informative, and the differential diagnosis and treatment strategies in cases of unsatisfactory results are not standardized, leading to potential intraoperative challenges. We present a case study of a patient with a thyroid nodule that was ultimately diagnosed with a schwannoma of the neck according to core-needle biopsy.

Keywords: thyroid; schwannoma; fine-needle aspiration; core-needle biopsy; tumours; nervous system

1. Introduction

Schwannomas are benign nerve sheath tumours that exhibit a slow rate of growth. In the vast majority of cases, schwannomas manifest as asymptomatic masses. The presence of symptomatic lesions may necessitate surgical removal [1]. The incidence of schwannomas ranges from 4.4 to 5.23 cases per 100,000 population, accounting for approximately 7% of all primary tumours in the central nervous system [2,3]. There is a limited number of case reports describing schwannomas outside the central nervous system. They usually appear during the 5th-6th decade with no sex predisposition. Approximately 20–50% of schwannomas arise in the head and neck region; however, schwannoma may be located anywhere in the body. Of these, 10–30% originate from Schwann cells of the vagus nerve, while another 10–20% arise from the sympathetic nervous system [4–6]. Despite the fact that the head and neck are one of the primary sites of occurrence, only 250 patients have been reported in the literature [7]. These cases primarily involve schwannomas affecting cranial nerves (such as V, VII, IX, X, XI, and XII), as well as sympathetic or peripheral nerves [6,8]. High-volume surgical centres typically see from 30 to 50 such cases every 8–9 years [5,6]. In rare instances, schwannomas may originate at the level of the thyroid gland.

In such cases, incidental neck schwannomas may be mistaken for thyroid or parathyroid tumours due to their anatomical closeness to these structures [9–15].

Thyroid cancer incidence rates have increased in many countries and settings. Globally, in 2020, the incidence of thyroid cancer was 10.1 per 100,000 women and 3.1 per 100,000 men [16]. This increase in the number of thyroid cancer cases resulted in close attention being paid to all thyroid nodules, both benign and malignant. Thyroid nodules are detected in up to 65% of autopsies, with only 4–6.5% being cancerous [15–18]. Thyroid tumours are typically diagnosed by USG; however, they are often revealed incidentally during neck CT or MRI for other conditions. To rule out malignancy, tumour verification is required. The modern diagnosis of thyroid cancer relies on fine-needle aspiration biopsy (FNA) and cytology, which is classified according to the Bethesda classification system [19].

However, not all FNAs are informative, and the differential diagnosis and treatment strategies in cases of unsatisfactory results are not standardized, leading to potential intraoperative challenges. We present a case study of a patient with a thyroid nodule that was ultimately diagnosed with a schwannoma of the neck according to core-needle biopsy (CNB).

2. Case Description

During an annual medical examination in 2022, a patient, a 32-year-old male, was found to have a proliferative mass in the neck area. Ultrasound examination of the thyroid gland revealed an oval hypoechoic heterogeneous formation with a size of 18 × 21 × 31 mm, clear, well-defined boundaries, and areas of abnormal blood flow in the projection of the left inferior parathyroid gland along the posterior surface of the left lobe of the thyroid gland (see Figure 1). Magnetic resonance imaging showed a volumetric formation with clear boundaries and heterogeneous contents measuring 33 × 24 × 25 mm on the lateral posterior surface of the left lobe of the thyroid gland, which looks hyperintensive on the T2-weighted image and has no signs of limited diffusion (see Figure 2).

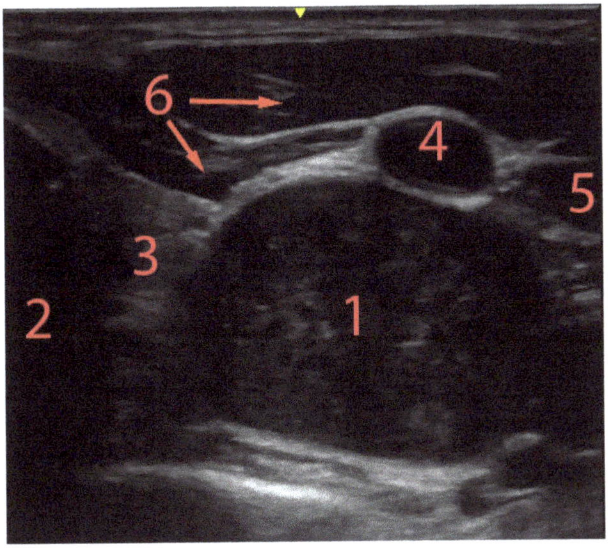

Figure 1. USG of the neck region at the level of the thyroid gland. 1—tumour, 2—trachea, 3—thyroid, 4—carotid artery, 5—jugular vein, 6—pretracheal muscles.

The computed tomography scan also revealed a mass with a size of 21 × 24 × 25 mm with a density of 18 Hounsfield units that accumulated contrast agent and was situated between the thyroid gland and the vertebral column (Figure 3). The parathyroid hormone level was 4.06 pmol/L, and the ionized calcium concentration was 1.22 mmol/L. Thyroid-stimulating hormone T3 and T4 were also within the normal range and comprised 2.7 mIU/L, 1.7 nmol/L and 89 nmol/L concurrently. Therefore, the patient had normal thyroid and parathyroid function. Also, there were no other laboratory deviations recorded at the time of hospitalization. The patient did not have any previous medical conditions and considered himself healthy.

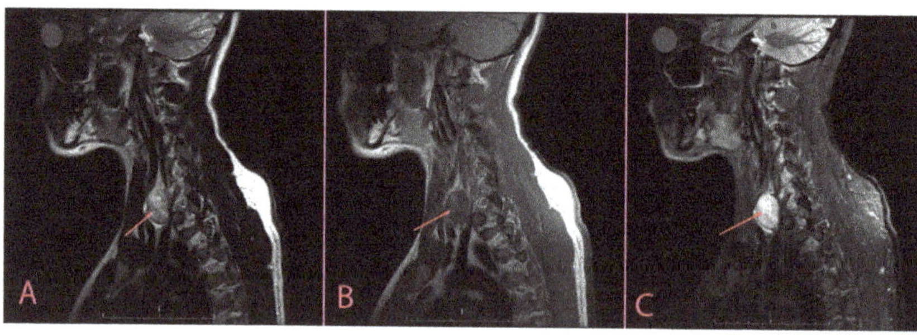

Figure 2. Soft tissue MRI (arrow indicates the tumour). (**A**)—T2, (**B**)—T1, (**C**)—T2 TIRM.

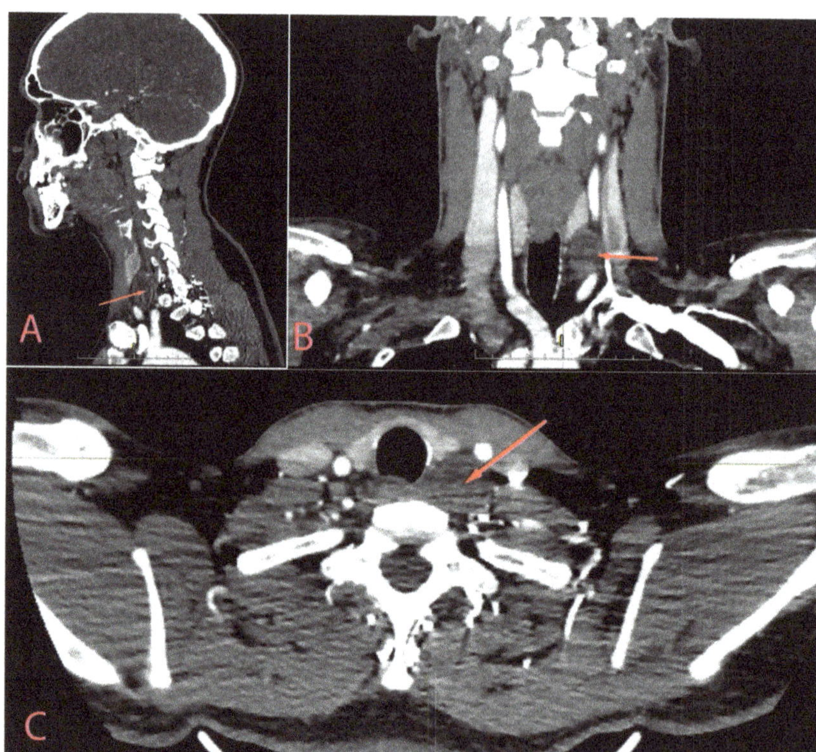

Figure 3. Contrast-enhanced CT scan of the neck at the level of the thyroid gland (arrow indicates the tumour). (**A**)—sagittal plane, (**B**)—frontal plane, (**C**)—axial plane.

The results of FNA were unsatisfactory and classified as Bethesda category I. A subsequent FNA was also non-diagnostic. To make a decision regarding diagnostic hemithyroidectomy, the patient was referred to an endocrine surgeon. Due to uncertainty about the diagnosis, the patient underwent CNB of the cervical region mass upon admission. Histopathological analysis revealed a schwannoma (Figure 4). Biopsy specimens contained spindle-shaped cells with areas of myxoid structure. Apart from that, characteristic palisade patterns of nuclei (Verocay bodies) and rare mitoses were noted (WHO grade I tumours).

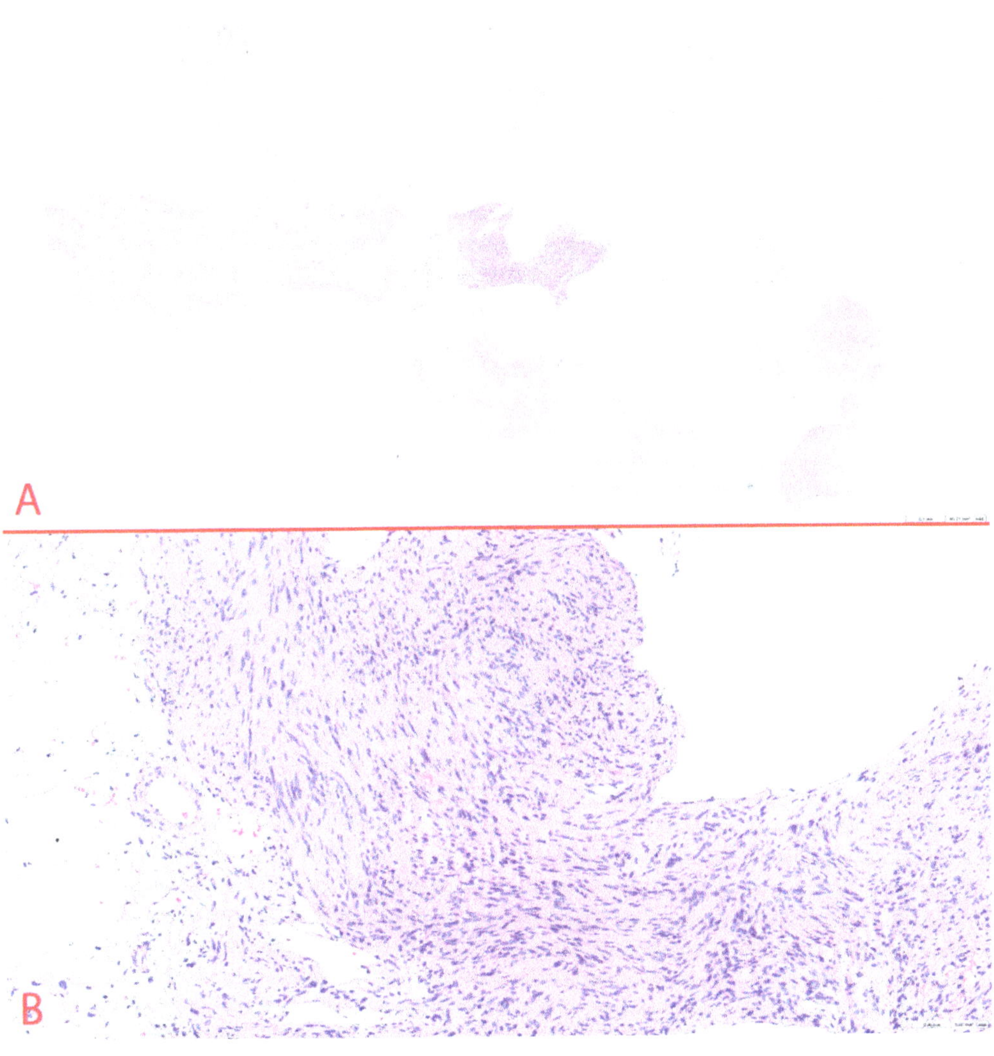

Figure 4. Histology of the specimens. (**A**)—CNB specimens (×5; H&E staining), (**B**)—CNB histology (×20 H&E staining).

The surgical procedure was conducted in aseptic conditions, under general anesthesia. Following meticulous marking, a small incision in the form of a collar was made on the left side of the neck, in the vicinity of the mass. The skin, subcutaneous fat, and platysma were accurately dissected, allowing for the identification of the sternocleidomastoid muscle and the common carotid artery, along with an adjacent volumetric mass measuring approximately 3 cm in diameter (see Figure 5).

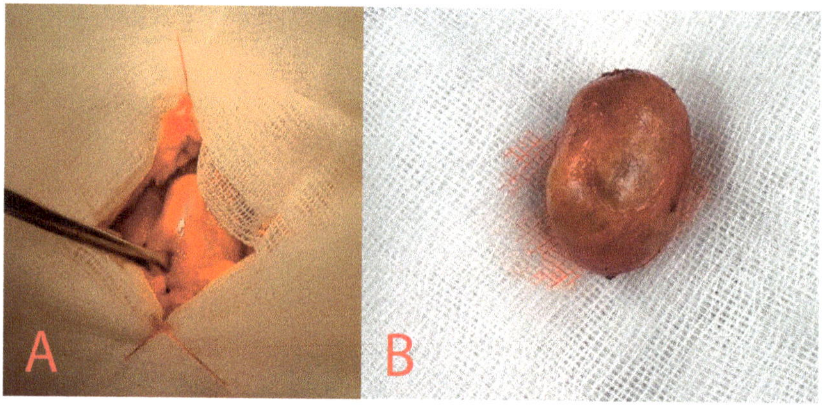

Figure 5. Macroscopic tumour appearance. (**A**)—intraoperative image of the tumour, (**B**)—postoperative specimen.

The apical margin of this formation was positioned at the level of the left lobe of the thyroid gland, while its inferior border approached the jugular notch. Laterally, the mass extended towards the left carotid artery, while its distal margin came into contact with the body of the lumbar vertebrae. Utilizing a dissector and cautery pencil, the mass was meticulously excised. A flexible drainage tube was inserted into the tumour bed, followed by the creation of a contraperture to facilitate the removal of any exudate. Once haemostasis was achieved in the surgical area, skin sutures were applied, and a sterile dressing was secured over the wound. The catheter was removed one day after the surgical procedure, and the patient was discharged two days later without any complaints.

The postoperative histological examination confirmed the findings of the CNB. Immunohistochemical analysis revealed that the tumour exhibited a positive reaction to S100 (100%) and a negative response to CD34 and SMA markers. The Ki67 index was 2%.

Following a two-year follow-up period, no signs of tumour recurrence or neurological deficits were observed.

3. Discussion

In up to 90% of cases, schwannomas are usually solitary and sporadic; however, they can be associated with type 2 neurofibromatosis or other genetic conditions [20]. Schwannomas of the cervical region stem from the vagus nerve in approximately 11–20% of cases. They can also originate from the sympathetic chain, which comprises 11–34% of cases, or the cervical plexus and the brachial plexus, which account for 3–50% and 17% of cases, respectively. In rare instances, schwannomas may result from the hypoglossal nerve (3–6%). Moreover, in some cases they can originate from the greater auricular nerve (5.6%), the hypoglossal nerve (3–5.55%), or even the recurrent laryngeal nerve (3%). The latter can lead to a misdiagnosis, as these tumours can be closely adjacent to the thyroid gland. In up to 17% of cases the exact origin of the nerve cannot be determined [5,6]. Figure 6 demonstrates the nerves, possible origins of schwannoma, and other neoplasms, which are located in close proximity to the thyroid. Tumours arising from some of these nerves can only be misidentified when they are large, with one of the tumour poles situated close to the thyroid gland. Schwannomas must be differentiated from paragangliomas and other nerve-associated tumours, such as neurofibromas, granular cell myoblastomas, neurogenic sarcomas, and melanomas [21].

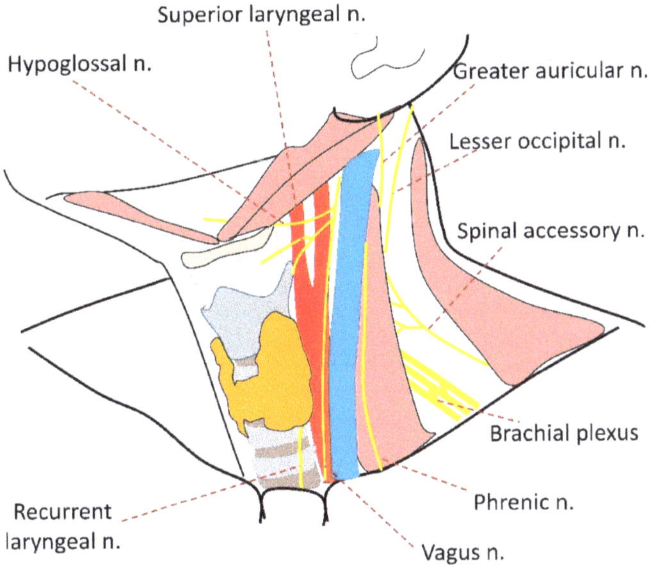

Figure 6. Nerves of the neck region that can potentially develop into schwannomas in proximity to the thyroid gland.

The first case report of a primary schwannoma of the thyroid gland was published in 1964 by Delaney and Fry [22]. Approximately 60% of tumours in the neck region present as asymptomatic, palpable masses, and 10% are incidentally discovered in imaging studies. Schwannomas are usually asymptomatic and can show no signs of disease for more than 10 years. On average, the growth rate of these lesions does not exceed 1–3 mm each year [1]. In 20% of cases, patients present with neurological deficits, and in 10% of cases, pain and obstruction of the neck veins are the prevalent symptoms. There have been a limited number of reports regarding thyroid schwannomas (Table 1). The vast majority of patients are 30–35-year-old females, who are typically concerned with a neck mass. Reports of male patients affected are less common. Progressive swelling in the neck region and Horner's syndrome may indicate malignancy but can also occur in benign tumours [21,23]. Furthermore, as the neoplasm expands, surgical excision of the tumour may give rise to a variety of complications, including the so-called first-bite syndrome [1]. First-bite syndrome (FBS) is a rare complication that occurs after damage to the sympathetic chain's superior cervical ganglion (SCG). With destruction of the SCG, the patient can develop FBS and Horner syndrome. This condition can be seen in patients who undergo parapharyngeal space surgery and can result in the development of severe parotid gland pain at the first bite of food [24].

In non-contrast computed tomography (CT) scans, schwannomas often exhibit a decreased density compared to muscle tissue, appearing hypodense. Schwannomas consist of spindle cells that have two growth patterns: Antoni type A and Antoni type B. In contrast-enhanced CT images, schwannomas predominantly exhibiting the Antoni A pattern manifest as solid, intensely enhancing, heterogeneous, and hypodense masses. Schwannomas characterized by the predominance of Antoni B typically present as pseudocysts, with minimal or no enhancement in contrast-enhanced images. On MRI, these lesions exhibit varying levels of intensity, ranging from low to equal intensity of normal tissue on T1-weighted sequences and high intensity on T2-weighted images, depending on their cellular composition. Contrast-enhanced T1-weighted MRI reveals moderate to significant enhancement of these lesions. The appearance of these lesions is generally homogeneous for smaller ones and becomes heterogeneous as they increase in size. In certain occasions, the pronounced hyperintense signal observed on T2-weighted MRI scans serves as a means of distinguishing the mass from the adjacent, less hyperintense structures such as the thyroid gland. The existence of a discernible boundary between the mass and the thyroid gland is indicative of the presence of an independent neoplasm [25].

The FNA biopsy of a tumour located near the thyroid gland is often inconclusive, as in most cases, the cytology reports fall into categories I, II, III, or IV according to the Bethesda system [9,10,12,13]. The specificity of FNA and imaging studies for diagnosing schwannomas is approximately 20% and 38%, respectively [6]. Table 1 presents a comparison of FNA results, indicating that in the prevalent number of cases, they are inconclusive.

During cytological evaluation, these tumours can be mistaken for other spindle cell lesions of the thyroid, such as smooth muscle tumours and spindle cell lesions [23]. The differential diagnosis of spindle cell tumours is a broad field that encompasses a diverse range of entities. These include neural-derived tumours, such as schwannomas, as well as mesenchymal neoplasms like leiomyomas and solitary fibrous tumours. Hemangiopericytomas are also included in this category. Epithelial tumours, such as anaplastic thyroid carcinomas, medullary thyroid carcinomas, thymomas, and spindle epithelial tumours with thymus-like features (SETTLE), are part of the spectrum as well. Moreover, hyalinizing trabecular adenomas deserve consideration. Immunohistochemical staining for S-100 protein has proven to be highly valuable for preoperative diagnosis of these neoplasms, especially in the case of schwannomas [10].

It is worth noting that non-thyroid lesions can sometimes be misdiagnosed as primary thyroid neoplasms if the FNA biopsy includes thyroid tissue, due to the trajectory of the needle through the gland prior to reaching the target lesion [26]. Consequently, the preoperative diagnosis is seldom established based on these investigations. Nonetheless, some experts advocate for CNB, as it can detect schwannomas more accurately.

Table 1. Thyroid schwannoma cases.

Age, Sex	Cytology	Clinical Picture	Reference
87, female	Bethesda III	Radiating pain after aspiration	[9]
70, male	Bethesda IV	Palpable mass, hoarseness, neck discomfort	[10]
30, female	Bethesda I	Swelling in the neck	[12]
47, male	Bethesda II	Progressive swelling in the neck	[13]
31, male	Schwannoma	Growing nodule in the neck	[3]
60, female	Schwannoma	Dysphagia and a significant increase in goitre size	[25]
33, female	Bethesda I	Palpable neck mass	[27]
33, female	Bethesda I	Large palpable mass, compression	[28]
26, female	Bethesda I	Neck mass	[29]
35, female	Bethesda I	Neck mass, Horner's syndrome	[21]
63, female	Bethesda I	Foreign body sensation with swallowing	[30]
23, female	Paucicellular sample with occasional follicular cells of equivocal diagnostic value	Neck mass	[31]
32, male	Bethesda I	Neck mass	Current case

The imaging of neck tumours that may be associated with thyroid cancer can involve various techniques, such as ultrasonography (USG), CT with contrast enhancement, MRI with contrast enhancement, and positron emission tomography (PET) or scintigraphy. A comparative analysis of these imaging modalities can be found in Table 2.

Table 2. Comparison of imaging technologies in schwannoma diagnostics.

Modality	Disease	Description	Reference
USG	Schwannoma	Hypoechoic mass, regular margins, contextual anechoic areola, multiseptate hypoechoic lesion, macro- and microcalcifications. Contrast-enhanced ultrasonography may be another possibility to distinguish schwannomas; however, data are limited to several case reports. The tumour usually appears as strong, inhomogeneous enhancement both in early and in late phases. Elastography usually indicates dense stiff tissue.	[3,9,10,12,13,25,27,29,31]
	Thyroid cancer	Hypoechoic mass, ill-defined margin, irregular shape, heterogeneity, absence of cystic lesion and/or halo sign, presence of calcification and invasion to other anatomical structures.	
CT	Schwannoma	Mass that can extend to intervertebral foramen. Contrast enhancement may be helpful as thyroid gland tends to accumulate iodine contrast and may reveal separate plane between gland and tumour.	
	Thyroid cancer	Mass with ill-defined borders, extra-thyroid extension, lymph node involvement, or invasion of surrounding structures.	
MRI	Schwannoma	Solid low-intensified and high-intensified tumour by T1- and T2-weighted images, respectively; can be connected to the cervical spinal cord. MRI can delineate mass as distinct from less hyperintense thyroid and enhanced T1-weighted images and demonstrate plane of separation between lesion and thyroid gland.	
	Thyroid cancer	Malignant nodules usually have lower apparent diffusion coefficient value and lower intensity ration on T2-weighted imaging. Similarly, invasion to adjacent structures is indication of malignancy.	
Sci	Schwannoma	Cold nodule in nature or normal thyroid scan.	
	Thyroid cancer	Cold nodule in nature or normal thyroid scan.	

There are several publications that suggest CNB of the thyroid gland is a safe procedure that can provide valuable additional information in cases when cytology results are inconclusive [32,33]. This is particularly relevant in instances of rare thyroid gland tumours or tumours that mimic thyroid tumours. Specific diagnoses, such as "suspicious schwannoma" and "consistent with schwannoma", can be made in up to 96.6% of CNB samples, while FNA yields such diagnoses in only 19.2% of cases ($p < 0.001$) [34].

Immunohistochemistry is crucial in this context, as the tumour should be positive for S-100 protein and negative for calcitonin, carcinoembryonic antigen (CEA), thyroglobulin, thyroid transcription factor 1 (TTF1), melan-A, and melanoma-associated antigen (HMB45), which helps to rule out schwannomas, medullary thyroid cancers, and well-differentiated thyroid cancers [25].

However, CNB remains somewhat controversial due to the potential risks of neuropathic pain or neurological deficits resulting from axonal damage [35]. Some experts recommend intracapsular resection of schwannomas with electrical nerve monitoring to reduce the risk of nerve injury [36].

A complete excision is strongly advised in order to prevent both the progression and recurrence of schwannomas [1,7]. These are slow-growing tumours that have a propensity to displace adjacent fascicles. Failure to excise them can result in their continued growth, leading to a myriad of clinical manifestations, including nerve dysfunction and paresthesia.

However, in certain cases, it is hard to distinguish between an extra-thyroidal mass and an intrathyroidal lesion, leading to unnecessary thyroid surgery. Frozen section pathology during surgery might be helpful in such situations to guide the surgeon [10]. Partial resection carries a high risk of recurrence (greater than 50%), as well as the possibility of malignant transformation (4%). A complete excision is strongly advised to prevent both progression and recurrence. Additionally, an increase in size can lead to potential hemorrhage, cystic degeneration, and necrosis, as reported in the literature [1,7,37].

Therefore, in this particular case of thyroid neoplasia, the patient had undergone several FNAs with no diagnostic result and was referred for hemithyroidectomy. CNB allowed us to obtain preoperative diagnosis and, since the tumour was not within the thyroid gland, abstain from hemithyroidectomy. The multidisciplinary approach that involved a medical ultrasonographer, radiologist, pathologist, and surgeon enabled us to obtain the diagnosis and choose adequate treatment tactics.

4. Conclusions

Schwannoma of the thyroid is a rare pathological condition, with only a handful of cases reported in the scientific literature. FNA is the standard method for diagnosing thyroid malignancies in the presence of suspicious nodules. However, its accuracy in the context of rare tumours is often limited. In such cases, CNB often provides more reliable results, albeit with a higher risk associated with the procedure. The benefit of a CNB is that the obtained histological specimen provides a tissue sample, unlike FNA, and the specimen can be studied by means of immunohistochemistry. The decision to proceed with CNB must be carefully balanced against the importance of obtaining a definitive diagnosis prior to surgery.

Author Contributions: Conceptualization, S.C. and A.B.; methodology, A.S., I.K., A.E. and E.Z.; formal analysis, S.C., A.B., A.E. and A.S.; resources, I.K. and E.Z.; data curation, S.C., A.B. and I.K.; writing—original draft preparation, S.C. and A.B.; writing—review and editing—A.B., A.E. and A.S.; visualization, I.K., E.Z. and S.C.; supervision, S.C. and A.E. All authors have read and agreed to the published version of the manuscript.

Funding: This research received no external funding.

Institutional Review Board Statement: Not applicable.

Informed Consent Statement: Written informed consent has been obtained from the patient to publish this paper.

Data Availability Statement: Data is available on personal request.

Conflicts of Interest: The authors declare no conflicts of interest.

References

1. Xing, M.H.; Sandler, M.L.; Tuttle, R.M.; Khorsandi, A.; Samankan, S.; Mundi, N.; Urken, M.L. Abnormal growth rate of a benign cervical sympathetic chain schwannoma. *Otolaryngol. Case Rep.* **2021**, *19*, 100295. [CrossRef]
2. Aoki, T.; Kumeda, S.; Iwasa, T.; Inokawa, K.; Hori, T.; Makiuchi, M. Primary neurilemoma of the thyroid gland: Report of a case. *Surg. Today* **1993**, *23*, 265–268. [CrossRef] [PubMed]
3. Mikosch, P.; Gallowitsch, H.; Kresnik, E.; Lind, P. Schwannoma of the Neck Simulating a Thyroid Nodule. *Thyroid®* **1997**, *7*, 449–451. [CrossRef]
4. Batsakis, J.G. *Tumours of the Peripheral Nervous System*, 2nd ed.; Williams and Wilkins: Baltimore, MD, USA, 1979.
5. Leu, Y.S.; Chang, K.C. Extracranial Head and Neck Schwannomas: A Review of 8 Years Experience. *Acta Oto-Laryngol.* **2002**, *122*, 435–437. [CrossRef]
6. Liu, H.L.; Yu, S.Y.; Li, G.K.; Wei, W.I. Extracranial head and neck Schwannomas: A study of the nerve of origin. *Eur. Arch. Oto-Rhino-Laryngol.* **2011**, *268*, 1343–1347. [CrossRef]
7. Boros, M.J.; Wysong, S.T. Syndromes after resection of a cervical schwannoma. *Ear Nose Throat J.* **2011**, *90*, 431–433. [CrossRef]
8. Tryggvason, G.; Barnett, A.; Kim, J.; Soken, H.; Maley, J.; Hansen, M.R. Radiographic association of schwannomas with sensory ganglia. *Otol. Neurotol.* **2012**, *33*, 1276–1282. [CrossRef]
9. Oka, K.; Iwamuro, M.; Otsuka, F. Neck schwannoma mimicking a thyroid tumor. *J. Gen. Fam. Med.* **2017**, *18*, 473–474. [CrossRef] [PubMed]
10. Gambardella, C.; Docimo, L.; Candela, G.; Cozzolino, G.; Mongardini, F.; Serilli, F.; Nesta, G.; Pignatelli, M.F.; Ferrandes, S.; Gambardella, A.; et al. Thyroid-Bed Schwannoma Mimicking a Thyroid Neoplasm: A Challenging Diagnosis: Report of a Case and Literature Review. *Medicina* **2022**, *24*, 58. [CrossRef]
11. Beute, J.E.; Seo, G.T.; Saturno, M.; Xing, M.H.; Mundi, N.; Dowling, E.M.; Matloob, A.; Chen, H.; Khorsandi, A.S.; Steinberger, J.; et al. Central compartment neoplasms masquerading as thyroid tumors: Presentation of two unusual cases and review of the literature. *Otolaryngol. Case Rep.* **2022**, *25*, 100471. [CrossRef]

12. Pillai, S.; Agarwal, A.C.; Mathew, M.; Nayak, D.R. Ancient schwannoma mimicking a thyroid mass with retrosternal extension. *BMJ Case Rep.* **2013**, *2013*, bcr2013200608. [CrossRef] [PubMed]
13. Dhar, H.; Dabholkar, J.P.; Kandalkar, B.M.; Ghodke, R. Primary thyroid schwannoma masquerading as a thyroid nodule. *J. Surg. Case Rep.* **2014**, *2014*, rju094. [CrossRef] [PubMed]
14. Fiore, R.; Gombert, E.; La Rosa, S.; Dunet, V.; Sykiotis, G.P.; Gorostidi, F. Esophageal schwannoma mimicking non-functional parathyroid adenoma on 99mTc-sestamibi imaging: A case report. *Front. Endocrinol.* **2024**, *15*, 1258233. [CrossRef] [PubMed]
15. Manzanedo-Romero, I.; García-Muñoz-Najar, A.; Acín-Gándara, D.; Carrión-Álvarez, L.; Urbasos-Pascual, M.; Pereira-Pérez, F. Schwannoma de la cadena simpática cervical asociado a adenoma paratiroideo [Cervical sympathetic chain schwannoma associated with parathyroid adenoma]. *Cir Cir* **2015**, *83*, 409–413. (In Spanish) [CrossRef]
16. Pizzato, M.; Li, M.; Vignat, J.; Laversanne, M.; Singh, D.; La Vecchia, C.; Vaccarella, S. The epidemiological landscape of thyroid cancer worldwide: GLOBOCAN estimates for incidence and mortality rates in 2020. *Lancet Diabetes Endocrinol.* **2022**, *10*, 264–272. [CrossRef]
17. Dean, D.S.; Gharib, H. Epidemiology of thyroid nodules. *Best Pract. Res. Clin. Endocrinol. Metab.* **2008**, *22*, 901–911. [CrossRef]
18. Zamora, E.A.; Khare, S.; Cassaro, S. Thyroid Nodule. In *StatPearls [Internet]*; StatPearls Publishing: Treasure Island, FL, USA, 2024. Available online: https://www.ncbi.nlm.nih.gov/books/NBK535422/ (accessed on 10 September 2024).
19. Ali, S.Z.; Baloch, Z.W.; Cochand-Priollet, B.; Schmitt, F.C.; Vielh, P.; VanderLaan, P.A. The 2023 Bethesda System for Reporting Thyroid Cytopathology. *Thyroid®* **2023**, *33*, 1039–1044.
20. Agnihotri, S.; Jalali, S.; Wilson, M.R.; Danesh, A.; Li, M.; Klironomos, G.; Krieger, J.R.; Mansouri, A.; Khan, O.; Mamatjan, Y.; et al. The genomic landscape of schwannoma. *Nat. Genet.* **2016**, *48*, 1339–1348. [CrossRef]
21. Cashman, E.; Skinner, L.J.; Timon, C. Thyroid swelling: An unusual presentation of a cervical sympathetic chain schwannoma. *Medscape J. Med.* **2008**, *10*, 201. [PubMed]
22. Delaney, W.E.; Fry, K.E. Neurilemoma of the thyroid gland. *Ann. Surg.* **1964**, *160*, 1014–1017. [CrossRef]
23. Aron, M.; Kapila, K.; Verma, K. Neural tumours of the neck presenting as thyroid nodules: A report of three cases. *Cytopathology* **2005**, *16*, 206–209. [CrossRef] [PubMed]
24. Mandel, L.; Syrop, S.B. First-bite syndrome after parapharyngeal surgery for cervical schwannoma. *J. Am. Dent. Assoc.* **2008**, *139*, 1480–1483. [CrossRef] [PubMed]
25. Nagavalli, S.; Yehuda, M.; McPhaul, L.W.; Gianoukakis, A.G. A Cervical Schwannoma Masquerading as a Thyroid Nodule. *Eur. Thyroid J.* **2017**, *6*, 216–220. [CrossRef]
26. Scherl, S.; Alon, E.E.; EKarle, W.; Clain, J.B.; Khorsandi, A.; Urken, M.L. Rare Tracheal Tumors and Lesions Initially Diagnosed as Isolated Differentiated Thyroid Cancers. *Thyroid®* **2012**, *23*, 79–83. [CrossRef] [PubMed]
27. Kang, J.Y.; Yi, K.S.; Cha, S.H.; Choi, C.H.; Kim, Y.; Lee, J.; Son, S.M. Schwannoma of the thyroid bed: A case report and review of the literature. *Medicine* **2020**, *99*, e18814. [CrossRef]
28. Ledgard, C.; Dickson, S.; Pochin, R. Surgical excision of a schwannoma mimicking a thyroid nodule. *ANZ J. Surg.* **2023**, *93*, 369–371. [CrossRef]
29. Donatini, G.; Iacconi, P.; De Bartolomeis, C.; Fattori, S.; Pucci, A.; Puccini, M.; Miccoli, P. Neck lesions mimicking thyroid pathology. *Langenbeck's Arch. Surg.* **2009**, *394*, 435–440. [CrossRef]
30. De Paoli, F.; Giugliano, G.; Casadio, C.; Tredici, P.; Bruschini, R.; De Fiori, E. Schwannoma of thyroid bed. A case report and considerations on interdisciplinary collaboration. *Acta Otorhinolaryngol. Ital.* **2005**, *25*, 250–252; discussion 253–254.
31. Badawi, R.A.; Scott-Coombes, D. Ancient schwannoma masquerading as a thyroid mass. *Eur. J. Surg. Oncol.* **2002**, *28*, 88–90. [CrossRef]
32. Jung, C.K.; Baek, J.H.; Na, D.G.; Oh, Y.L.; Yi, K.H.; Kang, H.C. 2019 Practice guidelines for thyroid core needle biopsy: A report of the Clinical Practice Guidelines Development Committee of the Korean Thyroid Association. *J. Pathol. Transl. Med.* **2020**, *54*, 64–86. [CrossRef]
33. Dolidze, D.D.; Covantsev, S.; Chechenin, G.M.; Pichugina, N.V.; Bedina, A.V.; Bumbu, A. Core needle biopsy for thyroid nodules assessment-a new horizon? *World J. Clin. Oncol.* **2024**, *15*, 580–586. [CrossRef] [PubMed]
34. Ahn, D.; Lee, G.J.; Sohn, J.H.; Jeong, J.Y. Fine-needle aspiration cytology versus core-needle biopsy for the diagnosis of extracranial head and neck schwannoma. *Head Neck* **2018**, *40*, 2695–2700. [CrossRef] [PubMed]
35. Guedes, F.; Henriques, V.M.; Torrão, F.L.; Haikal, N.P.; Sanches, G.E.; Barbosa, D.A.N.; Marsicano, F.G.; Rosa, L.A.N.; Siquara, A.C.; Malessy, M.J.A. When biopsy goes wrong: A case series of misdiagnoses and complications from biopsies of masses of unknown origin potentially originating from a peripheral nerve. *J. Neurosurg.* **2024**, *140*, 480–488. (In English) [CrossRef] [PubMed]
36. Ijichi, K.; Kawakita, D.; Maseki, S.; Beppu, S.; Takano, G.; Murakami, S. Functional Nerve Preservation in Extracranial Head and Neck Schwannoma Surgery. *JAMA Otolaryngol.–Head Neck Surg.* **2016**, *142*, 479–483. [CrossRef]
37. Agarwal, S.K.; Munjal, M.; Rai, D.; Rao, S. Malignant Transformation of Vagal Nerve Schwannoma in to Angiosarcoma: A Rare Event. *J. Surg. Tech. Case Rep.* **2015**, *7*, 17–19. [CrossRef]

MDPI AG
Grosspeteranlage 5
4052 Basel
Switzerland
Tel.: +41 61 683 77 34

Diagnostics Editorial Office
E-mail: diagnostics@mdpi.com
www.mdpi.com/journal/diagnostics

www.ingramcontent.com/pod-product-compliance
Lightning Source LLC
Chambersburg PA
CBHW061621210926
51850CB00009B/2394
9783725850433